Augmentative and Alternative Communication

Challenges and Solutions

Augmentative and Alternative Communication

Challenges and Solutions

BILLY T. OGLETREE, PhD, CCC-SLP

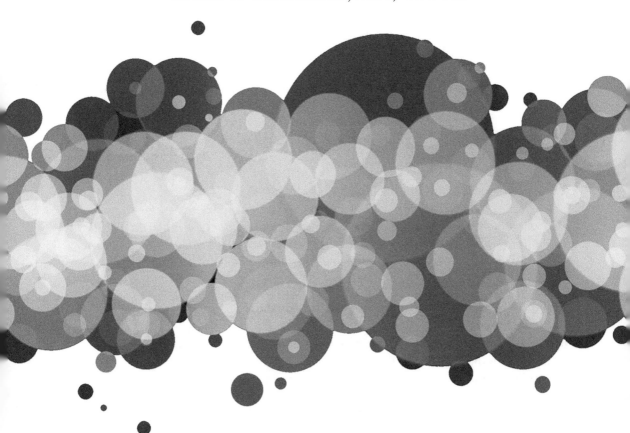

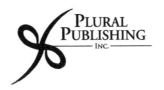

PLURAL
PUBLISHING
INC.

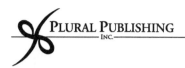

5521 Ruffin Road
San Diego, CA 92123

e-mail: information@pluralpublishing.com
Web site: https://www.pluralpublishing.com

Typeset in 10.5/13 Garamond by Flanagan's Publishing Services, Inc.
Printed in the United States of America by Integrated Books International

For permission to use material from this text, contact us by
Telephone: (866) 758-7251
Fax: (888) 758-7255
e-mail: permissions@pluralpublishing.com

*Every attempt has been made to contact the copyright holders for material originally
printed in another source. If any have been inadvertently overlooked, the publisher
will gladly make the necessary arrangements at the first opportunity.*

Library of Congress Cataloging-in-Publication Data:
Names: Ogletree, Billy T., editor.
Title: Augmentative and alternative communication : challenges and
  solutions / [edited by] Billy T. Ogletree.
Other titles: Augmentative and alternative communication (Ogletree)
Description: San Diego, CA : Plural Publishing, Inc., [2021] | Includes
  bibliographical references and index.
Identifiers: LCCN 2020048150 | ISBN 9781635502862 (paperback) | ISBN
  1635502861 (paperback) | ISBN 9781635502961 (ebook)
Subjects: MESH: Communication Aids for Disabled | Nonverbal Communication |
  Communication Disorders--rehabilitation | Interpersonal Relations |
  Needs Assessment
Classification: LCC RC428.8 | NLM WL 340.2 | DDC 616.85/503--dc23
LC record available at https://lccn.loc.gov/2020048150

◼ Contents

Preface   vii
Contributors   ix

PART I. Introduction

1 **Challenges and Solutions in Augmentative and Alternative**   3
Communication (AAC)
Billy T. Ogletree

PART II. AAC Challenges and Solutions: Childhood

2 **Earlier Is Better: Challenges to Implementing AAC During**   21
Early Intervention
Rose A. Sevcik, MaryAnn Romski, Casy Walters, and Gal Kaldes

3 **AAC in Preschool: Navigating Challenges in Language and**   41
Literacy Instruction
Andrea Barton-Hulsey, Marika King, and Jennifer Lyons-Golden

4 **AAC in Schools: Mastering the Art and Science of Inclusion**   81
Nancy B. Robinson and Gloria Soto

5 **Supporting Participation and Communication in Employment**   117
and Volunteer Activities for Adolescents With Complex
Communication Needs
David McNaughton and Salena Babb

PART III. AAC Challenges and Solutions: Adult Disorders

6 **AAC Interventions in Persons with Aphasia**   141
Tiffany Chavers, Cissy Cheng, and Rajinder Koul

7 **Decision-Making for Access to AAC Technologies in**   169
Late Stage ALS
Deirdre McLaughlin, Betts Peters, Kendra McInturf, Brandon Eddy,
Michelle Kinsella, Aimee Mooney, Trinity Deibert, Kerry Montgomery,
and Melanie Fried-Oken

8 Access to AAC for Individuals with Acquired Conditions: **199**
Challenges and Solutions in Early Recovery
Susan Koch Fager, Jessica E. Gormley, and Tabatha L. Sorenson

PART IV. AAC Challenges and Solutions:
Special Populations and Issues

9 Challenges in Providing AAC Intervention to People With   **229**
Profound Intellectual and Multiple Disabilities
Jeff Sigafoos, Laura Roche, and Kathleen Tait

10 The Challenge of Symbolic Communication for School-Aged
Students with the Most Significant Cognitive Disabilities   **253**
Karen Erickson, Lori Geist, Penny Hatch, and Nancy Quick

11 Implementing the Visual Immersion System™ in a Classroom   **283**
for Children with Autism Spectrum Disorder: Challenges
and Solutions
Ralf W. Schlosser, Howard C. Shane, Anna A. Allen, Christina Yu,
Amanda M. O'Brien, Jackie Cullen, Andrea Benz, Lindsay O'Neil,
Laurel Chiesa, and Lisa Miori-Dinneen

12 Fostering Communication About Emotions: Aided Augmentative   **313**
and Alternative Communication Challenges and Solutions
Krista M. Wilkinson, Ji Young Na, Gabriela A. Rangel-Rodriguez, and Dawn
J. Sowers

13 AAC and Multiculturalism: Incorporating Family Perspectives   **339**
for Improved Outcomes
Mary Claire Wofford and Rachel Hoge

PART V. Final Thoughts

14 Becoming a Solution-Oriented AAC Provider   **369**
Billy T. Ogletree and Kelsey Williams

Glossary   *383*
Index   *385*

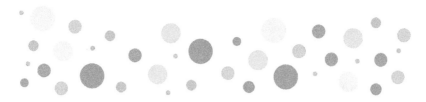

■ Preface

I met my first nonspeaking person during the summer after my freshman year of college. I was spending long days at a local department store, where I had been assigned the unpleasant job of sidewalk sales, pushing merchandise and running a register. This may not sound too bad as summer jobs go, but I was in south Mississippi, and it was very hot.

One afternoon, I noticed a well-dressed man approaching me from the parking lot. He walked in a determined yet labored manner and held a coat hanger. I was helping other customers but turned to him expecting to answer a quick question. Instead, I realized that he could not speak. He tried to offer a few words but struggled to do so. As his frustration grew, the man motioned with the coat hanger, indicating that his keys were locked in his car. I quickly found someone from the store to assist him, but I could not stop thinking about our encounter.

That brief storefront interaction changed my life forever. I declared my college major the next fall—Speech-Language Pathology. After three more years of undergraduate training and two years of graduate school, I found myself working with children and young adults with intellectual disabilities (ID). Each day, I was face-to-face with people who could not speak intelligibly. Some struggled to form speech sounds or words, others did not speak at all but communicated through conventional or unconventional forms. The field of augmentative and alternative communication (AAC) was in its early years, and I was unprepared to meet the needs of those I served.

I returned to graduate school, where I found myself drawn to populations with the most challenging communicative disorders. This led me to individuals with severe ID and began my interest in AAC. Over the past 30 years, I have worked increasingly in AAC assessment and intervention, serving on AAC teams in medical centers, and providing consultations for schools, institutional settings, and community group homes. I've also taught, published about, and served in the area of AAC in my position as a university professor. My experiences have been both rewarding and trying: rewarding in that I've been a part of AAC solutions that changed the lives of people with complex communication challenges, trying, because I've encountered challenges that have, at times, hindered or prevented positive outcomes.

When the staff at Plural Publishing contacted me about the possibility of a textbook, I was initially reluctant. There are excellent existing general resources on AAC, and I was uncertain about my ability to contribute something either new or meaningful. Then the idea of a book dedicated to challenges and solutions came to mind—a reference in which experts in the field of AAC could share a few of their professional challenges and the solutions they have used or considered in the face of these barriers. A book that also includes voices from individuals who use AAC and their stakeholders.

This effort is the product of authors with prominent reputations as AAC researchers and providers—individuals who collectively have hundreds of years of professional experience. Most chapters offer voices of those using AAC and of the people in their lives—all propose ideas useful in frontline AAC service delivery.

The book closes with a charge for all involved in AAC to show grit and resilience—to use these attributes to become solution-oriented AAC providers. My experience with the nonspeaking man at that department store years ago sparked a career dedicated to those with severe communication disorders. It is my hope that this book may do the same for you.

Billy T. Ogletree, PhD, CCC-SLP

■ Contributors

Anna A. Allen, PhD, CCC-SLP
Chapter 11
Director of Clinical Care and Research
Puddingstone Place, LLC
Post-Doctoral Research Affiliate
Autism Language Program
Boston Children's Hospital
Boston, Massachusetts

Salena Babb, MEd
Chapter 5
PhD Student in Special Education
Penn State University
Centre County, Pennsylvania

Andrea Barton-Hulsey, PhD, CCC-SLP
Chapter 3
Assistant Professor
School of Communication Science and
    Disorders
Florida State University
Tallahassee, Florida

Andrea Benz, MS, CCC-SLP
Chapter 11
Speech-Language Pathologist
Fayetteville-Manlius School District
Manlius, New York

Tiffany Chavers, MS, CCC-SLP
Chapter 6
Doctoral Student
University of Texas at Austin
Austin, Texas

Cissy Cheng, MS
Chapter 6
Doctoral Student

University of Texas at Austin
Austin, Texas

Laurel Chiesa, MA
Chapter 11
Director of Instructional Technology
Fayetteville-Manlius Central School
    District
Manlius, New York

Jacqueline Cullen, MS, CCC-SLP
Chapter 11
Speech Language Pathologist
Fayetteville-Manlius Schools
Fayetteville, New York

Trinity Deibert, MS, CCC-SLP
Chapter 7
Speech-Language Pathologist
Providence Home Health Care
Portland, Oregon

Brandon Eddy, MA, CCC-SLP
Chapter 7
Research Associate
Oregon Health and Science University
Portland, Oregon

Karen Erickson, PhD
Chapter 10
Director, Center for Literacy and
    Disability Studies
David E. and Dolores "Dee" J. Yoder
    Distinguished Professor
Department of Allied Health Sciences
University of North Carolina at Chapel
    Hill
Chapel Hill, North Carolina

Susan Koch Fager, PhD, CCC-SLP
Chapter 8
Director, Communication Center of
    Excellence
Institute for Rehabilitation Science and
    Engineering
Madonna Rehabilitation Hospital
Lincoln, Nebraska

Melanie Fried-Oken, PhD, CCC-SLP
Chapter 7
Speech-Language Pathologist
Professor of Neurology, Pediatrics,
    Biomedical Engineering, and
    Otolaryngology
Oregon Health & Science University
Portland, Oregon

Jessica E. Gormley, PhD, CCC-SLP
Chapter 8
Assistant Professor
Speech-Language Pathology
    Department, Munroe-Meyer Institute
University of Nebraska Medical Center
Omaha, Nebraska

Lori A. Geist, PhD, CCC-SLP
Chapter 10
Research Assistant Professor
Center for Literacy and Disability Studies
Department of Allied Health Sciences
University of North Carolina at Chapel
    Hill
Chapel Hill, North Carolina

Penelope Hatch, PhD
Chapter 10
Research Assistant Professor
Center for Literacy and Disability
    Studies
Department of Allied Health Sciences
University of North Carolina at Chapel
    Hill
Chapel Hill, North Carolina

Rachel Hoge, MA, CCC-SLP
Chapter 13
Speech-Language Pathologist and
    Doctoral Candidate
School of Communication Science and
    Disorders
Florida State University
Tallahassee, Florida

Gal Kaldes, MEd, CCC-SLP
Chapter 2
Georgia State University
Atlanta, Georgia

Marika King, PhD, CCC-SLP
Chapter 3
Assistant Professor
Communicative Disorders and Deaf
    Education
Utah State University
Logan, Utah

Michelle Kinsella, BS, OTR/L
Chapter 7
Research Associate
Oregon Health and Science University
Portland, Oregon

Rajinder Koul, PhD
Chapter 6
Department Chair and Professor
Department of Speech, Language, and
    Hearing Sciences
University of Texas at Austin
Austin, Texas

Jennifer Lyons-Golden
Chapter 3
Assistive Technology and AAC
    Implementation Specialist
Fulton County Schools
Atlanta, Georgia

Kendra McInturf, MS, CCC-SLP
Chapter 7

Speech-Language Pathologist
Providence Home Health Care
Portland, Oregon

Deirdre McLaughlin, MS, CCC-SLP
Chapter 7
Speech-Language Pathologist and
    Research Associate
Oregon Health and Science University
Portland, Oregon

David McNaughton, PhD
Chapter 5
Professor of Special Education
Penn State University
Centre County, Pennsylvania

Lisa Miori-Dinneen, BS, MS, CAS
Chapter 11
Assistant Superintendent for Special
    Services
Fayetteville-Manlius School District
Manlius, New York

Kerry Montgomery
Chapter 7
Individual with ALS

Aimee Mooney, MS, CCC-SLP
Chapter 7
Assistant Professor
Oregon Health and Science University
Portland State University
Portland, Oregon

Ji Young Na, PhD, CCC-SLP
Chapter 12
Assistant Professor
Department of Communication Disorders
Korea Nazarene University
Cheonan, South Korea

Amanda M. O'Brien, MS, CCC-SLP
Chapter 11
PhD Student

Progam in Speech and Hearing,
    Bioscience and Technology
Harvard University
Cambridge, Massachusetts

Lindsay O'Neill, MSED, BSED
Chapter 11
Special Education Teacher
Fayetteville-Manlius School District
Manlius, New York

Billy T. Ogletree, PhD, CCC-SLP
Chapters 1 and 14
Catherine Brewer Smith Professor of
    Communication Sciences and Disorders
Western Carolina University
Cullowhee, North Carolina

Betts Peters, MA, CCC-SLP
Chapter 7
Research Associate
Oregon Health and Science University
Portland, Oregon

Nancy Quick, PhD
Chapter 10
Research Assistant Professor
Center for Literacy and Disability Studies
Department of Allied Health Sciences
University of North Carolina at Chapel
    Hill
Chapel Hill, North Carolina

Gabriela A. Rangel-Rodriguez, MA
Chapter 12
Psychologist and Consultant
CATIC
PhD Candidate in Psychology of
    Communication and Change
Autonomous University of Barcelona
Bellaterra, Spain

Nancy B. Robinson, PhD, CCC-SLP
Chapter 4
Professor Emerita

Department of Speech, Language, and
   Hearing Sciences
San Francisco State University
San Francisco, California

Laura Roche, PhD
Chapter 9
Post-Doctoral Research Fellow
University of Queensland, Faculty of
   Medicine
Centre for Children's Health Research
South Brisbane, Australia

MaryAnn Romski, PhD, CCC-SLP
Chapter 2
Regents Professor of Communication,
   Psychology, and Communication
   Sciences and Disorders
Georgia State University
Atlanta, Georgia

Ralf W. Schlosser, PhD
Chapter 11
Full Professor
Department of Communication Sciences
   and Disorders
Northeastern University
Boston, Massachusetts
Director of Clinical Research
Communication Enhancement Center
Boston Children's Hospital
Boston, Massachusetts
Extraordinary Professor
Centre for Augmentative and Alternative
   Communication
University of Pretoria
Pretoria, South Africa

Rose A. Sevcik, PhD
Chapter 2
Regents Professor of Psychology
Georgia State University
Atlanta, Georgia

Howard C. Shane, PhD
Chapter 11
Director, Autism Language Program
Director, Center for Communication
   Enhancement
Boston Children's Hospital
Associate Professor of Otology and
   Laryngology
Harvard Medical School

Jeffrey S. Sigafoos, PhD
Chapter 9
Professor
Victoria University of Wellington

**Tabatha L. Sorenson, OTD, OTR/L,
CAPS**
Chapter 8
Occupational Therapist
Assistive Technology Specialist
Madonna Rehabilitation Hospital
Lincoln, Nebraska

Gloria Soto, PhD
Chapter 4
Professor
Department of Speech, Language and
   Hearing Sciences
San Francisco State University
San Francisco, California

Dawn J. Sowers, MA, CCC-SLP
Chapter 12
Doctoral Candidate
The Pennsylvania State University
Centre County Pennsylvania

Kathleen Tait, PhD, MBPsS, SFHEA
Chapter 9
Academic Program Director, Special
   Education
Macquarie University
Sydney, Australia

Casy Elyse Walters, MA, CCC-SLP
Chapter 2
Doctoral Candidate Developmental
  Psychology
Georgia State University
Atlanta, Georgia

Krista M. Wilkinson, PhD
Chapter 12
Professor
Communication Sciences and Disorders
The Pennsylvania State University
Centre County, Pennsylvania

Kelsey Williams, BS, CSD
Chapter 14

Graduate Student
Western Carolina University
Cullowhee, North Carolina

Mary Claire Wofford, PhD, CCC-SLP
Chapter 13
Assistant Professor
Western Carolina University
College of Health and Human Sciences
Cullowhee, North Carolina

Christina Yu, MS, CCC-SLP
Chapter 11
Speech-Language Pathologist
Boston Children's Hospital
Boston, Massachusetts

*This book is dedicated to those who use or could benefit
from augmentative and alternative communication and the
individuals who serve and communicate with them daily.*

PART I
Introduction

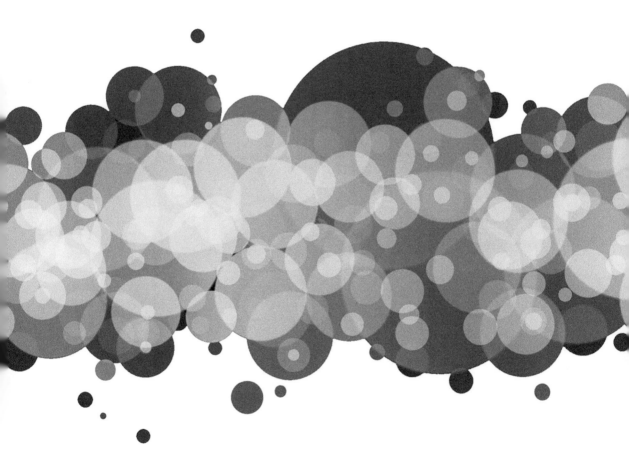

Challenges and Solutions in Augmentative and Alternative Communication (AAC)

Billy T. Ogletree

This book came to be, in part, because the application of AAC is fraught with challenges. In fact, the process of assisting someone with **complex communication needs (CCN)** is nothing if not challenging. Challenges occur during efforts to understand the potential abilities, needs, and preferences of people who rely on AAC. Challenges extend to complexities related to these individuals' communicative environments and partners. Challenges can even emerge specific to interpersonal or ideological differences within an AAC care team. If this is not enough, individual **AAC solutions** often unfold over years, creating ongoing challenges related to life changes.

In addition to these specific assessment and intervention challenges, researchers have been increasingly frustrated by the lack of evidence behind long-held AAC-practice assumptions. Questions have arisen specific to what **symbol forms** are best for children and adults and how these symbols should be arrayed on devices (Fried-Oken & Light, 2012). More questions have been posed about variables

confounding AAC use, such as cognitive and visual-processing abilities and preferences (Fried-Oken & Light, 2012; Wilkinson, Light, & Drager, 2012). Researchers have even found themselves challenged by evolving societal issues such as the ubiquitous presence of technology and the increasing diversity of people who rely on AAC with respect to language and culture (Higginbotham & Fager, 2012; Ogletree, McMurry, Schmidt, & Evans, 2018).

In sum, **AAC practitioners** and **researchers** frequently find themselves grappling with challenges. As individuals charged with serving those with CCN, we can be either deterred or motivated by this fact. If deterred, people who rely on AAC may never enjoy optimal AAC solutions. In contrast, the provider or stakeholder motivated to overcome challenges will often find him- or herself at the center of processes resulting in creative and innovative AAC applications.

This introductory chapter briefly describes AAC as a dynamic, team-based practice that requires the following of providers: knowledge of a rapidly changing field, competence with myriad disabilities impacting communication, and a personal commitment that transcends inevitable setbacks and disappointments. It also sets the stage for subsequent chapters by discussing the reality of challenges in one's professional life and the need to demonstrate professional grit and resilience. This chapter ends by introducing the book's chapter authors, commenting on challenges presented in this text, and foreshadowing future content by encouraging solution-driven AAC practices.

Although AAC is a field addressed by many professional disciplines, this book is primarily written by speech-language pathologists (SLPs). Therefore, much of what follows in this chapter and beyond will address challenges specific to that discipline and its participation in AAC services. It should be noted, however, that AAC challenges cross disciplinary boundaries, and solutions rely upon the expertise of dedicated, collaborative teams.

■ AAC Basics: Knowledge Assumed by the Authors of This Text

This book provides a platform for established AAC researchers/practitioners, people who rely on AAC, and other stakeholders to discuss challenges they have encountered in the field. Some draw from decades of AAC service provision or scholarship; others address challenges from very personal perspectives. All assume a level of reader knowledge that exceeds that of entry-level providers. This section serves as a simple review for many readers and an introduction to AAC for others. It is written to set the stage for the chapters

that follow. Critical AAC terms are highlighted in the text and defined in a glossary provided at the end of the book.

■ Defining AAC

The American Speech-Language Hearing Association's Practice Portal (ASHA, 2019) defines Augmentative and Alternative Communication (AAC) as "an area of clinical practice that addresses the needs of individuals with significant and complex communication disorders characterized by impairments in speech-language production and/or comprehension, including spoken and written modes of communication." Four things can be gleaned from this definition.

First, AAC is but one area of clinical practice. There are many subspecialties available to today's educational and allied health care providers. Of these areas, AAC may be the broadest in terms of services rendered and populations served. The ideal practice of **AAC assessment and intervention** requires a diverse range of **stakeholders** and professionals (team members) who possess unique contributions yet are dedicated to a singular outcome—the establishment and growth of effective communication for people who rely on AAC, leading to everyday inclusion and participation across all realms of life. The AAC team members include, but are not limited to, people who rely on AAC, family representatives, peers, medical personnel, educators, rehabilitation specialists, occupational therapists, physical therapists, psychologists, visual-impairment specialists, social workers, and speech-language pathologists. The composition of AAC teams is driven by the needs of the person who relies on AAC, and AAC teams can choose to function within more or less collaborative team structures (e.g., **multidisciplinary**, **interdisciplinary**, or **transdisciplinary teams**). AAC, as an area of clinical practice, then, is team driven. It's also incredibly expansive with respect to individuals served. That is, AAC has applications for both children and adults, and for individuals with a variety of developmental and acquired conditions.

Our second takeaway is that AAC is applied with myriad individuals presenting CCN. Beukelman and Light (2020) noted that there is no typical person who relies on AAC, but a group that crosses all age, socioeconomic, ethnic, and racial backgrounds and shares the need for "adaptive assistance for speaking and/or writing because their gestural, spoken, and/or written communication is temporarily or permanently inadequate to meet all of their communication needs" (p. 4). The communication needs of this group are often described as complex because their communicative efforts can be challenged by concomitant impairments in motor, sensory, intellectual, and other areas.

The third thing we learn from the portal definition (ASHA, 2019) is that AAC can be applied to address the needs of people who rely on AAC in both communication/language expression and comprehension. Too often, AAC has been highlighted for its remediation of expressive deficits. Whereas expression grabs attention due to its obvious visibility, many AAC applications relate to comprehension. For decades, AAC has been used as a means of communication and language input to promote receptive abilities and encourage communication success. In fact, some researchers have used

a primary AAC focus on comprehension as a bridge to gains in communication and language production (Sevcik, 2009).

Finally, ASHA's definition (ASHA, 2019) broadens the focus of AAC team members by including written modes of communication. This includes early attention to **emergent literacy** and a lifelong emphasis upon access to print wherever it may be found. For some, AAC efforts in the area of literacy may be limited to acquiring and using basic **sight words** associated with daily environments (Erickson, 2017). For others, there may be a significant focus upon writing and reading in varied contexts for complex purposes. In fact, today's AAC team member must be prepared to assist people who rely on AAC with access to expanding print experiences through growing social-media outlets (Caron & Light, 2015; McNaughton & Light, 2013; Paterson, 2017).

Where does this all leave us in terms of defining AAC? Let's sum it up by saying AAC is a team-based area of clinical practice (i.e., assessment and intervention) that has applications for many individuals with CCN. It addresses both communication/language expression and comprehension in all modalities, including writing. As stated earlier, AAC's primary focus is the establishment and growth of effective communication for people who rely on AAC, leading to everyday inclusion and participation across all realms of life.

■ Moving Past a Definition: Describing AAC Practices

So, what is involved in the frontline, day-to-day practice of AAC? AAC services have been described as a circular process involving assessment, **feature matching**, **device** or **system** procurement, implementation, and **follow-up** (Ogletree & Oren, 2006) (Figure 1–1). Each aspect of circular AAC service delivery is considered below.

The traditional AAC assessment process focuses on the consideration of current and future communication needs of people who rely on AAC and a critical review of their environments and partners (Beukelman & Light, 2020). This broad-based effort relies on the expertise of multiple team members. Ogletree and Oren (2006) suggest that assessments should involve the review of "physical competence" (e.g., vision, hearing, positioning, and seating), **access** to systems and devices (e.g., the ability to move in a way that allows for direct or alternative access), cognitive functioning, and

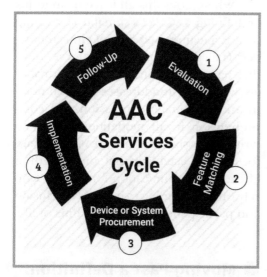

Figure 1–1. The Circular Process of AAC Services. Figure 1 From *Pro-Ed Series on Autism Spectrum Disorders: How to Use Augmentative and Alternative Communication* (p. 2), by Billy T. Ogletree and Thomas Oren, 2006, Austin, TX: Pro-Ed. Copyright 2006 by Pro-Ed, Inc. Reprinted with permission.

communication and language abilities" (p. 2). The communication and language assessment focus should include attention to residual speech capacity and potential (Beukelman & Light, 2020). Clearly, an assessment addressing targets mentioned thus far might involve physical and occupational therapists, psychologists, educators, and speech-language pathologists. This assessment will also involve the client him- or herself and stakeholders such as family members, peers, and other professionals (e.g., medical specialists, visual impairment (VI) experts, audiologists, social workers, rehabilitation engineers, and administrators).

It is worth noting that assessments for people who rely on AAC have more than one purpose. Frequently, the primary assessment question simply relates to the "in the moment" appropriateness of AAC for the client. This could be an initial evaluation or follow-up testing after an earlier team decision against AAC. The AAC assessment can also be conducted to determine if current AAC solutions remain effective or need to be changed. This type of assessment may involve the entire team, or subsets of team members critical to the question at hand. For example, a reevaluation due to an evolving visual impairment may involve a VI expert, an occupational therapist, and a speech-language pathologist, rather than the complete team.

Assessments for people who rely on AAC can be conducted in centers or in the various daily environments of the client. Most often, the assessment will, at least in part, extend beyond a specific center to natural environments. Conducting assessments in more than one context allows AAC teams to gather socially valid "real world" data on both the client and his/ her life environment and partners. Environmental and partner data collection may focus on communicative demands and opportunities, as well as any existing barriers to success (Beukelman & Light, 2020). Depending upon the AAC team's model of functioning, assessments can occur over one or several sessions. For example, a transdisciplinary team may involve all team members in one large collaborative assessment session, whereas a multi- or interdisciplinary team may assess over several discipline-specific sessions and offer a final team meeting for decision-making and sharing. Regardless of the team model, assessment of people who rely on AAC will typically depend on nonstandardized data collected via **informancy** and **observation**, although standardized, norm-referenced assessment measures can be useful (Beukelman & Light, 2020). **AAC environmental and partner assessment** will also rely more on informancy and observational data, although structured guidelines in this area are increasingly available (Blackstone & Hunt-Berg, 2012).

As the AAC assessment process moves past the data collection and sharing stage, the team shifts to feature matching. This is an action phase in which team members work to match client needs to possible AAC solutions. Several decision matrices have been developed to assist with feature matching (ASHA Practice Portal, 2019). Matched features can include, among other things, a device's **symbol capacity**, **vocabulary organization**, **linguistic features**, **voice options**, access possibilities, **display capacity**, **rate enhancement features**, and **operational demands** (ASHA Practice Portal, 2019; Beukelman & Light, 2020). As client needs and available solutions are compared, one or more AAC options can be selected for a **trial run** prior to procurement. Even-

tually, AAC teams may assist with the purchase of a chosen device or system. The procurement process can be time consuming, involving report writing for myriad funding sources.

The AAC implementation and team follow-up (see Figure 1–1) shift AAC services to intervention. Implementation involves all activities required to place a device or system, make it functional, and assure that it is responsive to changing needs. Implementation can be a protracted stage of AAC services and usually involves more than one team member (e.g., speech-language pathologists, occupational/physical therapists, educators, rehabilitation specialists) offering discipline-specific or cotreatment sessions (Sylvester, Ogletree, & Lunnen, 2017). Implementation will likely entail some initial training with the client and his or her stakeholders to troubleshoot operational competence, issues of access, and initial **message management** (e.g., the generation and use of messages to support communication in all its forms; Beukelman & Light, 2020). Once a device or system is in use, there will be inevitable follow-up with part or all of the AAC assessment team to address small adjustments or complete overhauls of initial assessment recommendations. These follow-up actions are often a first step to additional, broader team-based assessments, completing and reinitiating the AAC services circle (see Figure 1–1).

◼ The Evolving Nature of AAC Service Delivery

Current factors such as the ubiquitous nature of technology, the increasing heterogeneity of world populations, and the acceptance of interprofessional educational and practice philosophies are reshaping the AAC service-delivery process as it has been described above.

The Availability of Technology

The first three phases of the AAC service-delivery process (i.e., assessment, feature matching, and procurement) have been recommended practice for years (Beukelman & Light, 2020). Costello, Shane, and Caron (2013) describe these phases as "person first" and focused on identifying and matching current and anticipated client strengths and needs to feature sets available via various AAC solutions. Costello et al. go on to describe these actions as part of a meaningful and logical clinical process that recognizes and utilizes the knowledge and expertise of AAC practitioners and other stakeholders.

Increasingly, the "person first" process is being circumvented by what Costello et al. (2013) refer to as a "platform first" perspective. Here, decisions about AAC system/device appropriateness follow the selection of mobile devices and software by the client or his/her stakeholders. This is made possible due to the ubiquitous nature of technology, its ever-increasing affordability, and the presence of easily accessible information regarding purchase options. People who rely on AAC can now surf the Internet for mobile communication devices or software suggestions and pursue purchases at their local technology store or online. Costello and colleagues note that in a "platform first" orientation, decisions are often made based upon factors not central to the client's needs (e.g., device/software popularity or cost). Furthermore, with devices and software pre-

selected, AAC assessment teams may feel compelled to make purchases work for the client. Doing so jeopardizes the "person first" principle of prioritizing matching client needs to available systems and devices prior to procurement.

Ogletree et al.(2018) suggest that "platform first" influences on AAC services are unlikely to abate. If anything, these phenomena will gain traction in years to come. Ogletree et al. share that traditional AAC assessment processes must adapt to accommodate a "platform first" mentality. For example, an often-arduous and time-consuming traditional assessment process must become more efficient. One answer may be smaller "core" teams that triage referrals, reducing wait/decision times. Another could be concerted team efforts to inform referral networks (e.g., physicians, educators, allied health professionals) of the value of "person centered" AAC services. This idea could become a priority for national professional organizations, possibly resulting in Web-based and other tutorials easily assessable to those seeking AAC guidance. Finally, Ogletree at al. (2018) note that "platform first" procurement will inevitably occur, altering traditional AAC assessment processes. Given this fact, more effort should be made to encourage hard- and software development that accounts for the needs of individuals with CCN. Again, this may require advocacy from professional organizations representing the members of typical AAC teams.

The Changing Population of People Who Rely on AAC

Our world continues to change with respect to population growth and migration. Soto and Yu (2014) note that these variables are contributing to increased cultural and linguistic diversity in countries across the globe. As diversity grows, the likelihood increases of an individual encountering others who differ from the quickly fading "mainstream." This includes individuals who will use or need AAC solutions to communicate.

How will diversity, in all of its forms, impact AAC service delivery? An obvious answer is the need for AAC team members to honor the culture, language, and other differences of those they serve. Culture is defined as shared attitudes, values, goals, and practices (Spencer-Oatey, 2012). Culture can be honored by the application of cultural sensitivity, an aspirational concept at best, in AAC decision-making. In this chapter, AAC service delivery has been described as a circular process involving evaluation, feature matching, device/system procurement, follow-up, and, if needed, additional evaluation. At each step of this process, AAC team members should engage people who rely on AAC and their families to ensure that team actions are taken in ways consistent with cultural mores. For example, a client or family's cultural preference for collaboration should lead an AAC team to function within one of the more collaborative team models.

The AAC teams can honor language differences by featuring multiple languages on AAC systems and devices. Ogletree et al. (2018) recommend that AAC evaluations include the consideration of all languages to which the potential user is exposed. This will likely require teams to prioritize family stakeholders in the assessment process. Again, including stakeholders in AAC services will push teams to function more collaboratively, elevating the team status of people who rely on AAC and their family

members (Ogletree, 1999). Family members will be invaluable as the AAC team progresses through the other phases of AAC services (e.g., feature matching, procurement, implementation, and follow-up), as at each of these steps questions will arise specific to the language needs of the client.

Diversity is not limited to culture and language. It also includes other differences specific to racial or ethnic classifications, age, gender, religion, philosophy, physical abilities, socioeconomic background, and sexual orientation. Members of AAC teams must work to assure that devices and solutions represent all facets of the client he or she chooses to highlight. Although effective oral communicators may take the ability to share important personal information for granted, people who rely on AAC are dependent upon others for this.

Interprofessionality

Whereas the first two evolutionary variables in this chapter section—the ubiquitous nature of technology and the changing client population—present challenges that can make AAC service delivery more complex, the final variable, interprofessionality, may make it simpler. Interprofessionality is defined by D'Amour and Oandasan (2005) as

the process by which professionals reflect on and develop ways of practicing that provide an integrated and cohesive answer to the needs of the client/family population.... It involves continuous interaction and knowledge sharing between professionals, organized to solve and explore a variety of care issues all while seeking to optimize the patient's participation. . . .

Interprofessionality requires a paradigm shift, since interprofessional practice has unique characteristics in terms of values, codes of conduct, and ways of working. (p. 9)

The World Health Organization (2010) reported three core ideals central to interprofessional practice: patient and family centeredness, community-oriented care, and relationship-focused service delivery. These ideals can be learned during preservice training through interprofessional education (IPE), or acquired through continuing education and experience during professional practice. Whether through IPE, continuing education, or experience alone, the outcome of an interprofessional focus is seamless, integrated service delivery. Professionals and other stakeholders work side-by-side with a greater understanding and appreciation of each other's potential contributions and a collective commitment to the highest quality care for those they serve. The evidence supporting interprofessionality as a preferred educational and practice construct is growing (Deneckere et al., 2012; Zwarenstein, Goldman, & Reeves, 2009). Clearly, interprofessionality is worth consideration for AAC teams.

Early in this chapter, I mentioned that the effective team-based practice of AAC requires a personal commitment that transcends inevitable setbacks and disappointments. In my career, I have found AAC team members to be fully committed to identifying and supporting AAC solutions for individuals with CCN. Most often, this professional passion has emerged from personal experiences with people who rely on AAC, dedicated continuing-education efforts in AAC, or, more recently, exposure to AAC content in preprofessional academic/clinical

preparation. One can only imagine the possibilities for tomorrow's AAC providers if preprofessional training programs across disciplines commit to interprofessional AAC-related academic and clinical experiences.

It seems that the field of AAC lends itself to IPE. First, recommended practice is team-based. With this focus on teams, IPE efforts could involve joint preparation across disciplines typically involved in AAC assessment and intervention. With the use of distance instructional technology, universities without common AAC disciplines could join others to create ideal IPE experiences. IPE could be provided through a range of offerings, including cotaught classes, joint clinical experiences, or select exposure to integrated learning opportunities throughout more discipline-specific preparation. Finally, AAC and IPE would seem to be an ideal match given the complexities inherent in AAC service delivery and populations with CCN. Working together to solve complex problems during preservice training could only improve future frontline AAC practices.

To conclude, AAC services are changing. Traditional paradigms underlying assessment are evolving, populations are becoming more diverse, and new ideas specific to pre- and in-service professional training are gaining favor. We can only hope that the result of these changes will be improved services for individuals with CCN. One certainty is that AAC providers and researchers alike will continue to find their work challenging. There will undoubtedly be ups and downs as we all work to attain our ultimate goal—the establishment and growth of effective communication for people who rely on AAC leading to everyday inclusion and participation across all realms of life.

The reality of challenges in AAC service delivery brings into focus a need for professional and stakeholder grit and resiliency. Simply put, all involved in AAC will need motivation to find solutions when they are not apparent, to work hard on behalf of people who rely on AAC, and to be prepared to work harder as needed.

The Role of Grit and Resilience in Addressing AAC Challenges

Readers may be surprised to encounter terms like "grit" and "resilience" in a book on AAC. Remember, however, this is a text about challenges and solutions. There is a growing literature exploring the role of grit and resilience within health professions (Hammond, 2016; Howe, Smajdor, & Stockl, 2012; McCann et al., 2013). Whereas some debate the viability of these terms as measurable constructs, others are probing their importance as provider attributes (Crede, Tynan, & Harris, 2017; Stoffel & Cain, 2018). Emerging lines of inquiry have both examined the role of these traits as variables undergirding effective care and proposed the possibility of teaching or fostering grit and resilience as desirable professional qualities (Stoffel & Cain, 2018). What follows is an effort to clarify grit and resilience as potential important characteristics in AAC, and some general speculation about what may lead to the emergence of these attributes in AAC team members.

Stoffel and Cain (2018) collectively define grit and resilience as "the ability to persevere through hardships to meet goals" (p. 124). These concepts, however, have been considered individually. Personal grit has been described using terms such as perseverance, passion, and sustained commitment, and is often mentioned as an attribute necessary to achieve long-term goals (Duckworth, Peterson, Matthews, & Kelly, p. 207). Resilience, in turn, has typically referred to one's ability to "bounce back" after hardship (Tugade & Fredrickson, 2004). The presence of resilience has been associated with improved life quality and stress reduction (Tempski, Santos, & Mayer, 2015; Shi, Wang, YuGe, & Wang et al., 2015). Stoffel and Cain (2018) suggest that resilience is, in fact, "an inherent attribute of grit" (p. 125).

The concepts of grit and resilience resonate with allied health and educational professionals (Stoffel & Cain, 2018). That is, most in these fields have recognized grit and resilience in our best therapeutic efforts or the efforts of others we have observed. If we have worked for any length of time, we have also observed these traits in the efforts of dedicated parents/partners and other stakeholders. The explicit role of grit and resilience in AAC providers, however, has yet to be researched.

As a speech-language pathologist and AAC provider with well over thirty years of experience, I've served on my share of AAC teams. I've also encountered countless AAC practitioners and researchers within various professional circles. If my observations have any merit, grit and resilience are key attributes of successful AAC team members, people who rely on AAC, and stakeholders.

One of the interesting features of this book is the provision of the voices of people who rely on AAC and their stakeholders. To test the validity of my ideas about grit and resilience, I asked a few people who rely on AAC and stakeholders their thoughts about critical attributes of the best AAC professionals who have assisted them. I also asked what characteristics they have observed in other successful people who rely on AAC and stakeholders. Responses are provided below (Table 1–1).

The comments highlighted earlier certainly support grit and resilience as possible attributes of successful AAC providers, people who rely on AAC, and stakeholders. Descriptors such as "determinedness," "openness," "willingness," and "perseverance" occur repeatedly in quotes. One individual even includes the words "grit" and "resilience" in his responses.

Why might grit and resilience be so important? Could it be that the complexities of AAC often require the presence of these attributes? Again, collectively these terms have been defined as perseverance through hardship in the pursuit of goals. A successful circular process of AAC services involves many steps, environments, and individuals. Even in best-case scenarios, hardships arise. Policy, practice, knowledge, or operational **barriers** can impede optimal outcomes (Beukelman & Light, 2020). In addition, hardships may surface if AAC providers don't possess wide-ranging competencies in areas that change constantly (e.g., knowledge of disabilities, families, technology, funding). Finally, the complicated developmental or acquired conditions of people who rely on AAC, often occurring with concomitant cognitive, sensory, and behavioral sequelae, can be the source of hardships as AAC services unfold.

Clearly, complexities associated with AAC increase the probability of hardships as services are delivered. Simple exposure to hardship, however, does not ensure perseverance in the pursuit of goals. Hardship, personally or professionally, can also result in frustration, fatigue, and even failure. What promotes AAC grit and

resilience? More specifically, what is it that makes AAC providers, people who rely on AAC, and stakeholders persevere?

My experiences suggest that past AAC successes, even those that are quite limited, fuel perseverance. It may even be that an aspirational orientation toward success, defined as a hopeful attitude, is sufficient. I also feel professional perseverance can be driven by a healthy empathy, or the ability to understand and share the feelings of another. What AAC professional has not tried to understand and learn from the strengths and limitations of a person with CCN? In my personal experience, attempting to see the world through the eyes of a person who relies on AAC has been quite motivating.

Perseverance may have other sources as well, such as passion, spirituality, and encouragement within systems of support. Passion, for anything, can make humans push harder toward goals and persevere against hardships encountered during those efforts. As mentioned earlier, I have been a speech-language pathologist for over three decades and have participated in several areas of practice in my discipline and with other providers. In no other subspecialty of allied health disciplines have I observed a "practice passion" equal to that I've seen in AAC specialists and stakeholders.

Spirituality, however that may be defined, also seems to be a potential positive force in the face of adversity. I have observed considerable perseverance from individuals professing unifying personal belief systems. Their perseverance may stem from a sense of calling or a broader belief in order or purpose. Whatever the source, my experience suggests that spirituality can motivate perseverance.

Finally, encouragement can inspire perseverance. Let's face it, we all push

Table 1–1. Stakeholder and User Comments About Critical Aspects of Ideal AAC Users, Professionals, and Stakeholders

Stakeholder Comments	
About Users	"Ideal AAC users have a growth mindset . . . they are open to possibilities, determined, and willing to try new things."
	"I believe the most successful AAC users have the determination to learn how to communicate with a communication device."
	"I feel the most successful users have an ability to integrate life into the system. If it connects you to people, you win."
	"Ideal users are determined and lead the way with their communication. Their motivation is intrinsic."
	"Ideal users are curious and resilient."
About Professionals	Professionals must "learn the client, the device, the communicative needs and much more. Treat the client like a person first. Understand what they need and what is important in life. It is a marathon, not a sprint. A willingness to problem-solve is best."
	"The best professionals are willing to support users and open to possibilities. Openness is key as is a willingness to stick it out until solutions are found."
	"Ideal professionals persevere. They never let things drop or give up without a fight. They advocate to the end."
About Stakeholders	"The most successful stakeholders are those that fight for appropriate services."
	"The most successful stakeholders put LOVE first. If they feel supported, they can problem-solve issues, wait for complex answers on a device, learn how it works, help the device users grow their skills and much, much, much, more."
User Comments	
About Users	"AAC is going to be slow and it will take time to increase that rate of communication. This means many people will make assumptions of the person using an AAC device. It takes a lot of grit to prove those people wrong. You also have to be resilient to keep moving forward when people continue to put barriers in front of you. As a person who uses AAC, I believe more barriers are put in front of you both most people."
	"Everybody do it different."
About Professionals	"I believe the best AAC professionals are open to learn, to adjust, and to do what is best for the individual. They have to have the willingness also to do what is best for the individual. Many times, they may go into a situation thinking one way, but they may have to adjust and go in another direction. The best AAC professionals are able to do it."
	One user identified determination, willingness, and resilience in ideal AAC professionals noting that "Matt, Amy, Kathleen are my friends . . . we were good as AAC team."
About Stakeholders	"They love me so they will try fix."

harder when cheered on by those around us. In the world of AAC, cheers may come from fellow team members, other stakeholders, or the client him- or herself. With encouragement, those involved in AAC services are more likely to persevere than stumble when challenged.

So, what can be concluded about the role of grit and resilience in AAC service provision? Unfortunately, there is no specific literature to support that these traits inspire or drive successful AAC services. This likely is the result of difficulties inherent in defining grit and resilience, and not meant to imply that there is no effort to measure these attributes empirically in professionals, people who rely on AAC, and others involved with AAC. The lack of current empirical data, however, does not suggest that grit and resilience are not important; it simply means there is no currently published literature to support this. A positive role for grit and resilience in AAC is both appealing and intuitive. Definitive support, however, awaits further study.

■ AAC Challenges and Solutions: Introducing Authors and Describing Contributions

The remainder of this chapter has two purposes: (1) to introduce the authors and contributions that follow; and (2) to foreshadow content that is specific to developing and fostering a solution-oriented AAC perspective. Although comments will largely be directed to professional providers, they also have applicability to both people who rely on AAC and other AAC stakeholders. Before chapters are described, it is worth mentioning that the

scope of this text is limited to topics chosen by the authors. That is, authors were allowed the discretion to write about challenges they had experienced in practice, research, or both. This flexibility may have inevitably resulted in the omission of challenges you, as readers, may experience in your practice. Although I acknowledge this likelihood, I am pleased with the range of content provided, and I believe many of the solutions offered here may be applicable beyond their specific contexts.

The book opens with contributions related to challenges in childhood. Sevcik and colleagues discuss the challenges of AAC services in the first years of life. These authors are well known for their contributions to the field of AAC and provide innovative ideas specific to the very early application of AAC solutions. In their words, earlier is better. Barton-Hulsey, King, and Lyons-Golden continue a focus on childhood with a chapter on challenges specific to language and literacy instruction. As noted earlier, literacy is a primary area of concern for AAC providers. Barton-Hulsey et al. bring an exciting and creative perspective to language and literacy challenges facing AAC providers and stakeholders in early-education settings. Chapter 3 is authored by Nancy Robinson and Gloria Soto and dedicated to challenges experienced during the school years. Robinson and Soto are well qualified to present this content after authoring a book on AAC services in the schools in 2013 (Robinson & Soto, 2013). Their suggestions provide critical assistance to providers and stakeholders in school settings. The initial section of the book ends with McNaughton and Babb's forward-thinking chapter about AAC challenges for adolescents. These authors are known for their practical writings concerning AAC's role in closing gaps of all kinds for individuals with CCN. Their chapter is consistent with this theme, providing directions for solution-oriented practice specific to community and prevocational transitions.

Beginning with Chapter 6, content shifts to consider challenges encountered by adult people who rely on AAC and their stakeholders. Chavers, Cheng, and Koul review AAC applications for individuals with aphasia with a critical eye to challenges and solutions. These authors provide guidance for some persistent problems frequently encountered during work with this special population. The final two chapters in this section address adults with significant physical impairments and their many challenges related to AAC access. In Chapter 7, McLaughlin, Peters, McInturf, Eddy, et al. focus their efforts on AAC decision-making related to the later stages of ALS. This chapter provides creative and cutting-edge solutions that can help people who rely on AAC communicate in the face of challenging declines in volitional movement. In Chapter 8, Fager, Gormley, and Sorenson extend the access discussion by considering solutions applicable for a host of conditions impairing client movement. Solutions are current and provide potential communication options for individuals who heretofore have had little hope.

The third section of the book is dedicated to challenges and solutions more broadly related to either special populations or emerging practice issues. Sigafoos, Roche, and Tate focus on individuals with profound intellectual disabilities. These authors emphasize possibilities with a population that has too often been viewed as less than capable of using AAC. In Chapter 10, Ericson, Geist, Hatch, and Quick follow suit with a cogent argument for core vocabulary as a starting place for emergent communicators. These authors discuss the challenges faced by providers struggling to initiate AAC solutions and introduce core vocabulary as both an elegant and practical solution. In Chapter 11, Schlosser, Shane, Allen, Yu, et al. shift gears by addressing challenges associated with AAC services for students with autism. They present the Visual Immersion SystemTM as an AAC solution available for classroom use.

The final two chapters of this book take a deviation from traditional content by presenting broad challenges related to practice issues. Wilkinson and colleagues explore challenges specific to expressing emotion via AAC. These authors discuss strategies, ideas, and solutions applicable to people who rely on AAC across many diagnoses and settings. Finally, Wofford and Hoge present many of the AAC challenges emerging from the evolving multicultural nature of our society. They provide family-oriented solutions that are certain to be central to AAC efforts from this point forward.

The book ends with reflections on becoming a solution-oriented AAC provider. Never have I been so convinced that the successful application of AAC lays in the hands of solution-oriented providers—providers with grit and resilience who synthesize new and old ideas and embrace opportunities provided within emerging service-delivery paradigms—providers capable of sharing their AAC ideas and passions to build networks of support and success.

I believe that most people who rely on AAC, professionals and stakeholders want to be solution-oriented. But one question remains: "What gets us there?" The final chapter of this text provides directions for solution-oriented AAC practices. It examines this book's contributions for key ideas and common threads. It also revisits the concepts of grit and resilience and offers suggestions for how these attributes may be promoted in new or established individuals who rely on AAC, professionals, and stakeholders. Finally, it proposes a model of practice that assumes and provides guidelines for AAC success.

Although successful AAC services can be challenging, it is my hope, however, that the chapters that follow will illustrate successful practices and encourage them from all of us. People who rely on AAC and their stakeholders deserve nothing less.

■ References

American Speech Language Hearing Association. (2019). *Augmentative and alternative communication* [Practice portal]. Retrieved from https://www.asha.org/Practice-Portal/Professional-Issues/Augmentative-and-Alternative-Communication/

Beukelman, D., & Light, J. C., (2020). *Augmentative and alternative communication: Supporting children and adults with complex communication needs* (5th ed.). Brookes.

Blackstone, S. W., & Hunt-Berg, M. (2012). *Social networks: A communication inventory for individuals with complex communication needs and their communication partners*. Attainment Company.

Caron, J., & Light, J. (2015). "My world has expanded even though I'm stuck at home." Experiences of individuals with ALS who use AAC and social media. *American Journal of Speech-Language Pathology, 24,* 680–695.

Costello, J. M., Shane, K. C., & Caron, J. (2013). *AAC, mobile devices and apps: Growing pains with evidence-based practice*. Boston's Children's Hospital.

Crede, M., Tynan, M. C., & Harms, P. D. (2017). Much ado about grit: A meta-analytic synthesis of the grit literature. *Journal of Personality and Social Psychology, 113*(2), 492–511.

D'Amour, D., & Oandasan, I. (2005). Interprofessionality as the field of interprofessional practice and interprofessional education: An emerging concept. *Journal of Interprofessional Care, 19*(Suppl. 1), 8–20.

Deneckere, S., Euwema, M., Lodewijckx, C., Panella, M., Sermeus, W., & Vanhaecht, K. (2012). The European quality of care pathways (EQCP) study on the impact of care pathways on interprofessional teamwork in an acute hospital setting: Study protocol: For a cluster randomized controlled trial and evaluation of implementation processes. *Implementation Science, 7,* 47.

Duckworth, A. L., Peterson, C., Matthews, M. D., & Kelly, D. R. (2007). Grit: Perseverance and passion for long-term goals. *Journal of Personality and Social Psychology, 92*(6), 1011–1087.

Erickson, K. A. (2017). Comprehensive literacy instruction, interprofessional collaborative practice, and students with severe disabilities. *American Journal of Speech-Language Pathology, 26*(2), 193–205.

Fried-Oken, M., & Light, J. (2012, June 28). *Language and learning: Cognitive science considerations in the design of AAC technologies*. Presentation at the AAC-RERC Spread the Science Conference in Augmentative and Alternative Communication, Baltimore, MD.

Hammond, D. A. (2016). Grit: An important characteristic in learners. *Currents in Pharmacy Teaching and Learning, 9*(1), 1–3.

Higginbotham, J., & Fager, S., (2012, June 28). *Adaptive access: Key design considerations for people with communication, motor, and cognitive challenges*. Presentation at the AAC-RERC Spread the Science Conference in Augmentative and Alternative Communication, Baltimore, MD.

Howe A., Smajdor A., & Stockl, A. (2012). Towards an understanding of resilience and its relevance to medical training. *Medical Education, 46*(4), 349–356.

McCann, C. M., Beddoe, E., McCormick, K., Huggard, P., Kedge, S., Adamson, C., & Huggard J. (2013). Resilience in the health professions: A review of recent literature. *International Journal of Wellbeing, 3*(1), 60–81.

McNaughton, D., & Light, J. (2013). The iPad and mobile technology revolution: Benefits and challenges for individuals who require augmentative and alternative communication. *Augmentative and Alternative Communication, 29*(2), 107–116.

Ogletree, B. (1999). Introduction to teaming. In B. T. Ogletree, M. A. Fischer, & J.B. Schulz (Eds.), *Bridging the family-professional gap: Facilitating interdisciplinary services for children with disabilities* (pp. 3–11). Charles Thomas.

Ogletree, B. T., McMurry, S., Schmidt, M., & Evans, K., (2018). The changing world of AAC: Examining three realities faced by today's AAC provider. *ASHA SIG 12 Perspectives, 3*(Part 3), *113–117.*

Ogletree, B. T., & Oren, T. (2006). *How to use augmentative and alternative communication with individuals with autism spectrum disorders.* A series edited by Richard Simpson, Austin, TX: Pro-Ed.

Paterson, H. (2017). The use of social media by adults with acquired conditions who use AAC: Current gaps and considerations in research. *Augmentative & Alternative Communication, 33*(1), 23–31.

Robinson, N. B, & Soto, G. (2013). *AAC in the schools: Best practices for intervention.* Attainment Publishing.

Sevcik, R. (2009). Comprehension: An overlooked component in augmented language development, *Disability and Rehabilitation, 28*(3), 159–167.

Shi, M., Wang, X., YuGe, B., & Wang, L. (2015). The mediating role of resilience in the relationship between stress and life satisfaction among Chinese medical students: A cross-sectional study. *BMC Medical Education, 15*(16). https://doi.org/1086/s129 09-015-0297-2

Spencer-Oatey, H. (2012). What is culture? A compilation of quotations. *GlobalPAD*

Core Concepts. Available at GlobalPAD Open House. http://www.warwick.ac.uk/global padintercultural

Stoffel, J. M., & Cain, J. (2018). Review of grit and resilience literature within health professions education. *American Journal of Pharmaceutical Education, 82*(2), 124–134. https://doi.org/10.5688/ajpe6150

Sylvester, L., Ogletree, B. T., & Lunnen, K. (2017). Co-treatment as a vehicle for interprofessional collaborative practice: Physical therapists and speech-language pathologists collaborating in the care of children with severe disabilities. *American Journal on Speech Language Pathology,* 26, 206–216.

Tempski, P., Santos, I. S., Mayer, F. B., Enns, S. C., Perotta, B., Paro, H. B. M. S., . . . Martins, M.A. (2015). Relationship among medical student resilience, educational environment and quality of life. *PLoS ONE 10*(6), e0131535. https://doi.org/10.1371/journal .pone.0131535

Tugade, M. M., & Fredrickson, B. L. (2004). Resilient individuals use positive emotions to bounce back from negative emotional experiences. *Journal of Personality and Social Psychology, 86*(2), 320–333.

Wilkinson, K. M., Light, J., & Drager, K. (2012). Considerations for the composition of visual scene displays: Potential contributions of information from visual and cognitive sciences. *Augmentative and Alternative Communication,* 28, 137–147.

World Health Organization. (2010). *Framework for action on interprofessional education and collaborative practice.* Author. Retrieved from http://whqlibdoc.who.int/ hq/2010/WHO_HRH_HPN_10.3_eng.pdf ?ua=1

Zwarenstein, M., Goldman, J., & Reeves, S. (2009). Interprofessional collaboration: Effects of practice-based interventions on professional practice and healthcare outcomes. *Cochrane Database of Systematic Reviews.* https://doi.org/10.1002/14651858 .CD000072.pub2

PART II

AAC Challenges and Solutions: Childhood

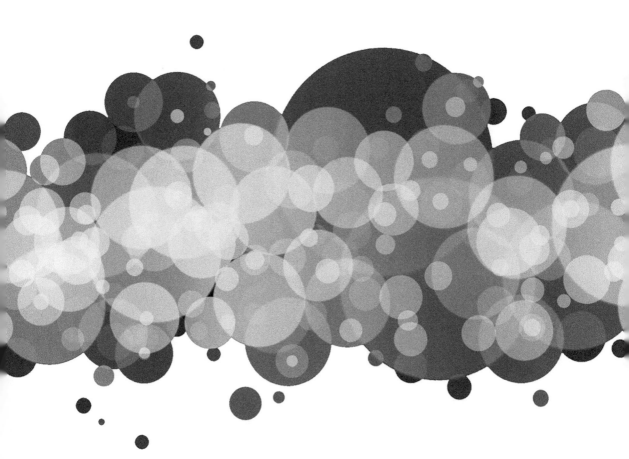

2

Earlier Is Better: Challenges to Implementing AAC During Early Intervention

Rose A. Sevcik, MaryAnn Romski, Casy Walters, and Gal Kaldes

> *Mrs. L told us: "If my son had had a communication system like the System for Augmenting Language (SAL) when he was 2 years old, I would have had different expectations for him as he developed."*

◾ Introduction

Mrs. L's message is strikingly powerful! It addresses the potential negative long-term effects of <u>not</u> providing a child with a way to communicate at a young age. We first met Mrs. L, and her late adolescent son JL who had a diagnosis of significant intellectual disability, when we began our school-aged study on the use of augmentative and alternative communication (AAC) at home and school (Romski & Sevcik, 1996). At 19, JL comprehended some single word spoken vocabulary, vocalized and gestured but used no spoken words. Upon the introduction of

his speech-generating device (SGD), he immediately began to use the symbols to communicate. He spontaneously took his SGD to church and his mom reported that other church members began to communicate with him independently. He sat in his bedroom and "practiced" repeatedly pressing each symbol to listen to each synthetic word paired with the symbol as it was spoken. JL also was extremely possessive of his SDG; he would not let anyone touch it including his Mom and carried its 16 pounds up and down the stairs at school. (Romski & Sevcik, 1996). We often wondered how his development would have progressed if he had had a SGD from the time he was two years old or younger. Mrs. L's message highlights how important the early inclusion of AAC could be to a child's long-term communication development and the family's perception of the child. If the young child does not have an immediate way to communicate, parents, family members, and teachers may not have appropriate short- and long-term expectations for the child's communication development. This is a disservice to the child and the family! Mrs. L advocated, in fact, she insisted, that we move our intervention research focus from school-aged children to preschoolers and toddlers (Romski & Sevcik, 1996). We listened and as we made this move, we encountered some longstanding influential myths about using AAC with young children: "The child is too young for AAC. AAC will stop the child from learning to talk." (Romski & Sevcik, 2005). Myths are widely held but false beliefs. These myths interfere with the use of AAC in early intervention services (Romski & Sevcik, 2005) even though the role AAC plays in early intervention has matured substantially over the last few decades (Romski, Sevcik, Barton-Hulsey, & Whitmore, 2015; Sevcik & Romski, 2016). In a 30-year review of the AAC early intervention literature, Romski et al. (2015) reported that there has been an increase in studies with preschool children, and to a lesser extent with children in the birth to three age group.

Looking back more than four decades, the field's thinking about what was "early" AAC intervention was at a very different place. When the use of AAC began in earnest in the late 1970s and early 1980s, the focus was on determining the age at which to provide AAC services. The literature presented a variety of different perspectives about how to utilize AAC depending on the disability with which the child presented. At that time, both Chapman and Miller (1981) and Shane (1981) argued for developmental candidacy models that included a chronological age dimension. Around eight years of age, was a starting point to consider AAC as an alternative to natural speech and only after the child had "failed" to develop natural speech. The concept of early intervention, encompassing birth to three, as

we know it today was different within that framework.

Since that time, clinicians, families, and individuals who use AAC have recognized that AAC is an important component of language intervention for children with disabilities who encounter difficulty learning to speak. In fact, AAC permits them to augment their existing communication skills and compensate for their lack of natural speech while their language skills are developing (e.g., Barton, Sevcik, & Romski, 2006; Beukelman & Light, 2020; Branson & Demchak, 2009; Romski & Sevcik, 1996; Sevcik & Romski, 2016). There also is support that AAC interventions increase vocal and speech development (e.g., Blischak, 1999; Blischak, Lombardino, & Dyson, 2003; Leech & Cress, 2011; Millar, Light, & Schlosser, 2006; Romski & Sevcik, 1996).

Amazingly, just a few weeks ago in 2020, as one of the authors was showing a self-advocate for intellectual and developmental disabilities a photo of young children using SGDs he asked: *"Don't these devices stop the child from talking? You have to be careful the child doesn't rely on it."* Luckily, we were readily able to convey to him the value of having a way to communicate from early on in development. Unfortunately, today the myths that argue that toddlers are too young to benefit from AAC and that AAC could hinder the child's ability to speak seem to recycle themselves and continue to re-emerge in a range of contexts as shown in the text box example.

> *During an initial consent session in which we explained what the interventions consisted of, one grandmother who accompanied her*

daughter and two-year-old grand-daughter, Mary, to the session said, "This will stop Mary from beginning to speak. Why are you giving up on Mary talking? You should not be part of this intervention." We offered an explanation about the data refuting such a claim, stated that we were not giving up on Mary talking, and answered the mom's questions. The family left us that day as mom said, "She would think it over." In a few days, mom called back to say her mother had convinced her that they should focus on Mary learning to talk and our intervention would not help her get there. Sadly, A few years later, mom called back to ask if we could help because Mary never started talking.

These myths hinder the implementation of Mrs. L's message. For very young children, not being able to communicate impacts all aspects of their immediate lives including their ability to participate in everyday childhood social and educational activities. Early communication experience that employs AAC to augment language experiences may facilitate communication development, including natural speech development (Romski, Sevcik, Barton-Hulsey, & Cheslock, 2017; Sevcik & Romski, 2016). At these young ages, it is certainly not clear that AAC will be the child's permanent form of communication. AAC also can be a temporary strategy during the early language development process. We have seen a number of children who use AAC to get started with communication while they are developing their spoken communication and language skills. As their natural speech

begins to emerge, their use of AAC slowly is supplanted with speech.

In order to ensure that AAC is included in early intervention services and supports, there must be solutions for two main challenges. The first challenge is providing practitioners and families with AAC language intervention strategies that can support beginning communication. The second challenge is discrediting the myths surrounding beginning AAC services and supports with very young children. In this chapter, we use the evidence-base from research and clinical practice to suggest solutions to these challenges. First, we present an evidence-based early language comprehension and production framework and interventions to facilitate the communication development for young children who may use AAC either temporarily or permanently from early in life. Next, we provide illustrations from our own clinical research experiences to highlight the use of these intervention strategies with young children. Following the case illustrations, we suggest potential solutions for how to adapt the interventions developed in these two studies to clinical and home environments. Finally, we return to the myths and offer solutions for clinicians to share with families and other professionals to refute these myths and change attitudes.

■ A Framework for Early Language Comprehension and Production Intervention

One important aspect of integrating AAC into early intervention services and supports is to provide clinicians and families with evidence-based intervention approaches that integrate AAC in every day environments. In order for young children to develop functional language and communication skills, they must be able to comprehend *and* produce language so that they can take on the roles of both listener and speaker in conversational exchanges (Sevcik & Romski, 2002). Comprehension is the ability to understand what is said to us so that we can function as a listener in communicative exchanges. Production is the ability to express information so that we can function as a speaker in communicative exchanges.

The communication development of children without disabilities provides an important framework for early language intervention incorporating AAC as presented in Romski, Sevcik, Barton-Hulsey, & Cheslock (2017). Young children without disabilities learn to speak before the age of 2 years. Well before beginning to speak, the stage is being set for their expressive language development through communication interactions and input from adults in environmental routines. Before actually uttering their first words, children typically comprehend about 50 words and develop a repertoire of intentional vocalizations and gestures that they use to request and to refer to objects and events in their world (Adamson, 1996). As Romski et al. (2017) articulated, speech comprehension typically precedes speech production during the emerging language development phase and builds the foundation for the development of first spoken words. By the time young Emily utters her first words at 15 months of age, she can, for example, carry out simple commands like "Bring Mommy her shoes," identify by name many objects, familiar people, and some body parts. Children begin to produce their first words after

spending more than a year of hearing spoken language input from their caregivers. They extract relevant information from the linguistic environment and associate it with their own developing vocal and nonvocal forms in order to express wants and needs (Baldwin & Markman, 1989; Golinkoff, Mervis, & Hirsh-Pasek, 1994; Mervis & Bertrand, 1993). Most children without disabilities build individual vocabularies over time composed of a range of words (e.g., objects, actions, emotions; Nelson, 1973). At about 18 to 20 months of age, they have a vocabulary growth spurt (Golinkoff et al., 1994). The rate of vocabulary growth then expands dramatically and the child quickly moves on to combine words and express early semantic relations. This early period, then, is rich with opportunities for the young child to develop a firm communication and language foundation even though he or she is not yet talking. This foundation includes opportunities to use the spoken input the child receives to develop language comprehension skills and begin communicating via vocalizations, gestures, and other means even before the child starts talking.

The literature on the communication and language development of children without disabilities strongly suggests that these early experiences are critical for the emergence of comprehension and production language skills. Most young children without disabilities quickly move on to producing words, phrases, and sentences and their comprehension of words, and even sentences, is taken for granted. Even with a base of vocalizations and gestures, a child with complex communication needs may not readily make the transition to spoken language without additional supports. AAC can provide those supports (Warren, Brady, Bredin-Oja, & Hahn, in press).

■ Designing Augmented Language Interventions for Early Intervention

We used this framework to create augmented language interventions that capitalize on the early relationship of receptive and expressive language development and on the parents' role in the process. Current evidence and perspectives suggest that the functions AAC can play in language and communication development are broader than providing an alternative output mode by which children can convey information (Romski et al., 2015). AAC also can provide an input mode as well as an output mode for communication for children with limited speech comprehension skills, augment existing speech and vocalizations, and serve as a tool to teach language (Romski & Sevcik, 1996).

In our clinical research program, we developed a set of parent-implemented augmented language interventions that varied the roles of comprehension and production to assess how they contributed to developing first words via symbols. We conducted two randomized control trial studies to examine these issues (Romski, Sevcik, Adamson, Cheslock, Smith, et al., 2010; Romski, Sevcik, Adamson, Barton-Hulsey, et al., manuscript in preparation). Table 2–1 describes the components of the four different interventions we examined in the two studies, highlighting their similarities and differences. As you can see, these interventions share many commonalities but each differs on one important dimension. Speech Communication Intervention (SCI) focuses only on developing the child's natural speech and was included as a contrast intervention. Augmented Communication Input (ACI) addresses communicative partner use of AAC symbols on the SGD to provide spoken and symbol word input models for the child. Augmented Communication Output (ACO) focuses on the child's production of symbols during routines. And, finally, the hybrid intervention, Augmented Communication Input/Output (ACIO), combines augmented input and output in one intervention to capitalize on the strengths of the two individual interventions.

Participants

The interventions were designed for toddlers at the beginning stages of language development. Each child had a spoken vocabulary of at most 10 intelligible words and a score of less than 12 months on the expressive language scale of the Mullen Scales of Early Learning (MSEL; Mullen, 1995). They had at least primitive intentional communication abilities; upper extremity gross motor skills that permit them to select the symbols on the SGD (though we did include a few children who had greater physical limitations (e.g., Romski, Krupa, Cheslock, Sevcik, & Adamson, 2008); and a primary disability other than delayed speech and language impairment or deafness/hearing impairment. One hundred and nine toddlers (24 to 36 months of age) and their mothers or fathers participated in these two clinical research studies and we randomly assigned them to one of the interventions.

Implementing Intervention Protocols

The children and their parents participated in 24, 30-minute sessions over approximately three months. The sessions coached parents to create communication

Table 2–1. Intervention Components and Studies Employed

INTERVENTION	SCI—Spoken Communication Intervention (Study 1)	ACI – Augmented Communication Input Intervention (Study 1)	ACO—Augmented Communication Output Intervention (Studies 1 & 2)	ACIO—Augmented Communication Input + Output Intervention (Study 2)
MODE	I/P and the child use speech to communicate	I/P uses SGD to provide communication input to child	Child uses SGD to communicate	I/P uses SGD to provide communication input to child
VOCABULARY	Individualized vocabulary of spoken words	Individualized vocabulary of visual-graphic symbols + words	Individualized vocabulary of visual-graphic symbols + words	Individualized vocabulary of visual-graphic symbols + words
STRATEGY	I/P encourages and prompts the child to produce spoken words	I/P provides vocabulary models to child using the SGD; symbols are positioned in the environment to mark referents	I/P encourages and prompts the child to produce communication using the SGD	I/P provides vocabulary models to child by using the SGD; symbols are positioned in the environment to mark referents; I/P encourages and prompts the child to produce communication using the SGD
COACHING AND RESOURCES	I provides resource and coaching for P	I provides resource and coaching for P	I provides resource and coaching for P	I provides resource and coaching for P

Note: I = interventionist/clinician; P = parent; SGD = speech generating device.

Source: Adapted from Fey, M. E., & Kamhi, A. G. (2017). *Treating language disorders in children, Second Edition* (p.165). As reprinted from Romski, M.A., & Sevcik, R.A. (1996). *Breaking the speech barrier: Language development through augmented means* (p. 77). Baltimore, MD: Paul H. Brookes Publishing Co.; reprinted by permission.

opportunities to support overall language development and specific strategies to communicate with the child via an SGD. Table 2–2 provides an overview of communication strategies that we employed during the study. We focused on SGDs instead of other forms of AAC (e.g., manual signs, communication boards, or books) because SGDs provide the child with a "voice." These permit familiar and unfamiliar communicative partners to hear the "speech" produced when the child activates a visual symbol on the SDG and immediately understands the message.

The SGD automatically links the child's visual symbol communication with a familiar auditory/spoken modality in social interactional contexts. It permits the child to use a multimodal form of communication, including a "voice" while retaining access to the visual modality. It also provides the child with a consistent model of spoken word production every time they use a symbol. (Romski et al., 2017, p. 170).

Table 2–3 summarizes the common protocol that we employed across all interventions.

Each 30-minute intervention session included three 10-minute routines—play, book, and snack—that targeted vocabulary words that the child did not yet comprehend or produce. Each routine activity has an overlay with specific vocabulary and additional vocabulary that appears on all the overlays (e.g., my turn). All interventions followed the same protocol that occurred within that naturalistic teaching routines and were readily able to be replicated in the family's home environment. These protocols included parent observation of the child, parent-coaching during intervention, and transfer from the clinical lab to the home communication environment. Table 2–4 provides an overview of guidelines for coaching parents during the intervention and Table 2–5 provides a list of areas on which to focus parent coaching.

Vocabulary

Prior to the first session, the speech-language pathologist (SLP) and parent worked together to choose target symbol and spoken vocabulary for use during the three routines. We represented the

Table 2–2. Communication Strategies to Use During Intervention Routines

Create Communication Opportunities:	Communicate With the Child by:
▪ Provide choices ▪ Disrupt the environment ▪ Give small amounts ▪ Briefly delay access ▪ Use pause time ▪ Use fill-in-the-blank activities	▪ Using parallel talk ▪ Using short, simple sentences ▪ Limiting questions ▪ Using key words ▪ Slowing rate of speech ▪ Immediately responding to child's communication attempts ▪ Following the child's lead ▪ HAVING FUN!

Table 2–3. Intervention Protocol Descriptions

24 Sessions	30-Minute Sessions	Parent-Implemented Focus
▪ 18 sessions in clinic ▪ 6 sessions generalization to home	▪ Three 10-minute blocks of play, book reading, snack ▪ Individualized vocabulary	▪ First 8 sessions parent observes with SLP ▪ Parent protocol manual with weekly materials ▪ Beginning with 9th session, parent backs into session with ongoing coaching by interventionist ▪ Beginning with 16th session, parent implements entire session ▪ Beginning with 19th session, intervention goes home; parent implements entire session

Table 2–4. Guidelines for Parent Coaching

- Be positive
- Present information in a manner that fits the parent's learning style (e.g., verbal and/or written feedback; demonstration/ modeling; video-tape review)
- Give specific and concrete examples
- Build feedback around what is needed most to support the child's progress and the parent's skill to implement the intervention
- Follow a consistent format
  - Ask parent for thoughts on the session
  - Give positive feedback first
  - Identify and give feedback on primary areas of needed support
  - Identify and give feedback on secondary areas, if needed and warranted
  - Ask parent if she or he has questions; Summarize with positive comments

vocabulary with Tobii-Dynavox's Board-maker® symbols (https://goboardmaker.com; Tobii-Dynavox, 2020). Six target words, which the child did not comprehend or produce, were chosen for each routine of play, book, and snack. For example, there was a combination of nouns and verbs (e.g., ball, doll, car, drink, bubbles, block, throw), as well as core vocabulary (e.g., my turn, all done, more) that overlapped across each routine. We used the Systematic Analysis of Language

Transcript software (SALT; Miller & Chapman, 2000) to code spontaneous target vocabulary use by the child. The mode of communication used by the child when expressing a target vocabulary word was coded as an augmented word (symbol), a spoken word, or both.

Table 2–5. Areas of Focus for Parent Coaching

- Creating a context for interaction and conversation
- Implementing the augmented language intervention protocol itself
- Modeling vocabulary
- Creating communication opportunities (e.g., choice-making, sabotage)
- Focusing child performance
- Addressing child behavior management issues (e.g., redirection, motivation, transitions)
- Modeling Interaction style (e.g., directive, passive)

■ Augmented Intervention Study Findings

In the first study, Romski and colleagues (2010) compared the effects of a spoken parent-implemented language intervention (SCI) with two augmented parent-implemented language interventions (ACI, ACO) on spoken and augmented vocabulary learning for 62 toddlers (24 to 36 months) and their parents. High school educated parents implemented the features of the three interventions equally well and it resulted in child vocabulary gains (Romski, Sevcik, Adamson, Cheslock, & Smith, 2007). As shown in Figure 2–1, both augmented interventions provided

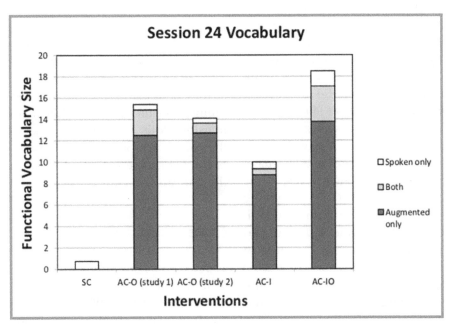

Figure 2–1. Mean functional vocabulary gains across all four interventions.

a way for the child to communicate via visual-graphic symbols + digitized spoken words after only 18 sessions of intervention. Augmented output, and to a lesser extent, augmented input, substantially increased the likelihood that children would produce natural spoken words after just 18 sessions of parent-implemented intervention than the spoken language intervention. The use of an SGD contributed positively to the intelligibility of child communicative utterances. These findings provide clear evidence against the myth that AAC use in early intervention will stop the child from talking. In fact, the findings, as shown in Figure 2–1, indicate that the two AAC interventions actually have better natural speech outcomes than the spoken communication intervention.

In the second study, we (Romski et al., 2020) compared the effects of the most successful parent-implemented augmented intervention from study one, augmented output, with a hybrid intervention that combined ACO with ACI on spoken and augmented vocabulary learning. This study also examined the effects of development on intervention outcomes. Without intervention, children did not develop expressive communication skills. It suggests that without an AAC intervention, these children would not have spontaneously developed expressive language skills. It provides evidence to dispel the myth about starting AAC at too young of an age. ACIO, the hybrid intervention that combined augmented input and output, provided a stronger outcome of augmented and spoken words than ACO alone. Figure 2–1 also presents the number of target augmented (symbol) and spoken words produced by the children across the four interventions and two

studies. This finding continues to dispel the myth about AAC hindering speech development.

■ How Do You Decide Which Intervention Approach to Use With an Individual Child?

We suggest a two-pronged solution-oriented approach when considering which intervention to implement with an individual child. It includes child assessment outcomes and parent-child dyad interactions. First, it is critical to determine what communication strengths and weaknesses a child brings to the intervention task. In particular, it is important to include assessment of early communication (e.g., vocalizations, gestures) and speech comprehension skills. Understanding the environments and routines that the child participates in is also important. If the child's comprehension skills are just emerging, either the augmented input intervention (ACI) or the hybrid intervention (ACIO) may be a good choice as they both incorporate augmented communication input. If the child's comprehension skills are fairly well developed, the augmented output intervention (ACO) or the hybrid intervention (ACIO) may be the appropriate choice.

Case Illustrations

These case illustrations provide examples of intervention challenges and successes of children at two different ends of the continuum in terms of speech comprehension. The two children, Franklin and Jennifer, profiled below, participated in our parent-implemented AAC interventions using SGDs. They illustrate the use of the different augmented language interventions.

Franklin

Franklin had just turned three (38 months) when he and his mother began the ACO intervention. Around 2 years of age, his parents first became concerned about his delayed expressive language, and he received a diagnosis of developmental delay. He did not regularly use spoken words to communicate. He typically used vocalizations and gestures to make simple requests and respond to his parents and twin brother. Franklin had hearing and visual acuity within normal limits, and he was able to point and walk without difficulty. At the beginning of intervention, his mother reported that he comprehended 229 words on the McArthur Bates Communication Development Inventory (MCDI; Fenson et al., 2007). However, he used 10 spoken words that included mostly food and body related nouns (e.g., "a-le" for apple, "eye," "more"). On the MSEL (Mullen, 1995), he received receptive and expressive age equivalent scores of 34 and 24 months, respectively.

As he began the 12-week intervention, he received a *CheapTalk (Enabling Devices)* SGD, and the first overlays on it included 18 words—comprised of nouns, adjectives, and verbs (e.g., "music," "on," "off," "jumping"). According to intervention notes, he quickly demonstrated comprehension and use of these new spoken words/symbols on the SGD. He used augmented and spoken-target words most frequently to make requests for preferred activities and snacks. At session 8, more complex language was added to support

the development of multiword utterances including pronouns, conjunctions, and articles (e.g., "you," "me," "and," "the"). Intervention notes identified that targeting pronouns was difficult for Franklin to navigate on the SGD and in spoken language. For example, the interventionist said, "you turn page" and Franklin would imitate "you turn page" but would intend "I turn page." When the interventionist said, "I turn page" Franklin would imitate "I turn page" but would intend "you turn page." Although it took him longer to master comprehension and use of these words, by the end of the 24th Session, he produced these targeted words accurately most of the time.

Figure 2–2 illustrates the number of different augmented and spoken target words Franklin used at 6, 12, 18, and 24th intervention sessions. These augmented and spoken words expanded rapidly to 19 and 27 words by session 24, respectively. He also produced 10 by session 24. Franklin used 24 different augmented words by session 12 after which his use of these augmented words decreased slightly across the remaining sessions as his spoken target words increased.

Franklin's mean length of utterance (MLU) increased slightly from 1.02 to 1.35 by the end of intervention, and his percent of intelligible utterances, which included utterances produced on the SGD, increased from 13% to 71%. This upward trend of language development was confirmed on the Sequenced Inventory of Communication Development (SICD; Hendrick, Prather, & Tobin, 1984). Franklin made gains of 4 and 16 months on the receptive and expressive language scales, respectively. Additionally, the MCDI revealed that both the number of words Franklin understood and produced

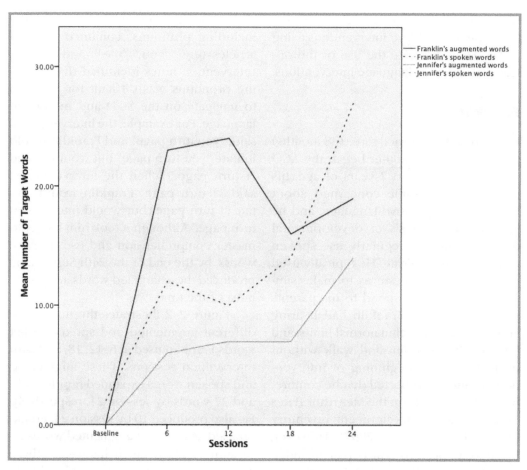

Figure 2–2. Franklin and Jennifer's target vocabulary gains across the 24 sessions.

increased to 370 and 364, respectively. This substantial gain in expressive language suggests that this intervention was successful in supporting Franklin's language development. Franklin's relatively high receptive language skills at the start of intervention made the augmented output intervention a very good fit and provided opportunities for him to express himself across multiple modalities. It demonstrated that AAC intervention can support spoken language development and rejects the myth that early AAC intervention may prevent children from learning to talk.

Jennifer

Thirty-month-old Jennifer and her mother participated in the AC-IO hybrid intervention. Her hearing was within normal limits. Jennifer was independently mobile but demonstrated overall lack of coordination and weakness of gross motor skills such as walking, reaching, and grabbing. Jennifer was identified with a developmental delay at 2 years of age through Babies Can't Wait, which is an early intervention program in Georgia that provides a variety of services for infants and toddlers. Jennifer was receiving speech, occupational, and physical therapy services once a week when she began the study but these services did not incorporate AAC.

During the baseline phase of the study, Jennifer's mother reported that Jennifer mainly communicated through crying and vocalizing. According to the MCDI, Jennifer comprehended a total of ten words, which consisted mostly of food items and toys. She produced two spoken words: "mama" and "ball," but did not use them often to functionally communicate. Her age equivalent scores on the receptive and expressive subtests of the MSEL were 9 and 10 months, respectively, both well below average for children without disabilities her age.

Jennifer began intervention with a *Cheaptalk* SGD that had a display of three different overlays that included 5 words on each overlay for a total of 15 spoken words + visual-graphic symbols. The words included a variety of nouns, adjectives, and verbs. In addition, some short phrases were included as single words (e.g., myturn). Practice on the SGD provided Jennifer with opportunities for expressive language output. Jennifer's mother and the project's interventionist observed that Jennifer demonstrated some physical weaknesses and lack of coordination when using the SGD during the initial phases of the intervention. Jennifer began physically exploring the SGD during Session 2, and her mother frequently modeled symbols on the SGD when Jennifer appeared to look in the direction of the symbols. Jennifer's mother thought that Jennifer began to gaze longer at the target vocabulary symbols as her comprehension improved. Her mother also used hand-over-hand modeling to increase her motor coordination with the SGD. Jennifer showed emerging signs of using the SGD to intentionally communicate during

Session 5 by using symbols appropriately during snack time (e.g., using the symbol "cookie" to request a cookie and waiting for her mother to respond accordingly). According to the interventionist's observations, Jennifer's frequency of using the device spontaneously increased around Session 15. By Session 24, Jennifer was able to use 14 of her 15 aided symbol vocabulary for expressive communication purposes. Jennifer's progress suggested that the type of augmented language input she received in the hybrid intervention supported her ability to build an understanding of the words and a sense of how to use them appropriately. As shown in Figure 2–2, Jennifer's functional vocabulary (i.e. total number of spoken words and symbols) increased from 0, to 5, 7, 7, and 14 across baseline, Session 6, Session 12, Session 18, and Session 24, respectively.

Other measures collected from language sample data and standardized assessments paralleled Jennifer's progress during intervention. Jennifer made high overall receptive vocabulary gains. On the receptive language subtest of SICD, Jennifer's score increased from 12 months at baseline to 24 months at Session 24. On the MCDI, her receptive vocabulary increased to 41 words. Jennifer's expressive language abilities modestly improved. On the SICD expressive language subtest, her score increased from 8 months at baseline to 12 months at Session 24. She demonstrated an expressive vocabulary of 15 words on the MCDI. Her MLU changed from 0.96 at baseline to 1.32 at the end of intervention. Jennifer's percent of intelligible utterances substantially increased from 0% at baseline to 46% at the end of intervention due to the inclusion of an SGD as an additional modality for expressive language. Although Jennifer did not develop any spoken words during the 24-session intervention, the SGD importantly provided her a way to communicate by the time she was two and a half years old.

Summary

Together, these two cases illustrated how these AAC language interventions worked for children with initial distinctive communication profiles. Franklin and Jennifer began intervention with very different receptive language skills that resulted in unique profiles during intervention. Both children increased their receptive and expressive language skills over the course of the intervention. Franklin began intervention with relatively high receptive language skills and the SGD provided a way to visualize new advancing vocabulary and gave him an outlet to express himself as he built his spoken language skills. Jennifer, who began the intervention with beginning receptive language skills, dramatically improved her receptive language. She also modestly increased her expressive abilities via the SGD. It may be that providing augmented input, that is modeling targeted symbol and spoken vocabulary on the SGD, supported her comprehension of spoken words by providing visual symbols and repeated representation of specific words on the SGD. These case illustrations highlight how children with distinct language profiles benefit from using SGDs during language intervention, and we have shared some of the unique solutions that may arise with different language profiles.

It is always important to consider the length and intensity of these interventions because they can influence the outcomes. Built for a study, our intervention protocols were administered in a relatively concise time frame: 24 sessions ideally twice a week for approximately 3 months. Individual children may need different lengths and intensities of intervention. Consistently implement the same strategies week after week and document progress over time. There clearly are degrees of success and success can vary based on how it is measured and how long the intervention has been underway. One notable caution that we would emphasize is do not stop intervention too soon when success appears to be slow. Provide ample time for a child to demonstrate success. For some children, it may take an extended time before there are visible gains. It is important to consider the notion of success along a continuum rather than as an all-or-none phenomenon (Romski et al., 2016).

■ Challenging Myths That Limit Early Communication Success

There are both empirical intervention and clinical success data that dispel myths about early AAC use. Yet, these myths still rear their ugly heads just when you think they are no longer a concern. How do we develop solutions to fight the propagation of these myths so that we can consistently facilitate early communication success? We argue that clinical myths are derived from individual professionals' beliefs or assumptions, sometimes without any empirical support or despite empirical evidence to the contrary (Romski & Sevcik, 2005). A modest research base, along with the immediate demands of providing clinical services, have fostered practices that rely more on a professional's clinical intuition than on current evidence (Brady et al., 2016; Cress & Marvin, 2003). These beliefs grow out of information expressed in the past clinical literature that current empirical evidence does not support. Regrettably, the myths remain and find their way into clinician and family perspectives about early intervention AAC supports and services as illustrated in Table 2–6. These clinician views come from comments made in response to an online early intervention presentation the

Table 2–6. AAC Stakeholder Clinicians' Comments About Early Communication Intervention Myths

Clinician #1	*Right now, I have the most experience implementing and assessing AAC for students in preschool, middle, and high school with autism. This helped me understand how AAC can still apply to children at very young developmental stages—and provided me with specific insights to use for parent coaching and training in EI. I feel confident in explaining how AAC can augment and even assist facilitation of speech and language development for the birth to 3 population, and specific laws/research bodies/and studies where I can reference to back these claims.*
Clinician #2	*The citations provided in this presentation were very helpful. I can use these resources as a starting point for sharing empirical evidence to support the use of AAC with parents/colleagues that may be resistant to my recommendation for a device.*
Clinician #3	*I recently had to debunk the myth that a 2-year-old is too young for AAC, and figure out how to navigate funding for evaluation and device. This presentation is very useful for exactly those situations. I was happy to see the trend growing for AAC in EI so even though there are still people out there that continue the myths, maybe there are more advocates now.*
Clinician #4	*I have encountered all of these myths in my work as an early intervention evaluator. It is helpful to know that the evidence is on the side of using AAC and not waiting to use it as a last resort. Parents often do balk at the idea of signs or pictures because they are convinced that means their child will never talk. I will continue to try to encourage AAC use early on by sharing that it can actually encourage speech and language development, not hinder it.*
Clinician #5	*I do not have a lot of experience with AAC devices; however, this session helped make me aware that even young children can often benefit significantly with their use. I have used PECS and manual signs with young children on my caseload, and even then, there are myths that parents will call to my attention. The one I hear the most is that expressive language will be delayed even more if their child relies on pictures or signs. I have one parent who not only gets EI services for her son, but also pays privately for another SLP. This SLP does not believe in AAC so the mother has had negative feelings about using any alternative communication. Sometimes, as you stated over and over again in your presentation, we just have to advocate and show others the research! I appreciate all of your efforts in this area and the research you both have done!*

first two authors gave this past year (Romski & Sevcik, 2019). They highlight the challenges clinicians face when working to debunk these myths.

There are a number of advocacy solution options for clinicians and families to use to debunk these myths. First, share examples of child success using AAC with other clinicians and parents. These examples could be verbal descriptions of your own experiences, including video clips with the examples that can visually illustrate a child's success. Second, ask families who have positive experiences with AAC use speak with a family who is having difficulty accepting the approach or who has questions and or concerns. We have had, for example, a parent who was supportive of using AAC with his young child write a brief article including FAQs for a parent newsletter. Third, provide abstracts, quotes, or publications of research studies that illustrate that AAC does not hinder speech development in young children. The National Joint Committee (NJC) on the Communication Needs of Individuals with Severe Disabilities has a range of materials including the 15-item Communication Bill of Rights they developed (Brady et al., 2016). Sharing the Bill of Rights with clinicians and families can provide a starting point for a discussion about why it is important to use AAC for beginning communication. Another area for advocacy is to ensure that preprofessional training programs provide accurate information in classes and in student clinical experiences. Some preprofessional training programs still do not present current information about AAC or incorporating it into early language intervention. Sometimes student clinical placements have clinical supervisors who also do not have the most current information about AAC and provide misinformation. One

potential solution to this issue is to have clinicians with early intervention expertise volunteer to provide a presentation about AAC and early intervention to a child language disorders class or another appropriate class.

Obviously, clinicians and families are the best advocates for the child. As a clinician, examine your own perceptions and attitudes regarding AAC and early intervention to determine if they are solutions oriented. Assess how many children you serve who may benefit from AAC services and support and act on it using the AAC language intervention strategies described. It is important to note that sometimes you may not be able to find a solution to debunk the myth on the first try. Correcting misinformation may take time and effort. Used in conjunction with providing early augmented language interventions, these suggested advocacy solutions can aid in dispelling myths that challenge the implementation of AAC in early intervention services and supports.

■ Conclusions

In conclusion, it is never too early to begin AAC intervention! In fact, it is a first line of defense against not being able to communicate with family, friends, and the community at large. Unfortunately, some myths continue to challenge access to AAC intervention services and supports. A SGD is a tool, a means to an end—language and communication skills—not the end. Debunking myths requires having solutions that illustrate how to incorporate AAC into early intervention. New evidence, technologies, and interventions about communication outcomes provide viable solutions for clinicians and families to challenge myths about AAC and its use during early intervention. We must be actively solutions-oriented to debunk these myths to ensure that all children have early access to communication.

Acknowledgments. The contributions of the first two authors, Sevcik and Romski, are equal. We extend our sincere thanks to Mrs. L for her support and encouragement over the course of our early studies. The authors thank the children and families whom we worked with in these studies and helped us defy myths about AAC and early intervention.

■ References

Adamson, L. B. (1996). *Communication development during infancy*. Westview.

Baldwin, D., & Markman, E. (1989). Establishing word-object relations: A first step. *Child Development, 60*, 381–399.

Barton, A., Sevcik, R. A., & Romski, M. A. (2006). Exploring visual-graphic symbol acquisition by pre-school age children with developmental and language delays. *Augmentative and Alternative Communication, 22*(1), 10–20.

Barton-Hulsey, A., Sevcik, R. A., Romski, M. A. & Cheslock, M. A. (2018). Communication development in children with multiple disabilities: The role of augmentative and alternative communication. In B. B. Shulman & N. Capone (Eds.), *Language development: Foundations, processes and clinical applications* (3rd ed.). Jones and Bartlett.

Beukelman, D., & Light, J. (2020). *Augmentative and alternative communication* (5th ed.). Brookes.

Blischak, D. M. (1999). Increases in natural speech production following experience with synthetic speech. *Journal of Special Education Technology, 14*(2), 44–53.

Blischak, D., Lombardino, L., & Dyson, A. (2003). Use of speech-generating devices: In support of natural speech. *Alternative and Augmentative Communication, 19*(1), 29–35.

Brady, N. C., Bruce, S., Goldman, A., Erickson, K., Mineo, B., Ogletree, B. T., . . . Wilkinson, K. (2016). Communication services and supports for individuals with severe disabilities: Guidance for assessment and intervention. *American Journal on Intellectual and Developmental Disabilities, 121*, 121–138.

Branson, D., & Demchak, M. (2009). The use of augmentative and alternative communication methods with infants and toddlers with disabilities: A research review. *Augmentative and Alternative Communication, 25*(4), 274–286.

Chapman, R. S., & Miller, J. F. (1981). Analyzing language and communication in the child. In R. L. Schiefelbusch (Ed.), *Nonspeech language and communication analysis and Intervention* (pp. 159–196). University Park Press.

Cress, C., & Marvin, C. (2003). Common questions about AAC services in early intervention. *Augmentative and Alternative Communicataion, 19*, 254–272.

Fenson, L., Marchman, V. A., Thal, D. J., Dale, P. S., Reznick, J. S., & Bates, E. (2007). *MacArthur-Bates Communicative Development Inventories: User's guide and technical manual* (2nd ed.). Brookes.

Golinkoff, R., Mervis, C., & Hirsh-Pasek, K. (1994). Early object labels: The case for lexical principles. *Journal of Child Language, 21*, 125–155.

Hendrick, D., Prather, E., & Tobin, A. (1984). *Sequenced Inventory of Communication Development*. Western Psychological Services.

Leech, E. R. B., & Cress, C. J. (2011). Indirect facilitation of speech in a late talking child by prompted production of picture symbols or signs. *Augmentative and Alternative Communication, 27*(1), 40–52. https://doi.org/10.3109/07434618.2010.550062

Mervis, C., & Bertrand, J. (1993). Acquisition of early object labels: The role of operating principles. In S. F. Warren & J. Reichle (Series Eds.), A.P. Kaiser & D. Gray (Vol.

Eds.), Communication and language intervention series: Vol. 2. *Enhancing children's communication: Research foundations for intervention* (pp. 287–316). Brookes.

Millar, D. C., Light, J. C., & Schlosser, R. W. (2006). The impact of augmentative and alternative communication intervention on the speech production of individuals with developmental disabilities: A research review. *Journal of Speech, Language, and Hearing Research, 49*(2), 248–264. https://doi.org/10.1044/1092-4388(2006/021)

Miller, J., & Chapman, R. (2000). *Systematic analysis of language transcripts* (Version 6). University of Wisconsin, Language Analysis Lab.

Mullen, E. (1995). *Mullen Scales of Early Learning.* American Guidance Service.

Nelson, K. (1973). Structure and strategy in learning to talk. *Monographs of the Society for Research in Child Development, 38*(1–2), Serial No. 139.

Romski, M. A., Krupa, J. H., Cheslock, M., Sevcik, R. A., & Adamson, L. B. (2008). Language and communication changes in a child with holoprosecephaly: A case report. *Medical Journal of Speech Language Pathology, 14,* 10–19.

Romski, M. A., & Sevcik, R. A. (1996). *Breaking the speech barrier: Language development through augmented means.* Brookes.

Romski, M. A., & Sevcik, R. A. (2005). Early intervention and augmentative communication: Myths and realities. *Infants and Young Children, 18,* 174–185.

Romski, M. A. & Sevcik, R. A. (2019, May). *AAC myths and realities.* Invited presentation and e-chat at the American Speech Language Hearing Association Online Conference on Birth to Three: Working Together to Serve Children and Families.

Romski, M. A., Sevcik, R. A., Adamson, L. B., Barton-Hulsey, A., Smith, A., Barker, M., . . . Bakeman, R. (Manuscript in preparation). *Parent-coached early augmented language interventions for toddlers with developmental delays: A randomized comparison.*

Romski, M. A., Sevcik, R. A., Adamson, L. B., Cheslock, M., & Smith, A. (2007). Parents can implement AAC interventions: Ratings of treatment implementation across early language interventions. *Early Childhood Services, 1,* 249–259.

Romski, M. A., Sevcik, R. A., Adamson, L. B., Cheslock, M. A., Smith, A., Barker, R. M., & Bakeman, R. (2010). Randomized comparison of parent-implemented augmented and non-augmented language intervention on vocabulary development of toddlers with developmental delays. *Journal of Speech, Language, and Hearing Research, 53,* 350–364.

Romski, M. A., Sevcik, R. A., Barton-Hulsey, A., & Whitmore, A. S. (2015). Early intervention and AAC: What a difference thirty years makes. *Augmentative and Alternative Communication, 31,* 181–202.

Romski, M. A., Sevcik, R. A., Cheslock, M., & Barton, A. (2017). The system for augmenting language: AAC and emerging language intervention. In R. McCauley, R. Gilliam, & M. Fey (Eds.), *Treatment of language disorders in children: Conventional and controversial intervention,* (2nd ed., pp. 155–186). Brookes.

Sevcik, R. A., & Romski, M. A. (2002). The role of language comprehension in establishing early augmented conversations. In J. Reichle, D. Beukelman, & J. Light (Eds.), *Implementing an augmentative communication system: Exemplary strategies for beginning communicators* (pp. 453–474). Brookes.

Sevcik, R. A., & Romski, M. A., (2016). Communication interventions for individuals with severe disabilities: Research and practice gaps, opportunities and future directions. In R. A. Sevcik & M. A. Romski (Eds.), *Communication interventions for individuals with severe disabilities: Exploring research challenges and opportunities* (pp. 327–340). Brookes.

Shane, H. C. (1981). Decision making in early augmentative communication system use. In R. L. Schiefelbusch & D. D. Bricker

(Eds.), *Early language: Acquisition and intervention* (pp. 389–425). University Park Press.

Tobii Dynavox LLC. (2020). *Boardmaker*®. Retrieved from https://goboardmaker.com

Warren, S. F., Brady, N., Bredin-Oja, S., & Hahn, L. (in press). Language and communication. In J. A. Burack, J. Edgin, & L. Abbeduto (Eds.), *Oxford handbook of Down syndrome and development*. Oxford University Press.

3

AAC in Preschool: Navigating Challenges in Language and Literacy Instruction

Andrea Barton-Hulsey, Marika King, and Jennifer Lyons-Golden

For children, the transition to preschool is inherently complex, filled with new routines, communication partners, and contexts in which they are expected to continue to grow their language skills. Prior to entering preschool, children may have had a range of experiences that include being at home with a parent or caregiver or attending daycare. These experiences may or may not have included consistent routines. Some children may have experience with more or less formal daycare programs that either do or do not assist in the preparation for the transition to preschool. Regardless, the primary focus of settings prior to preschool usually are centered on the physical, social and emotional care of the child, with little formalized demand placed on the child to gain academic skills. However, the transition to preschool often means an increase in structure and social and learning demands. In the United States, all states have developed Early Learning Developmental Guidelines (ELDGs)

for preschool children (National Center on Early Childhood Quality Assurance, 2019). These guidelines vary from state to state, but generally include recommendations across the following developmental and learning domains: Physical Development and Health, Approaches to Learning, Social and Emotional Development, Language and Literacy, Mathematical Thinking, Scientific Inquiry, Social Study, and Creative Arts. The ELDGs identify key skills which lay the foundation for Kindergarten readiness, and outline expectations for all children regardless of their differences in development, culture, home environment, and learning styles.

For children who are typically developing, extant language comprehension and social skills usually support a smooth transition from their prior daily routines to those of the preschool classroom. Approximately 6.99% of children between 3 to 17 years of age, however, have a diagnosed developmental disability that may hinder this transition in a number of ways

(Zablotsky, Black, & Blumberg, 2017). Children with developmental disabilities may have significant impairments in language comprehension and production that impact their ability to navigate, and successfully participate in the preschool classroom. Recent estimates in the United States indicate that over 40% of students in special education classrooms do not have their communication needs met using spoken language alone (Andzik, Schaefer, Nichols, & Chung, 2018). Furthermore, Binger and Light (2006) found that 12% of preschoolers receiving special education services required the use of Augmentative and Alternative Communication (AAC) supports. The transition to preschool may be even more complex for children who require AAC. In this chapter, we will primarily focus on speech generating device (SGD) AAC systems that provide a child access to both visual and auditory modalities of language. Romski and Sevcik, (1996) suggest that the voice-output component of an SGD is a critical aspect of AAC intervention. Voice-output provides the child with a spoken model that highlights their turn in the conversation, giving them a clear voice in the interaction, and may facilitate greater understanding of the purpose of an AAC system when learning to communicate symbolically. Although early intervention services (birth to 3 years of age) have advanced significantly in the past 30 years to better incorporate AAC (Romski, Sevcik, Barton-Hulsey, & Whitmore, 2015), preschool is often a time when families are continuing to explore the range of AAC systems that are available to best meet their child's communication needs. Families are either developing transition plans to adapt AAC intervention strategies used in early intervention to the preschool setting, or

introducing these systems to their children for the first time with the support of preschool staff that includes their teacher, speech-language pathologist, and other related service providers such as para-educators, occupational and/or physical therapists. A number of challenges exist for children who use AAC during this critical developmental period of 3 to 5 years of age.

In this chapter we describe challenges in providing *access* to AAC services for children in preschool, challenges that are specific to *language and literacy instruction* using AAC in preschool, and challenges with *including families* in the AAC assessment and intervention process during preschool. We follow each challenge with suggestions of evidence-based solutions, and include examples from our own research and clinical experiences.

■ Access Challenges

Access challenges can include difficulties related to the physical access of an AAC system, but also less tangible barriers such as beliefs, attitudes, and policies that prevent a child from acquiring or using AAC. Issues such as teacher bias against the introduction of AAC, limited training in the use of AAC, and inadequate team based supports to evaluate and implement an AAC system for a child have all been found to limit the introduction of AAC to children in preschool. In a survey of 40 preschool teachers of children with significant developmental disabilities, Barker, Akaba, Brady, and Thiemann-Bourque, (2013) found that only 25% of teachers received training in the use SGDs, with the majority of teachers (80%) receiving training in the Picture Exchange Communication System (PECS). The AAC systems were reported to be infrequently used by teachers or other adults in the classroom, with AAC-based instruction occurring only two or three times per day. In our own experience within preschool settings, teachers have communicated the need for more systematic training and follow-up regarding AAC service provision to feel competent using the resources at hand. Lack of education on the part of practitioners, whether it be the student's lead teacher, classroom aid, speech-language pathologist, or school administrator, creates a barrier at the outset of service provision, and will limit physical access to AAC services in preschool.

Additionally, a number of AAC myths identified originally by Romski and Sevcik (2005) continue to surface, suggesting that children must have a certain set of prerequisite skills to use AAC, have tried all other speech options and failed, or that AAC may hinder the development of speech. These myths continue to limit access to AAC in preschool. Finally, the expert model of waiting for the assistive technology (AT) team to evaluate the child is a common barrier to accessing AAC in preschool. Team-based assistive technology supports may not be readily available for some school districts, requiring children to wait an extended amount of time before they are provided access to an evaluation and appropriate AAC system. The child's local teacher and speech-language pathologist (SLP) may not have access to AAC technology for use with children until the AT team provides it. Solutions exist that allow for preschool teachers and SLPs to work in concert with AT teams to provide AAC resources to children without delaying service provision and are detailed in the following section.

Solutions to Access Challenges

1. How Do We Work With Team Members Who Are Against the Introduction of AAC in Preschool?

Preschool team members may bring with them a number of biased perspectives that reduce access to AAC for a child. The authors of this chapter have heard preschool staff communicate thoughts such as: *"He just isn't ready"* or *"She's making progress in speech, so we decided to just work on speech for a while," "we have to get his behavior under control first,"* and *"it's just too hard to manage an AAC device with all the other kids in the classroom."* Romski and Sevcik (2005) address many of these perspectives in their article on myths and realities related to the introduction of AAC during early intervention. Many of these myths remain as children transition to preschool, with the solutions presented still applicable. The teacher who thinks *"he just isn't ready"* may be subscribing to a commonly held belief that a child has to either be of a certain age to benefit from AAC, have a certain skill set of abilities, or understand a representational hierarchy in order to benefit from AAC. During in-service trainings, informal or formal team meetings, team members could be pointed to the work of Romski and Sevcik (2005), who debunk each of these myths with evidence that suggests there are no pre-requisite skills necessary to introduce AAC to a child. AAC is an intervention approach in itself that we discuss in detail in our next section. No child should be expected to come to an AAC system with the knowledge and skills to use it proficiently the first time it is introduced. Learning to use an AAC system takes time, and is a process. The SLP who says *"she's making progress in speech, so we decided to just work on speech for a while,"* is subscribing to the myth that AAC should be used as a last resort after all other communication intervention options have failed (Romski & Sevcik, 2005). Evidence to date suggests that AAC actually supports speech development, and provides the child with a means of continued language development when speech is difficult (Millar Light, & Schlosser, 2006; Romski & Sevcik, 1996; Romski et al., 2010). And finally, the team member who suggests *"we have to get his behavior under control first"* and *"it's just too hard to manage in the classroom"* may need further in-service training regarding the evidence to date that suggests child behaviors may often be rooted in communication difficulty (Reichle & Wacker, 2017). The AAC may in fact help the routines of the classroom to run more smoothly, allowing the child greater access to communication, supporting language learning, development, and access to the academic curriculum. Training regarding ways to embed AAC supports within natural routines in the preschool classroom, and infuse AAC with all children as an additional support for learning could be provided. The included case example provides suggested ways that AAC can be used across children to encourage language development regardless of speech ability.

2. What If My Team Members Have Little Training in the Use of AAC and Access to Equipment?

It may be the case that a barrier for a child in accessing AAC intervention is due to a number of team members' limited experience, or limited training in evidence-based AAC intervention approaches as well as the physical tools to provide that instruction. Although preservice education in AAC across disciplines is becoming more available, there remains a need to provide in-service professional development to many team members. Team members should advocate to school administrators to support professional development opportunities around AAC to ensure that all team members are knowledgeable. In order to provide federally mandated supports and services for assistive technology, school districts should employ staff trained in AAC service delivery, even if that staff is centralized and provides training and support to local schools for implementation. However, centralizing AT supports using the expert model of waiting for the AT team to evaluate the child is a common barrier to accessing AAC in preschool. The child's teacher and SLP may not have access to AAC technology until the AT team provides it, requiring children to wait an extended amount of time before they are provided access to an evaluation and appropriate AAC system.

One solution to these training needs, as well as the barriers that an expert model of AT service delivery can create, has been developed by a school district in Fulton County, Georgia. Teachers, paraprofessionals, and speech-language pathologists are provided a broad-based, general AAC training before the school year starts, with monthly specialty trainings offered thereafter. All teachers and support staff who attend the initial training are provided access to a reproducible and customizable set of digital materials to print and use with students (Fulton County Assistive Technology Team, 2019a), as well as access to the voice-output software program Chat Editor (PRC-Saltillo, 2019), used in conjunction with the TouchChat® (PRC-Saltillo, 2019) and Words for Life™ apps (PRC-Saltillo, 2019). All teachers have SMART® boards in their classrooms so they are able to use the visual and/or auditory supports if used in conjunction with NOVAChat® (PRC-Saltillo, 2019) with their entire class, not just children who have limited speech. This training and initial set of materials allows the teacher, paraprofessionals, and local speech-language pathologist/s to (1) have access to a team of professionals that can address questions related to negative bias they may have that limits their use of AAC, (2) have access to education on best practices to support language development using AAC, and 3) direct access to equipment and the autonomy to provide intervention to children who are in need of AAC systems without waiting for an expert team to arrive.

The local teachers are provided a set of digital materials that contain customizable visual supports to use daily in their classrooms (Lyons-Golden & Seeley, 2020). These materials contain the same core vocabulary as the systems for instruction during training. Appendices 3–A and 3–B contain examples of classroom based social scripts for teachers, SLPs, paraprofessionals or other support staff to use when providing children instruction using their AAC system. Appendix 3–A represents a sample script that support staff are taught to use during the initial morning meeting of the preschool classroom. The first page contains a list of topics that are typically discussed during morning meeting such as greeting their peers, the day of the week, weather, lunch options, class jobs, and current events. Support staff are provided the series of symbols to use to model the teacher's communication about

each of those topics. On subsequent pages, a series of symbols to navigate possible answers from the child are provided in order for the teacher to support modeling the use of the child's communication system, and then allowing time for the child to respond. Appendix 3–B provides a similar set of social scripts that support staff can use when transitioning to activities outside of the classroom such as physical education, lunch, the playground, and other related services. Support staff can use the scripts contained here to model for the child social communication about each of these activities when going to and from the classroom.

Each local team of support staff is provided follow-up meetings with the centralized AT team for specific needs of children who require a dedicated, individualized system and more extensive supports in the areas of access and intervention. Additionally, local speech-language pathologists are seen as a critical part of the AT evaluation process, and provide evaluation of communication skills and knowledge of symbolic communication. One way they do this, is by using the Test of Aided Symbol-Communication Performance (TASP; Bruno, 2010). The TASP provides an initial understanding of a child's knowledge of symbol-referent relationships for communication, and should not be used as a tool to deny a system, but rather allows the speech-language pathologist to understand the child's current abilities so that intervention using an AAC system can be designed appropriately. This information is used as part of a comprehensive communication evaluation, is discussed with the AT team and family, and an appropriate AAC system is chosen to use to support the child.

Assessing the efficacy of AAC training programs such as the one described here is an important research need. Recently Hanline, Dennis, and Warren, (2018) conducted a study to understand the impact of providing professional development to preschool teachers across a number of rural counties to best support successful use of AAC. Seventeen preschool teachers, paraprofessionals, and SLPs providing services to 3- to 5-year-old children across four rural school districts participated. Service providers agreed that the most helpful components of the professional development programming was the ability to view videotapes of how to implement AAC, participate in workshops that allowed time to develop materials to be used in their classroom, and that they were given access to individual coaches that supported their AAC instruction and problem solving in the classroom.

Anecdotally, we have also received positive feedback and promising reports of increased participation and interaction in classrooms following formal trainings. For example, when asked about the value of the AT training in the Fulton County Schools, a teacher responded:

"Attending [assistive technology] AT training has always been an important part of my educational career. Before I attended AT training with the core vocabulary, I was inadvertently limiting the ways my students could communicate with me. . . . During training I had an aha moment. I realized how much more my students could talk to me. At first it was difficult to switch my mindset and difficult to learn the board. I tried explaining to my assistants, but it wasn't sinking in. Then my assistant went to training

and I saw the increased communication in my classroom. My assistant and I were trying to use the board frequently (very clumsily at first until we became proficient) and saw the students responses. During free time in the classroom, the students would explore the big Velcro board. They would touch the boards and move the Velcro pieces. Each child made progress differently using the board. Some students still worked on a single word. Some students started using two words. Some would do more. Once we all learned the core vocabulary board it was so easy to use it in every area of the classroom. We knew we could carry the board from circle time to the table to the kitchen and be able to use it everywhere. Using core vocabulary helped increase everyone's communication, but the training for my assistant and I made it possible."

Instructional Challenges

Instructional challenges during preschool exist such that providing evidence-based strategies to support language and literacy development for children in preschool who use AAC are often extremely difficult. Teachers are only one part of the instructional team. Teaching assistants or paraprofessional educators are often present in the preschool classroom to support the additional needs of students with AAC needs. Barker et al. (2013) found that preschool teachers reported they received little training regarding ways in which to support AAC use in the classroom, much less their paraprofessionals. Furthermore, Binger and Light (2006) reported that preschoolers needing AAC came from diverse backgrounds, may include bilingual needs, and represent a wide variety of disabilities resulting in a range of support needs for instruction. No two children with AAC needs are alike. Furthermore, when it comes to literacy instruction, a common component of the academic curriculum in preschool, we are still understanding how to best use AAC systems to support early reading instruction. Given the evidence to date (Barton-Hulsey, 2017; Barton-Hulsey, Sevcik, & Romski 2018; Caron Light, Holyfield, & McNaughton, 2018; Erickson, Hanser, Hatch, & Sanders, 2009; Fallon, Light, McNaughton, Drager, & Hammer, 2004), the implementation of early literacy instruction using AAC by practitioners in the preschool setting is relatively new. Preschool is a critical time for language and literacy development, and the preschool experience lays the foundation on which children build their social, language and literacy skills. For many children, the preschool years may be the first time they are in a classroom setting with other children their age. The social, language, and literacy skills they develop are key to later academic success.

Solutions to Instructional Challenges

In this section we present evidence-based solutions to the following challenges that face practitioners who work with preschool-age children who use AAC: (1) How do we provide evidence-based interventions to support language development in preschool? (2) How do we introduce AAC with preschool children who are bilingual? (3) How do we support

early literacy skills in preschool children who use AAC? The strategies discussed here are not specific to a particular SGD AAC system or child with a specific communication profile; rather the findings are a synthesis of current best practices to support preschool children with a range of abilities who use AAC.

1. How Do We Provide Evidence-Based Interventions to Support Language Development?

The first step in providing evidence-based AAC interventions is to complete a comprehensive AAC evaluation that includes a thorough speech and language assessment. The goals of an AAC evaluation are to assess current abilities and to recommend AAC strategies (including both non-electronic AAC systems and electronic SGD AAC systems) that meet the child's communication needs across environments and communication partners and that support language development. Considerations for AAC device selection may include access needs, the individual's current language/cognitive/social skills, family/school support, funding, and cultural appropriateness. A comprehensive discussion of AAC evaluation practices is beyond the scope of this chapter; however, there are several key considerations that are particularly important for preschool age children.

Given the importance of the preschool years for establishing foundational language and social skills, practitioners working with preschool-age children who use AAC systems should have the expectation that the system will grow with the child and will support development across language domains (e.g., semantics, syntax/morphology, pragmatics). Another key consideration for preschool children is ensuring that the AAC system supports functional communication with vocabulary that can be integrated across environments and within classroom activities. Reichle, York, and Sigafoos, (1991) provide helpful guidelines for ensuring that vocabulary selection is ecologically valid and Fallon, Light, and Paige, (2001) provide recommendations for selection of developmentally appropriate vocabulary for preschool-age students based on language sample analysis. A final consideration in the AAC assessment process is to incorporate family values and perspectives to support the generalization of the child's communication skills using AAC beyond the preschool classroom. In the next section, we describe evidence-based AAC intervention strategies with the assumption that the child has received a comprehensive AAC evaluation, that the AAC team has selected an appropriate system for the child, and that progress monitoring is ongoing and will continue to inform intervention.

Language Modeling Using Aided AAC. Providing children with linguistic input is central to supporting their language and communication development in terms of both the quality and quantity of language input (e.g., Hart & Risley, 1995; McDuffie & Yoder, 2010). However, children who use AAC receive considerably less input in the modality with which they are expected to communicate (i.e., AAC). This phenomenon is described as an "input-output" mismatch (Smith & Grove, 2003) and the result is that children who use AAC rarely see others communicate using the same modality as them. This input-output asymmetry experienced by children who use AAC contributes to the challenges in learning language. Thus, many intervention approaches include

providing language models using AAC modalities (sometimes referred to as augmented input, aided language stimulation, and aided language modeling).

The AAC interventions that use aided AAC modeling are by far the most researched and practiced intervention approaches for children who use AAC. There is substantial research evidence indicating that aided AAC modeling can improve language outcomes across language domains including morphosyntax, semantics, and pragmatics. Brady, Herynk, and Fleming (2010) found that aided and unaided adult communication input (e.g., initiation, prompt, response) was significantly related to the frequency of communication by children using AAC in a preschool classroom. Surprisingly, classroom characteristics (e.g., space and furnishings, personal care routines, language reasoning, activities, interaction, program structure, and parents and staff) did not correlate with child communication rate.

Recently, three systematic reviews independently evaluated intervention studies that used aided AAC input approaches (Allen, Schlosser, Brock, & Shane, 2017; Biggs, Carter, & Gilson, 2018; O'Neill, Light, & Pope, 2018) to improve language and communication outcomes for children and adults who use AAC. Across the three reviews, 16 of the 64 studies that met inclusion criteria included preschool-aged children. These reviews evaluated the best research currently available, and the findings suggested that augmented input approaches can be effective for supporting development across language domains. Table 3–1 summarizes the findings from the studies of preschool-aged children included in the reviews, and presents the evidence for AAC interventions to support development across language domains.

Table 3–1. Summary of Studies Using Augmented Input Interventions With Preschool Children

Study	Intervention Procedures	Intervention Target/s	Setting/ Contexts
VOCABULARY DEVELOPMENT			
Drager et al., (2006); Harris and Reichle (2004)	Modeled vocabulary	Target symbol vocabulary	Home/School, play (D)
King, Hengst, & DeThorne, (2013)	Modeled SGD (natural speech drill, prompting, responsivity)	Spoken words, AAC use	Clinic, shared reading, play (D)
Angelo and Goldstein (1990)	Modeled within least-to-most prompting hierarchy during structured trials (+prompting, reinforcement)	Questions with targeted wh- words	School (D)
MULTIWORD COMBINATIONS			
Iacono, Mirenda, & Beukelman, (1993)	Modeled two-word combinations using mand-modeling during structured trials (+prompting, signed models)	Two-word combinations	School (D)
Binger and Light (2007)	Modeled multisymbol messages	Multisymbol messages	Home/School, play (D)
Binger, Kent-Walsh, Berens, Del Campo, & Rivera, (2008); Binger, Kent-Walsh, Ewing, & Taylor, (2010)	Modeled within least-to-most cuing hierarchy and to respond to child communication (expectant delay, open-ended questions)	Multisymbol messages	NR (C), school, shared book reading (D)
Binger, Kent-Walsh, King, & Mansfield (2017); Binger, Kent-Walsh, King, Webb, & Buenviaje (2017); Kent-Walsh, Murza, Malani, & Binger (2015)	Provided concentrated models at the beginning of a session and augmented input through models and recasts (+responsivity, expectant delay, open-ended questions, prompting)	Semantic-syntactic messages; Declarative word combinations, Interrogative word combinations	Clinic, play (D)

continues

Table 3–1. *continued*

Study	Intervention Procedures	Intervention Target/s	Setting/ Contexts
SOCIAL COMMUNICATION			
Johnston, Nelson, Evans, & Palazolo (2003); Johnston, McDonnell, Nelson, & Magnavito (2003); Schepis, Reid, Behrmann, & Sutton (1998)	Peers and/or teachers modeled target behavior within least-to-most prompting hierarchy (+creating communication opportunities, prompting, reinforcement)	Requests (i.e., entrance to play groups)	School, play (C)
-	Modeled vocabulary in the first session (+expectant delay, open-ended questioning, prompting)	Communicative turns	School (C)
Kent-Walsh (2003); Kent-Walsh, Binger, & Hasham (2010)	Modeled within least-to-most cuing hierarchy and to respond to child communication (expectant delay, open-ended questions)	Communicative turns, Number of different concepts	NR, book-reading (C)/ Home, shared reading (C)
Trembath, Balandin, Togher, & Stancliffe (2009)	Modeled SGD during interactive play (+peer interaction strategies)	Communicative turns	School (C)
Kasari et al. (2014)	Modeled vocabulary and provided aided recasts/expansions (+creating communication opportunities, prompting)	Spontaneous communication, number of word roots, comments	Clinic (D)

Note. C = contextualized (i.e., within regular activities/settings); D = decontextualized (i.e., outside regular activities/settings). Table adapted from systematic reviews by Allen et al. (2017); Biggs et al. (2018); O'Neill et al. (2018). Studies included here were published in peer-reviewed journals and included 4- to 5-year-old participants who used aided AAC and had a variety of communication impairments and disabilities (e.g., Autism Spectrum Disorder, Down syndrome, Intellectual Disability, Apraxia of Speech, Cerebral Palsy). Intervention procedures that were used in conjunction with aided AAC modeling are listed in parentheses.

Augmented input strategies appear to be particularly effective for increasing expressive language via AAC; however, considerably fewer studies have investigated using AAC to improve language comprehension (Allen et al., 2017; Romski & Sevcik, 1993; Sevcik, 2006) including comprehension of the graphic or orthographic symbols at single-symbol and multisymbol levels. Children typically comprehend language forms before they use them expressively (Goodwin, Fein, & Naigles, 2012; Petretic & Tweney, 1977). Furthermore, between the ages of 4 and 6 is a key period of development for vocabulary growth and syntactic development. Aided input is critical during this stage to teach children symbol-referent relationships regardless of the symbol type, and can increase symbol comprehension in children who use AAC (Barton, Sevcik, & Romski, 2006; Dada & Alant, 2009; Drager et al., 2006; Harris & Reichle, 2004; Wolf Heller et al., 1995). Overall, the available research investigating aided AAC input, indicates that for preschool-age children, providing rich language input (including aided AAC input) and frequent opportunities for communication, are effective in supporting language development and communication using AAC. See Table 3–1 for specific contexts and strategies for providing aided input during preschool classroom activities.

Peer Interactions in the Preschool Classroom. Preschool is a time when peer interactions take a prominent role as children begin spending more time in groups and their language and conversational skills develop. Peer interactions are a context in which rich language instruction and learning can occur. Conversational competence becomes increasingly important to peer interactions, and influences the extent to which children interact successfully with and are accepted by their peers (Hay, Payne, & Chadwick, 2004). Yet children who use AAC tend to be more passive and use fewer communication functions and initiate communication less frequently than peers. In a study of 30 children using AAC in a preschool setting, Brady et al. (2010) found that children who used AAC initiated communication only 0.133 times per minute and primarily interacted with adults. Language development during preschool may also be supported by increasing the opportunity for peer interactions. To increase interactions between peers and children who use AAC, peers must be educated on how best to communicate with students who use AAC and educators must facilitate opportunities for interactions between children who use AAC and their peers on a regular basis (King & Fahsl, 2012). The following strategies (adapted from King & Fahsl, 2012) may be particularly beneficial for increasing peer interactions among children who use AAC in preschool settings.

- Discuss how people communicate in many different ways other than speech (e.g., gestures, sign language, speech-generating AAC, pictures, eye gaze). Create picture symbols for each of these communication modalities and have children role-play communication using different nonspeech modalities.
- Add picture symbols to word-walls to demonstrate how pictures can be used to communicate.
- Read and discuss books about people who use AAC.

- Teach students to count to 10 to make sure they are providing plenty of time for their peer who uses AAC to comprehend and formulate their message.
- Assign the students who use AAC classroom jobs that require them to ask questions or engage in conversation with peers.
- Include specific opportunities for one-on-one communication during circle/sharing time.
- Introduce core words during circle times and modify songs for core word practice. (Zangari, Lloyd, & Vicker, 1994)

2. How Do We Introduce AAC With Preschool Children Who Are Bilingual?

There is a scarcity of empirical data related to AAC services and supports for children and adults from culturally and linguistically diverse backgrounds. Several studies have investigated culturally and linguistically appropriate symbols and core vocabulary across various languages and cultures (e.g., Andres, 2006; Blake Huer, 2004; Bornman, Alant, & Du Preez, 2009; Robillard, Mayer-Crittenden, Minor-Corriveau, & Bélanger, 2014). Other studies have examined perspectives of AAC through ethnographic interviews and surveys with families and students from culturally and linguistically diverse backgrounds (see Kulkarni & Parmar, 2017 for a recent review).

To date, no published research has investigated AAC assessments or interventions for bilingual children. A recent unpublished master's thesis (Stewart, 2017) described an intervention case study of a bilingual adolescent with Down syndrome who used AAC. The participant communicated in English at school and Spanish at home, and findings supported the efficacy of AAC intervention in the home language in improving overall communication outcomes. In a paper discussing general considerations for provision of services to bilingual children who use AAC, Soto and Yu (2014) advocated for a sociocultural approach to AAC service delivery that supports a bilingual child's communication development across both languages. Soto and Yu highlighted the urgent need for more research in this area and acknowledged that due to the lack of empirical research current recommendations are largely speculative.

Bilingual children are a heterogeneous group, and the rate and trajectory of development across the languages they regularly are exposed to is highly varied and depends on a constellation of intrinsic and extrinsic factors. Research evidence from typically developing bilingual children indicates that language input and current use predict vocabulary and syntactic skills across both languages (e.g., Bedore, Peña, Griffin, & Hixon, 2016; Bedore et al., 2012; Hoff, Core, Place, Rumiche, Señor, & Parra, 2012; Hoff, Quinn, & Giguere, 2018; Paradis, Nicoladis, Crago, & Genesee, 2011; Ribot, Hoff, & Burridge, 2018). For many bilingual children who use AAC, the preschool classroom may be the first time they are receiving consistent exposure to a second language. Research investigating language abilities of bilingual children with language impairments indicates that bilingual children are no more delayed than their monolingual peers with language impairments (Kay-Raining Bird, Genesee, & Verhoeven,

2016). This research suggests that learning more than one language does not exacerbate, increase, or cause a language impairment.

Furthermore, many bilingual children grow up in bilingual communities where it is necessary for them to communicate in more than one language. For young bilingual children, bilingual communication may be an important aspect of their connection with family, culture, and community. Several studies have documented the harmful effects on family socialization and cohesion when, on the advice of professionals, parents of children with disabilities stop speaking to their child in their native language (Fernandez y Garcia, Breslau, Hansen, & Miller, 2012; Jegatheesan, 2011; Yu, 2013).

Like typically developing bilingual preschool children, bilingual preschoolers who use AAC are shifting between language environments and speakers at home and school, and in their communities. It is critical then, that bilingual children who use AAC are able to communicate across these diverse environments, and have access to vocabulary in the different languages they are regularly exposed to. Family members of bilingual children who use AAC have expressed frustration that AAC devices do not include their home language (McCord & Soto, 2004). However, in the last decade, device manufacturers have developed AAC software applications that support bilingual communication with vocabulary layouts in different languages, and speech-output options that include bilingual child voices (Dukhovny & Kelly, 2015).

Most of the bilingual AAC systems that are commercially available require that the user be able to functionally dif-ferentiate between the language layouts in order to switch between languages. The ability to switch between languages according to the language of the communication partner is present in typically developing 2-year-old bilingual children (e.g., Comeau, Genesee, & Lapaquette, 2003; Genesee, Boivin, & Nicoladis, 1996; Lanza, 1992; Reyes, 2004). However, 2-year-old bilingual children may not yet understand, on a conceptual level, that they are communicating in two different languages. Switching between languages using AAC on the other hand, presumably requires the user to be aware that languages can be separated into categories that are represented either by language-specific visual characteristics (e.g., background color, specific images) or are housed in a different location on an AAC system. Preliminary research suggests that the preschool years may be an important developmental period for language differentiation using AAC. In a study of 4- to 6-year-old Spanish-English bilingual children, King (2019) found that younger children had more difficulty switching between languages using bilingual speech-output devices than older bilingual children. However, the author concluded that bilingual 4- to 6-year- old children with and without language impairments were able to successfully switch between languages using bilingual speech-output devices, indicating that these children were able to discriminate between the Spanish and English vocabulary layouts on the speech-output devices.

Although research with bilingual preschool children who use AAC is very limited, AAC intervention with bilingual children should draw on our understanding of bilingual language development as well as research evidence from intervention and assessment of bilingual children with language impairments. We recommend the following considerations to support language development in both languages for bilingual preschool children who use AAC.

- Ensure the AAC system includes functional vocabulary in both languages.
- Provide frequent, quality language input (including aided language input) in both languages.
- Consider that younger children or children with developmental delays may need to be explicitly taught how to differentiate languages on their AAC system.
- Ensure that graphic symbols and vocabulary items are culturally and linguistically appropriate.
- Provide culturally competent services by working with families and ensuring that their values are respected and included in the assessment and intervention process.

3. How Do We Support Early Literacy Skills in Preschool Children Who Use AAC?

Early literacy skills in preschool and kindergarten form the foundation for learning to read in the school-age years. Literacy is critical for academic achievement and vocational success. However, learning to read is a complex skill which presents additional challenges for children with limited speech. Traditionally, reading instruction involves teaching phonics skills (letter-sound relationships) that rely heavily on verbal production of sounds.

Furthermore, children with limited speech who use AAC to communicate do not have the same opportunities to participate in reading assessment and instruction as their peers with typical development. Phonological awareness, or explicit knowledge of the sound structure of a language is a critical foundational skill for learning to read (McCardle & Chhabra, 2004; Perfetti, 1985). Activities that involve rhyming, identification of the first sound of a word, and identifying words that all begin or end with the same sounds are activities that promote phonological awareness and begin in preschool. These activities inherently involve speech to participate. In a study examining the role of speech ability in the development of phonological awareness, however, Barton-Hulsey et al., 2018 found that receptive language skills, rather than productive speech ability, was a better predictor of phonological awareness skills in preschool-aged children with developmental disabilities. Even with limited speech ability, children were able to use their extant comprehension skills to identify pictures of words that rhymed, pictures of words that began with the same initial and final sounds, and blend individual sounds they heard to identify corresponding pictures. Advances in technology such as electronic keyboards that speak the names and sounds of letters, as well as new intervention and assessment techniques for children with minimal speech, show promise for supporting literacy skills. Barton-Hulsey (2017) describes a number of strategies to encourage early reading development during preschool using AAC approaches. Table 3–2 identifies a number of tools that can be used to encourage participation in reading instruction for children with limited speech ability.

Table 3–2. Tools to Encourage Participation in Reading Instruction

Instruction Goal	Tool	Input Method	Output Method
Rhyming	**Eye gaze board** Words that rhyme are depicted as picture choices	Teacher/SLP looks to, points at, and says aloud the choices on board. Teacher provides answer by looking to and pointing at choice on the eye gaze board.	Student looks to choice OR Student points to choice
Phoneme isolation	Words that start with the same sounds are depicted in pictures		
Phoneme blending	Pictures of simple consonant-vowel-consonant (CVC) words are depicted in pictures. Teacher/SLP speaks each phoneme slowly.		
Letter recognition	**Dry erase board** Teacher/SLP writes 4 letters on dry erase board.	Teacher/SLP names letters as they point to them	Student looks to letter or circles letter. Can use dry erase board to write letters
	SGD touchscreen device Keyboard on SGD	Teacher/SLP uses SGD keyboard to identify letters.	Student uses SGD keyboard to name letters.
Letter-sound recognition	**Note cards** Teacher/SLP writes a single letter (s) or letter combination (sh), or morpheme (-ing) on a note card.	Teacher/SLP presents cards and names the sound the letter or letter combination makes.	Student chooses card, hands to teacher, picks from a group when the teacher/SLP says the sound of a letter or letter combination.
	SGD with paper overlays Teacher/SLP prints a single letter (s) or letter combination (sh), or morpheme (-ing) on buttons of the SGD and programs the SGD to speak the sound of the letter or letter combination when pressed.	Teacher/SLP uses SGD during group instruction to model the sound that each letter or letter combination makes.	Student uses SGD during group instruction to speak the sound the single letter or letter combination makes.

Source: Barton-Hulsey, 2017; in Challenges and Opportunities in Reading Instruction for Children with Limited Speech; *Seminars in Speech and Language*, pp. 253–262, Vol. 38, No. 4. © Georg Thieme Verlag KG)

■ Inclusion of Families

Transition from early intervention services to preschool can be challenging for parents as they may be faced with an unfamiliar system with different administrative structures and demands. However, including families in the decision making process from the outset is critical. Often times, families may not understand the need for AAC in preschool, what their role in this process is, and that they are a critical member of the team. Families may need to be informed about the role of AAC in language development and how it can support, and not hinder, their child's use of spoken communication. Families may believe a number of myths discussed earlier that need to be carefully navigated with their school team. In the United States, when a child with a disability enters preschool, the school team and parents create an Individualized Education Plan (IEP) for the student. Parent participation in the educational decision-making process for their children with disabilities is a fundamental aspect of the Individuals with Disabilities Education Act (IDEA, 2004). This Federal law (in the U.S.) is supported by research, and numerous studies confirm the importance of including families in the AAC assessment and intervention process (Calculator & Black, 2009; Parette, Brotherson, & Huer, 2000; Soto, Muller, Hunt, & Goetz, 2001). Carryover of their child's AAC system between home and school settings can be difficult when IEP goals are focused on academic skills alone. Finding time to teach families to use intervention strategies in home contexts to continue to build language and literacy may be difficult. There is evidence however, that parent involvement is criti-cal to successful AAC outcomes, citing key ways to encourage parent involvement (e.g., Granlund, Björck-Åkesson, Wilder, & Ylvén, 2008). Next, we explore this evidence to date, and provide practical solutions for the inclusion of families in AAC.

Solutions to Challenges in Including Families

1. How Do We Include Parents in the AAC Decision-Making Process?

Although professionals recognize the importance of including parents of children who use AAC in the assessment and intervention process, in practice, parent-involvement is often challenging for teachers and clinicians (Pickl, 2011). These difficulties may be due to language barriers, differing views on disability, education, and intervention, lack of knowledge about AAC, and time constraints/competing responsibilities. Furthermore, families may not expect to be involved in the decision-making process and may not disagree with professional recommendations even if those recommendations may not be beneficial given their home circumstances (McCord & Soto, 2004). The following suggestions outline ways to include parents throughout the AAC decision-making process:

■ *Elicit family input regarding AAC and other goals for their child, including the selection of methods of communication at school and at home* (Calculator & Black, 2009). The family should play an important and active role in the AAC assessment process, including the identification and prioritizing of communication needs at home.

- *Respect family values and expertise* (Bailey, Parette, Stoner, Angell, & Carroll, 2006; Calculator & Black, 2009; Goldbart & Marshall, 2004; McCord & Soto, 2004; Parette & Brotherson, 2004). Practitioners and school-based assessment and intervention teams should respect and incorporate the families' ideas, concerns and priorities when designing and implementing AAC programs.

- *Link AAC team-generated assessment and child and family evaluative information* (Parette & Angelo, 1996). Collect ongoing, formative feedback from family members and children who use AAC to continue to inform decision-making.

- *Offer parent training sessions on AAC through the school district.* One of our authors has found that parent training sessions have been a successful way to reach a number of families who have similar support needs when AAC is first being used with their child. Training sessions with families can be helpful in introducing parents to language intervention principles such as the importance of modeling when using AAC, as well as proving a time to address unique technical support needs of their child's SGD. School support staff at their child's local school can then provide additional, individualized support to parents to meet the needs of their child's AAC system, classroom contexts, and home environments.

Each of these suggestions are supportive of interprofessional collaborative practice (IPCP) models that keep the family and child at the center of all decisions that are made. IPCP draws on the individual strengths and expertise of team members from various backgrounds who by working together cooperatively, can provide the family and child with holistic, high-quality services (Ogletree, 2017). For young children who use AAC, IPCP is critical during assessment and intervention to ensure that the various stakeholders (including therapists, teachers, and family members) are involved and invested in the AAC decision making process and that each team member's perspective and expertise is valued and integrated in the plan of care. Ogletree and colleagues (2017) used the case of Mary, a young woman with severe disabilities, to underscore the real-life challenges of IPCP, but also to illustrate how team collaboration can result in holistic, family-centered care. The authors described how when IPCP formed the framework for Mary's plan of care, Mary and her family were empowered and both functional and academic goals were successfully promoted. However, the authors also described Mary's preschool years during which Mary's therapists worked individually on isolated goals and Mary's parents were not involved in the decision-making process related to her care. The absence of IPCP during these early years ultimately set Mary back and resulted in missed opportunities in providing appropriate services and left her parents feeling disengaged and discouraged.

One way that parents can be empowered and engaged in the decision-making process during the preschool years is to support them in writing a "communication vision" for their child. Recently, one of our authors had a conversation with Christine, the mother of a young woman with Angelman syndrome, about supporting parents of children who use AAC during the early years. Christine described how her child's SLP had asked her to write a communication vision to reflect on her long-term communication goals for her daughter.

> Christine remembered, *"[writing the communication vision] was a really hard and emotional thing to write, but it was also extremely powerful. It helped me think about my long-term goals and to see that the AAC I chose, PODD, is the best available path to get there."*

Christine's experience demonstrates how SLPs can elicit and incorporate parent's input regarding their child's communication goals by showing parents that their goals are respected and valued. Gaining parents' "buy-in" for AAC may be challenging, but it is essential if AAC systems and associated language and literacy strategies are to be incorporated at home.

2. How Do We Support the Carryover of AAC Supports in the Preschool Classroom to Home?

Providing parents and caregivers with training as mentioned above, as well as individualized strategies for supporting AAC device use at home, is key to promoting the generalization of language and literacy skills beyond the classroom. Furthermore, family participation is critical to ensuring that AAC devices are not abandoned (Dove Jones, Angelo, & Kokoska,

1998; Kemp & Parette, 2000; Parette, Brotherson, & Huer, 2000). Empirical evidence indicates that partner interventions (including parent-training programs) are highly effective in improving the communication outcomes in children who use AAC with a range of abilities (see Kent-Walsh et al., 2015 for a review). Teaching parents strategies such as modeling language using AAC, asking open-ended questions, and using expectant delay are elements of successful interventions.

In their curriculum, TELL ME: AAC in the Preschool Classroom, Zangari and Wise (2016) provide practical "home-extension activities" that include both training materials (e.g., explanations of strategies) but also implementation resources (e.g., picture symbols of core words, example scripts) for parents of preschool children who use AAC. The home-extension activities are designed so that preschool children can share what they are learning in the preschool classroom with their families and allow the child additional opportunities to practice language and literacy skills that were targeted in classroom activities. Zangari and Wise recommend beginning with home extension activities that are simple and place few demands on parents and then gradually introducing more information and activities as parents gain confidence and become more accustomed to the approach.

AAC teams must be aware of and sensitive to the needs and realities of family life when designing and implementing transition programs. Families of children with disabilities are faced with many challenges and demands on their finances, time, and energy. As Christine, the mother of a child with Angelman syndrome, explained, *"When I get home, I just want to collapse on the couch."* She described what she called *"AAC guilt"*—a nagging feeling that she should be modeling AAC and providing more frequent communication opportunities than she was able to. Although Christine feels *"AAC guilt,"* she is an incredibly supportive mom who recognized early on that AAC would be integral to her daughter's communication development and spent countless hours learning about AAC and creating communication boards for her daughter's communication system. Yet Christine still feels that she is not doing enough for her daughter, and that feeling weighs on her. When AAC teams ask parents to implement AAC strategies at home, it is critical that they work together with parents to find realistic options that are sensitive to parents' abilities and supportive of the child's needs.

Supporting parents of preschool children who use AAC involves having a training plan in place. Direct coaching from SLPs or other knowledgeable persons should be available if parents wish to learn how to incorporate AAC more effectively with their child at home. SLPs and teachers should be compassionate toward the unique challenges each family faces as they work to determine manageable ways to incorporate AAC at home within existing routines and structures. The AAC team should ensure that procedures are in place to coordinate AAC instruction between school and home. As mentioned prior, a solution for this need is to provide a centralized training that covers broad-based AAC implementation practices that all families would benefit from, and then each family's local SLP can provide individualized support for carryover of AAC at home. Just as teacher trainings were described earlier, a parent-training model (Fulton County Assistive Technology Team, 2019b) has been developed so

that parents can be provided direct training and resources for their child when first being introduced to AAC. This initial training is largely focused on fundamental principles of aided language input where intervention principles are discussed, examples are provided, and parents are given time to practice and/or role-play with the assistive technology team. Additional support is provided to families on an individual basis for technical needs of their child's AAC system, as well as specific vocabulary and/or access needs. Within this training, parents are also provided education regarding advocating for their child's AAC/AT needs on their IEP, and how to ensure AAC is documented so their child receives these services each year as they transition between support staff in the school district. Furthermore, training should be culturally and linguistically relevant, and the AAC team should be aware that the needs, abilities, and perceptions of AAC vary greatly among families. Within this model, the assistive technology team acknowledges the bilingual needs of families and addresses these needs as appropriate, with interpreters present at trainings to support and facilitate best communication between parents and the AT team. McCord and Soto (2004) provided suggestions for facilitating family involvement in AAC when working with families from culturally and linguistically diverse backgrounds. For example, the AAC team should be clear about their beliefs and expectations of the family, teach culturally relevant strategies, ensure that the vocabulary programmed on AAC devices is meaningful to the home environment and available in the languages spoken at home, and develop a collaborative plan for AAC use at home that incorporates the family's values and expectations.

The following suggestions summarize strategies to support the transition of AAC from the preschool classroom to the home environment:

- Ensure that procedures are in place to coordinate AAC instruction and implementation between school and home (Calculator & Black, 2009).
- Provide both generalized training and direct coaching to family members if they wish to learn how to incorporate AAC use more effectively and practically at home (Calculator & Black, 2009).
- Increase sensitivity to needs, demands, routines and realities of family life (Dove Jones et al., 1998; McCord & Soto, 2004; Parette & Angelo, 1996; Parette et al., 2000).
- Provide clear, accurate communication about beliefs and expectations (Angelo, 2000; McCord & Soto, 2004; Parette et al., 2000).
- Provide culturally relevant parent training (Angelo, Jones, & Kokoska, 1995; Bailey et al., 2006; Joginder Singh, Hussein, Mustaffa Kamal, & Hassan, 2017; McCord & Soto, 2004).

■ Case Illustration and Discussion

The following case illustration describes a hypothetical preschool classroom—highlighting three children—in which the challenges mentioned above in the areas of *access, instruction*, and *family involvement* for children in need of AAC may arise. We follow this case illustration with a discussion of how solutions mentioned

above may be applied given the unique needs each child brings.

Sara, Todd, and Josue were each 4 years of age and attended an inclusive, public preschool classroom of children both with and without developmental disabilities. Sara had a diagnosis of Down syndrome, and Todd and Josue did not yet have formal diagnoses, but were using limited speech for communication, and qualified for services under the diagnostic criteria of significant developmental delay. Three additional peers in their classroom also had developmental delay diagnoses, but used more developed spoken communication.

Sara had much stronger receptive than expressive language abilities, with her speech being 90% unintelligible to novel listeners due to significant motor speech impairments that often accompany Down syndrome. Todd mainly used gestures and vocalizations for expressive communication, with again, higher receptive than expressive language skills. Josue's parents immigrated from Mexico, and spoke primarily Spanish. Josue had an 8-year-old sister and a 14-year-old brother who spoke to him primarily in English. Sara, Todd and Josue all received early intervention services until they turned 3. Josue used approximately 10 spoken words in English and Spanish as well as several manual signs. Sara, Todd, and Josue were all ambulatory but presented with fine motor delays and global cognitive delays for their age. None of the children used AAC during early intervention, however, upon entry into preschool, the SLP at their school, suggested to each family that an SGD be introduced to support their communication development. Their teacher was initially hesitant to do so because: (1) Sara had recently made some progress in speech, (2) she had con-

cerns about Todd's behavior, and his ability to use an SGD was in question, and (3) an optimal approach for Josue was uncertain given his bilingual needs. Furthermore, there were other children in the classroom with developmental delays who used speech, and the teacher feared they would be distracted by the technology. Overall, the teacher was concerned that she could not support all of the children's unique communication needs with the demands of an SGD also being placed on her to incorporate during instruction, but she was willing to try.

The SLP, in consultation with the assistive technology team within their school district, provided an evaluation of receptive and expressive language for each child, and used the TASP (Bruno, 2010) to evaluate current symbolic awareness and use for communication. This information was communicated to the local assistive technology team, as well as the classroom teacher. The classroom teacher, two paraeducators, and the SLP attended a two-hour training on how to incorporate AAC in the classroom provided by the AT team at the start of the school year. The classroom teacher was provided a set of digital materials to use within the classroom with all students, and that were also able to be customized for each student with AAC needs. The teacher was provided access to Chat Editor with WordPower™ to use via the classroom SMART® Board with all children as a visual support when teaching academic concepts, and during typical routines of the day, such as circle time and shared book reading. The SLP collaborated with the teacher to use the digital resources to print communication boards using core and fringe vocabulary to be displayed around the room for communication support during center time and on daily visual schedules. All materials were provided in both Spanish and English so that Josue's paraprofessional could model vocabulary in Spanish.

Each child's family attended a half-day family training session provided by the school district's AT team to review fundamentals of AAC instruction using modeling, and identified ways to incorporate AAC into their home environment. Families were provided time to ask questions and further understand the operating system of their child's iPad and communication Application. The local SLP provided weekly follow-up support with each family to ensure that they understood how to target specific vocabulary within home settings and carry over the use of the AAC system.

■ Case Summary, Discussion and Conclusions

In the above case illustration, the AT team, in concert with each student's family and local SLP, worked together to determine the best AAC system for each Sara, Todd, and Josue. Sara and Todd were provided an iPad with both core and fringe vocabulary using NovaChat® with WordPower™, the same symbol set that the teacher used for classroom instruction. Josue was provided an iPad with an AAC app that also included core and fringe vocabulary, but had pages in both English and Spanish. Teacher and paraprofessional support was critical to making AAC work for each child. Josue's teacher spoke English, but he had a bilingual paraprofessional. The additional classroom paraprofessional supported Sara and Todd during various classroom routines, with a focused plan of instruction for target vocabulary and specific communication needs within each context. The AT team and resources provided by the district were critical at the outset to overcome the *access barriers* that included both attitudes from the teacher, and technology needs that the teacher and SLP needed at the local level to provide necessary communication supports.

During training, and with support from the local SLP, paraprofessionals were provided scripts that they used with each child during morning meetings with the children to model on each child's device the appropriate answers for questions, and allowed the child time to answer while other students were instructed to wait for their turn next. The teacher used the SMART® Board to model language during circle time, and provided students the vocabulary choices to answer. For example, when asked, "What is the weather like today?" she displayed choices of "sunny," "rainy," "cloudy," on the screen. Paraprofessionals worked together with the SLP to understand communication goals of each child, and had additional targeted times throughout the day that they provided focused modeling of target vocabulary, and provided children time to use the device. These times were during shared book reading, center activities of dramatic play, and lunch. The SLP came into the classroom weekly to provide support during focused literacy instruction and math. The teacher was able to carry over this support daily.

In the preschool classroom, decision making surrounding AAC often occurs within the classroom context which may include children without disabilities. The decisions made regarding solutions to *access challenges, instructional challenges*, and how to *include families* were made with the broader classroom dynamics and available resources in mind, and within the framework of the existing classroom structure. In evaluating the outcomes of teacher and paraprofessional training in AAC, and access to visual supports that were used with all students more broadly, AAC benefitted everyone. Best practices support the need for children who use AAC to be provided instruction in inclusive classrooms, alongside children who are typically developing, as well as peers with disabilities who have speech ability. In conclusion, we list a number of actions that could be taken to ensure that AAC service delivery is successful within a classroom, such as the one described above in order to overcome *access barriers, instructional barriers,* and *barriers to including families in the process*:

- *Overcoming Access Barriers*—
  Classroom staff are trained on operation of AAC devices and on modeling techniques in order to:
  - Use hardware and software applications competently.
  - Maintain the operation of the SGDs in the classroom.
  - Demonstrate familiarity with vocabulary organization on SGDs.
  - Program communication software on the SGD.
  - Set up students' SGDs and computers for participation in instructional activities.
  - Use multiple communication systems effectively during instructional activities.
  - Organize the day around "activities" or "experiences" rather than subjects.
  - Organize content in thematic units that reiterate core and fringe vocabulary.

◼ *Overcoming Instructional Barriers —Ways to Engineer the Classroom for Instruction*
  ◾ Educational materials are organized, accessible and labeled with text and picture symbol.
  ◾ Materials are organized so that students can easily access materials.
  ◾ Classroom schedules are posted with picture symbols.
  ◾ Classroom rules are posted with picture symbols.
  ◾ Bulletin boards contain visual supports for use during instruction.
  ◾ Access to communication display boards is provided with symbols and vocabulary layouts matching those used by students.
  ◾ Communication systems are provided in both the child's home language and in English
  ◾ AAC provides access to instruction and conversational turns during literacy instruction
◼ *Family involvement*
  ◾ Families are included in the decision-making process for an AAC SGD.
  ◾ Adequate training is provided so that parents feel comfortable with and understand intervention strategies using AAC.
  ◾ Each child's SLP follows up with parents to support unique needs of each child, and works with the family to ensure carryover of AAC at home.
  ◾ Families know who to contact for questions regarding the operating system of the SGD.

In conclusion, the strategies outlined in this chapter to overcome barriers to *access, instruction,* and *family inclusion*

using AAC during preschool can provide students with limited speech ability that is a strong foundation for continued development in Kindergarten and beyond. Furthermore, the tools used within the classroom in the above case example encouraged communication not only from children with limited speech ability, but have been reported to encourage children with speech ability to use even greater speech and more diverse vocabulary. A number of models exist to support inclusive instruction, with team teaching from a general education teacher and special education teacher alongside the SLP, which is a highly supportive model (Zurawski, 2014). Fortunately, in the preschool classroom, many of the same strategies used to support language and literacy development in children who use AAC can also be beneficial to children who have developmental disabilities and use speech. The evidence and practical solutions presented in this chapter provide teachers, SLPs, and related service providers the tools to support the inclusion of AAC at the earliest stage of a child's academic journey. It is critical that a child's school team be responsive to these barriers to *access, instruction,* and *family inclusion* so that children with AAC needs are allowed the opportunity to develop communication skills to their fullest potential.

◼ References

Allen, A. A., Schlosser, R. W., Brock, K. L., & Shane, H. C. (2017). The effectiveness of aided augmented input techniques for persons with developmental disabilities: A systematic review. *Augmentative and Alternative Communication, 33,* 149–159. https://doi.org/10.1080/07434618.2017.1338752

Andres, P. (2006). Developing an appropriate icon set for a Mandarin Chinese augmentative communication system. *International Journal of Computer Processing of Languages, 19,* 275–283. https://doi.org/10.11 42/s0219427906001499

Andzik, N. R., Schaefer, J. M., Nichols, R. T., & Chung, Y. C. (2018). National survey describing and quantifying students with communication needs. *Developmental Neurorehabilitation, 21,* 40–47. https://doi.org /10.1080/17518423.2017.1339133

Angelo, D. H. (2000). Impact of augmentative and alternative communication devices on families. *Augmentative and Alternative Communication, 16,* 37–47.

Angelo, D. H., & Goldstein, H. (1990). Effects of a pragmatic teaching strategy for requesting information by communication board users. *Journal of Speech and Hearing Disorders, 55,* 231–243. http://doi:10.1044/jshd.5502.231

Angelo, D. H., Jones, S. D., & Kokoska, S. M. (1995). Family perspective on augmentative and alternative communication: Families of young children. *Augmentative and Alternative Communication, 11,* 193–201.

Bailey, R. L., Parette, H. P., Stoner, J. B., Angell, M. E., & Carroll, K. (2006). Family members' perceptions of augmentative and alternative communication device use. *Language, Speech, and Hearing Services in Schools, 37,* 50–60. https://doi.org/10.1044 /0161-1461(2006/006)

Barker, R. M., Akaba, S., Brady, N. C., & Thiemann-Bourque, K. (2013). Support for AAC use in preschool, and growth in language skills, for young children with developmental disabilities. *Augmentative and Alternative Communication, 29,* 334–346. https:// doi.org/10.3109/07434618.2013.848933

Barton, A., Sevcik, R. A., & Romski, M. A. (2006). Exploring visual-graphic symbol acquisition by pre-school age children with developmental and language delays. *Augmentative and Alternative Communication, 22*(1), 10–20. https://doi. org/10.1080/07434610500238206

Barton-Hulsey, A. (2017). Challenges and opportunities in reading instruction for children with limited speech. *Seminars in Speech and Language, 38*(4), 253–262. https://doi.org/10.1055/s-0037-1604273

Barton-Hulsey, A., Sevcik, R. A., & Romski, M. (2018). The relationship between speech, language, and phonological awareness in preschool-age children with developmental disabilities. *American Journal of Speech-Language Pathology, 27,* 616–632. https:// doi.org/10.1044/2017_AJSLP-17-0066

Bedore, L. M., Peña, E. D., Griffin, Z. M., & Hixon, G. G. (2016). Effects of age of English dxposure, current input/output, and grade on bilingual language performance. *Journal of Child Language, 43,* 687–706. https:// doi.org/10.1017/S0305000915000811

Bedore, L. M., Peña, E. D., Summers, C. L., Boerger, K. M., Resendiz, M. D., Greene, K., . . . Gillam, R. B. (2012). The measure matters: Language dominance profiles across measures in Spanish–English bilingual children. *Bilingualism: Language and Cognition, 15,* 616–629. https://doi.org/10.1017/ S1366728912000090

Biggs, E. E., Carter, E. W., & Gilson, C. B. (2018). Systematic review of interventions involving aided AAC modeling for children with complex communication needs. *American Journal on Intellectual and Developmental Disabilities, 123*(5), 443–473. https://doi.org/ 10.1352/1944-7558-123.5.443

Binger, C., Kent-Walsh, J., Berens, J., Del Campo, S., & Rivera, D. (2008). Teaching Latino parents to support the multi-symbol message productions of their children who require AAC. *Augmentative and Alternative Communication, 24,* 323–338. https://doi. org/10.1080/07434610802130978

Binger, C., Kent-Walsh, J., Ewing, C., & Taylor, S. (2010). Teaching educational assistants to facilitate the multisymbol message productions of young students who require augmentative and alternative communication. *American Journal of Speech-Language Pathology, 19,* 108–120. https://doi .org/10.1044/1058-0360(2009/09-0015)

Binger, C., Kent-Walsh, J., King, M., & Mansfield, L. (2017). Early sentence productions of 3- and 4-year-old children who use augmentative and alternative communication. *Journal of Speech, Language, and Hearing Research, 60*, 1930–1945. https://doi.org/10.1044/2017_JSLHR-L-15-0408

Binger, C., Kent-Walsh, J., King, M., Webb, E., & Buenviaje, E. (2017). Early sentence productions of 5-year-old children who use augmentative and alternative communication. *Communication Disorders Quarterly, 38*(3), 131–142. https://doi.org/10.1177/1525740116655804

Binger, C., & Light, J. (2006). Demographics of preschoolers who require AAC. *Language, Speech, and Hearing Services in Schools, 37*(3), 200–208. https://doi.org/10.1044/0161-1461(2006/022)

Binger, C., & Light, J. (2007). The effect of aided AAC modeling on the expression of multi-symbol messages by preschoolers who use AAC. *Augmentative and Alternative Communication, 23*, 30–43. https://doi.org/10.1080/07434610600807470

Blake Huer, M. (2004). Examining perceptions of graphic symbols across cultures: Preliminary study of the impact of culture/ethnicity. *Augmentative and Alternative Communication, 16*, 180–185. https://doi.org/10.1080/07434610012331279034

Bornman, J., Alant, E., & Du Preez, A. (2009). Translucency and learnability of Blissymbols in Setswana-speaking children: An exploration. *Augmentative and Alternative Communication, 25*, 287–298. https://doi.org/10.3109/07434610903392456

Brady, N. C., Herynk, J. W., & Fleming, K. (2010). Communication input matters: Lessons from prelinguistic children learning to use AAC in preschool environments. *Early Childhood Services (San Diego, Calif.), 4*(3), 141-154.

Bruno, J. (2010). *Test of Aided Symbol Performance (TASP).* Tobii Dynavox LLC.

Calculator, S. N., & Black, T. (2009). Validation of an inventory of best practices in the provision of augmentative and alternative communication services to students with severe disabilities in general education classrooms. *American Journal of Speech-Language Pathology, 18*, 329–342. https://doi.org/10.1044/1058-0360(2009/08-0065)

Caron, J., Light, J., Holyfield, C., & McNaughton, D. (2018). Effects of dynamic text in an AAC app on sight word reading for individuals with autism spectrum disorder. *Augmentative and Alternative Communication, 34*, 143–154. https://doi.org/10.1080/07434618.2018.1457715

Comeau, L., Genesee, F., & Lapaquette, L. (2003). The Modeling Hypothesis and child bilingual codemixing. *International Journal of Bilingualism, 7*, 113–126. https://doi.org/10.1177/13670069030070020101

Dada, S., & Alant, E. (2009). The effect of aided language stimulation on vocabulary acquisition in children with little or no functional speech. *American Journal of Speech-Language Pathology, 18*(1), 50–64. https://doi.org/10.1044/1058-0360(2008/07-0018)

Dove Jones, S., Angelo, D. H., & Kokoska, S. (1998). Stressors and family supports: Families with children using augmentative and alternative communication technology. *Journal of Children's Communication Development, 2*, 37–44.

Drager, K. D. R., Postal, V. J., Carrolus, L., Castellano, M., Gagliano, C., & Glynn, J. (2006). The effect of aided language modeling on symbol comprehension and production in 2 preschoolers with autism. *American Journal of Speech-Language Pathology, 15*, 112–125. https://doi.org/10.1044/1058-0360(2006/012)

Dukhovny, E., & Kelly, E. B. (2015). Practical resources for provision of services to culturally and linguistically diverse users of AAC. *Perspectives on Communication Disorders and Sciences in Culturally and Linguistically Diverse Populations, 22*, 25–39.

Erickson, K., Hanser, G., Hatch, P., & Sanders, E. (2009). *Research-based practices for creating access to the general curriculum in reading and literacy for students with significant intellectual disabilities.* Monograph prepared for the Council for Chief State School Officers (CCSSO) Assessing Special Education Students (ASES) State Collaborative on Assessment and Student Standards (SCASS). https://doi.org/10.1017/CBO9781107415324.004

Fallon, K. A., Light, J., McNaughton, D., Drager, K., & Hammer, C. (2004). The effects of direct instruction on the single-word reading skills of children who require augmentative and alternative communication. *Augmentative and Alternative Communication, 24,* 1424–1439. https://doi.org/10.1080/07434610410001699690

Fallon, K. A., Light, J. C., & Paige, T. K. (2001). Enhancing vocabulary selection for preschoolers who require augmentative and alternative communication (AAC). *American Journal of Speech-Language Pathology, 10,* 81–94.

Fernandez y Garcia, E., Breslau, J., Hansen, R., & Miller, E. (2012). Unintended consequences: An ethnographic narrative case series exploring langauge recommendations for bilingual families of children with autism spectrum disorders. *Journal of Medical Speech-Language Pathology, 20*(2), 10–16.

Fulton County Assistive Technology Team. (2019a, August). AAC implementation. *Teacher and Support Staff Training for Augmentative and Alternative Communication.* Fulton County Schools, Fulton County, GA.

Fulton County Assistive Technology Team. (2019b , August). Assistive Technology Parent Training. *Parent Training for Augmentative and Alternative Communication.* Fulton County Schools, Fulton County, GA.

Genesee, F., Boivin, I., & Nicoladis, E. (1996). Talking with strangers: A study of bilingual children's communicative compentence. *Applied Psycholinguistics, 17,* 427–442.

Goldbart, J., & Marshall, J. (2004). "Pushes and pulls" on the parents of children who use AAC. *Augmentative and Alternative Communication, 20*(4), 194–208. https://doi.org/10.1080/07434610400010960

Goodwin, A., Fein, D., & Naigles, L. R. (2012). Comprehension of wh-questions precedes their production in typical development and autism spectrum disorders. *Autism Research, 5*(2), 109–123. https://doi.org/10.1002/aur.1220

Granlund, M., Björck-Åkesson, E., Wilder, J., & Ylvén, R. (2009). AAC interventions for children in a family environment: Implementing evidence in practice. *Augmentative and Alternative Communication, 24,* 207–219. https://doi.org/10.1080/08990220802387935

Hanline, M. F., Dennis, L. R., & Warren, A. W. (2018). The outcomes of professional development on AAC use in preschool classrooms: A qualitative investigation. *Infants and Young Children, 31*(3), 231–245. https://doi.org/10.1097/IYC.0000000000000120

Harris, M. D., & Reichle, J. (2004). The impact of aided language stimulation on symbol comprehension and production in children with moderate cognitive disabilities. *American Journal of Speech-Language Pathology, 13,* 155–167. https://doi.org/10.1044/1058-0360(2004/016)

Hart, B., & Risley, T. R. (1995). *Meaningful differences in the everyday experience of young American children.* Brookes.

Hay, D. F., Payne, A., & Chadwick, A. (2004). Peer relations in childhood. *Journal of Child Psychology and Psychiatry and Allied Disciplines, 45*(1), 84–108. https://doi.org/10.1046/j.0021-9630.2003.00308.x

Hoff, E., Core, C., Place, S., Rumiche, R., Señor, M., & Parra, M. (2012). Dual language exposure and early bilingual development. *Journal of Child Language, 39,* 1–27. https://doi.org/10.1017/S0305000910000759

Hoff, E., Quinn, J. M., & Giguere, D. (2018). What explains the correlation between growth in vocabulary and grammar? New evidence from latent change score analyses of simultaneous bilingual development. *Developmental Science, 21*(2), 1–16. https://doi.org/10.1111/desc.12536

Iacono, T., Mirenda, P., & Beukelman, D. (1993). Comparison of unimodal and multimodal

AAC techniques for children with intellectual disabilities. *Augmentative and Alternative Communication, 9,* 83–94. https://doi.org/10.1080/ 07434619312331276471

Jegatheesan, B. (2011). Multilingual development in children with autism: Perspectives of South Asian Muslim immigrant parents on raising a child with a communicative disorder in multilingual contexts. *Bilingual Research Journal, 34*(2), 185–200. https://doi.org/10.1080/15235882.2011.597824

Joginder Singh, S., Hussein, N. H., Mustaffa Kamal, R., & Hassan, F. H. (2017). Reflections of Malaysian parents of children with developmental disabilities on their experiences with AAC. *Augmentative and Alternative Communication, 33,* 110–120. https://doi.org/10.1080/07434618.2017.1309457

Johnston, S. S., McDonnell, A. P., Nelson, C., & Magnavito, A. (2003). Teaching functional communication skills using augmentative and alternative communication in inclusive settings. *Journal of Early Intervention, 25*(4), 263–280. https://doi.org/10.1177/105381510302500403

Johnston, S., Nelson, C., Evans, J., & Palazolo, K. (2003). The use of visual supports in teaching young children with autism spectrum disorder to initiate interactions. *Augmentative and Alternative Communication, 19,* 86–103. https://doi.org/10.1080/0743461031000112016

Kasari, C., Kaiser, A. P., Goods, K., Nietfeld, J., Mathy, P., Landa, R., . . . Almirall, D. (2014). Communication interventions for minimally verbal children with autism: Sequential multiple assignment randomized trial. *Journal of the American Academy of Child Adolescent Psychiatry, 53*(6), 635–646. https://doi.org/10.1016/j.jaac.2014.01.019

Kay-Raining Bird, E., Genesee, F., & Verhoeven, L. (2016). Bilingualism in children with developmental disorders: A narrative review. *Journal of Communication Disorders, 63,* 1–14. https://doi.org/10.1016/j.jcomdis.2016.07.003

Kemp, C. E., & Parette, H. P. (2000). Barriers to minority family involvement in assistive technology decision-making processes. *Education & Training in Mental Retardation & Developmental Disabilities, 35*(4), 384–392.

Kent-Walsh, J. (2003). *The effects of an educational assistant instructional program on the communicative turns of students who use augmentative and alternative communication during book reading activities* (Doctoral dissertation). The Pennsylvania State University, State College.

Kent-Walsh, J., Binger, C., & Hasham, Z. (2010). Effects of parent instruction on the symbolic communication of children using augmentative and alternative communication during storybook reading. *American Journal of Speech-Language Pathology, 19,* 97–107. https://doi.org/10.1044/1058-0360(2010/09-0014)

Kent-Walsh, J., Murza, K. A., Malani, M. D., & Binger, C. (2015). Effects of communication partner instruction on the communication of individuals using AAC: A meta-analysis. *AAC: Augmentative and Alternative Communication, 31*(4), 271–284. https://doi.org/10.3109/07434618.2015.1052153

King, M. (2019). *Language switching using augmentative and alternative communication: An investigation of Spanish-English bilingual children with and without language impairments* (Unpublished doctoral dissertation).

King, A. M., & Fahsl, A. J. (2012). Supporting social competence in children who use augmentative and alternative communication. *Teaching Exceptional Children, 45*(1), 42–49. https://doi.org/10.1177/004005991204500106

King, A. M., Hengst, J. A., & DeThorne, L. S. (2013). Severe speech sound disorders: An integrated multimodal intervention. *Language, Speech, and Hearing Services in Schools, 44,* 195–210. https://doi.org/10.1044/0161-1461(2012/ 12-0023)

Kulkarni, S. S., & Parmar, J. (2017). Culturally and linguistically diverse student and family perspectives of AAC. *Augmentative and Alternative Communication, 33,* 170–180.

https://doi.org/10.1080/07434618.2017.13
46706

Lanza, E. (1992). Can bilingual two-year-olds code-switch? *Journal of Child Language, 19*(3), 633–658. https://doi.org/https://doi
.org/10.1017/S0305000900011600

Lyons-Golden, J & Seeley, L. (2020). Unpublished handbook of AAC implementation materials, Fulton Co., Georgia.

McCardle, P. E., & Chhabra, V. E. (2004). *The voice of evidence in reading research*. Brookes.

Mccord, M. S., & Soto, G. (2004). Perceptions of AAC: An ethnographic investigation of Mexican-American families. *Augmentative and Alternative Communication, 20,* 209–227. https://doi.org/10.1080/07434610400
005648

McDuffie, A., & Yoder, P. (2010). Types of parent verbal responsiveness that predict language in young children with autism spectrum disorder. *Journal of Speech, Language, and Hearing Research, 53,* 1026–1039. https://
doi.org/10.1044/1092-4388(2009/09-0023)

Millar, D. C., Light, J. C., & Schlosser, R. W. (2006). The impact of augmentative and alternative communication intervention on the speech production of individuals with developmental disabilities: A research review. *Journal of Speech, Language, and Hearing Research, 49,* 248–264.

National Center on Early Childhood Quality Assurance. (2019, August). *Early Learning and Development Guidelines*. Administration for Children and Families, U.S. Department of Health and Human Services. Retrieved from https://childcareta.acf.hhs
.gov/sites/default/files/public/075_1907_
state_eldgs_web_final508.pdf

O'Neill, T., Light, J., & Pope, L. (2018). Effects of interventions that include aided augmentative and alternative communication input on the communication of individuals with complex communication needs: A meta-analysis. *Journal of Speech, Language, and Hearing Research, 61*(7), 1743–1765. https://doi
.org/10.1044/2018_JSLHR-L-17-0132

Ogletree, B. (2017). Addressing the communication and other needs of persons with severe disabilities through engaged interprofessional teams: Introduction to a clinical forum. *American Journal of Speech-Language Pathology, 26*(2), 157–162. https://doi.org/
10.1044/2017

Ogletree, B. T., Brady, N., Bruce, S., Dean, E., Romski, M., Sylvester, L., & Westling, D. (2017). Mary's case: An illustration of interprofessional collaborative practice for a child with severe disabilities. *American Journal of Speech-Language Pathology, 26*(2), 217–226. https://doi.org/10.1044/2017_AJSLP-15-0065

Paradis, J., Nicoladis, E., Crago, M., & Genesee, F. (2011). Bilingual children's acquisition of the past tense: A usage-based approach. *Journal of Child Language, 38*(3), 554–578. https://doi.org/10.1017/S030500
0910000218

Parette, H. P., & Angelo, D. H. (1996). Augmentative and alternative communication impact on families: Trends and future directions. *Journal of Special Education, 30*(1), 77–98. https://doi.org/10.1177/00
2246699603000105

Parette, H. P., & Brotherson, M. J. (2004). Family-centered and culturally responsive assistive technology decision making. *Infants and Young Children, 17*(4), 355–367.

Parette, H. P., Brotherson, M. J., & Huer, M. B. (2000). Giving families a voice in augmentative and alternative communication decision-making. *Education and Training in Mental Retardation and Developmental Disabilities, 35*(2), 177–190.

Parette, P., VanBiervliet, A., & Hourcade, J. J. (2000). Family-centered decision making in assistive technology. *Journal of Special Education Technology, 15*(1), 45–55. https://
doi.org/10.1177/016264340001500104

Perfetti, C. (1985). *Reading ability*. Oxford University Press.

Petretic, P. A., & Tweney, R. D. (1977). Does comprehension precede production? The development of children's responses to telegraphic sentences of varying grammatical adequacy. *Journal of Child Language, 4*(2), 201–209. https://doi.org/10.1017/S0
305000900001604

Pickl, G. (2011). Communication intervention in children with severe disabilities and multilingual backgrounds: Perceptions of pedagogues and parents. *Augmentative and Alternative Communication, 27*(4), 229–244. https://doi.org/10.3109/07434618.2011.630021

PRC-Saltillo. (2019). Chat Editor (Version 2.0) [Computer software].

PRC-Saltillo. (2019). NOVAChat® [Mobile application software].

PRC-Saltillo. (2019). TouchChat® [Mobile application software].

PRC-Saltillo. (2019). Words for Life™ [Mobile application software].

Reichle, J., & Wacker, D. (2017). *Functional communication training for problem behavior.* Guilford.

Reichle, J., York, J., & Sigafoos, J. (1991). *Implementing augmentative and alternative communication: Strategies for learners with severe disabilities.* Brookes.

Reyes, I. (2004). Functions of code switching in schoolchildren's conversations. *Bilingual Research Journal, 28*(1), 77–98. https://doi.org/10.1080/15235882.2004.10162613

Ribot, K. M., Hoff, E., & Burridge, A. (2018). Language use contributes to expressive language growth: Evidence from bilingual children. *Child Development, 89*(3), 929–940. https://doi.org/10.1111/cdev.12770

Robillard, M., Mayer-Crittenden, C., Minor-Corriveau, M., & Bélanger, R. (2014). Monolingual and bilingual children with and without primary language impairment: Core vocabulary comparison. *Augmentative and Alternative Communication, 30*, 267–278. https://doi.org/10.3109/07434618.2014.921240

Romski, M. A., & Sevcik, R. A. (1993). Language comprehension: Considerations for augmentative and alternative communication. *Augmentative and Alternative Communication, 9*(4), 281–285.

Romski, M. A., & Sevcik, R. (1996). *Breaking the speech barrier: Language development through augmented means.* Brookes.

Romski, M. A., & Sevcik, R. A. (2005). Augmentative communication and early interven-

tion: Myths and realities. *Infants & Young Children, 18*(3), 174–185.

Romski, M. A., Sevcik, R. A., Adamson, L. B., Cheslock, M., Smith, A., Barker, R. M., & Bakeman, R. (2010). Randomized comparison of augmented and nonaugmented language interventions for toddlers with developmental delays and their parents. *Journal of Speech, Language, and Hearing Research, 53*, 350–364. https://doi.org/10.1044/1092-4388(2009/08-0156)

Romski, M. A., Sevcik, R. A., Barton-Hulsey, A., & Whitmore, A. S. (2015). Early intervention and AAC: What a difference 30 years makes. *Augmentative and Alternative Communication, 31*(3), 1–22. https://doi.org/10.3109/07434618.2015.1064163

Schepis, M. M., Reid, D. H., Behrmann, M. M., & Sutton, K. A. (1998). Increasing communicative interactions of young children with autism using a voice output communication aid and naturalistic teaching. *Journal of Applied Behavior Analysis, 31*(4), 561–578. https://doi.org/10.1901/jaba.1998.31-561

Sevcik, R. A. (2006). Comprehension: An overlooked component in augmented language development. *Disability and Rehabilitation, 28*(3), 159–167. https://doi.org/10.1080/09638280500077804

Smith, M., & Grove, N. (2003). Asymmetry in input and output for individuals who use augmentative and alternative communication. In J. C. Light, D. R. Beukelman, & J. Reichle (Eds.), *Communicative competence of individuals who use augmentative and alternative communication* (pp. 163–195). Brookes.

Soto, G., Muller, E., Hunt, P., & Goetz, L. (2001). Clinical exchange professional skills for serving students who use AAC in general education classrooms: A team perspective. *Language Speech and Hearing Services in Schools, 32*, 51–56.

Soto, G., & Yu, B. (2014). Considerations for the provision of services to bilingual children who use augmentative and alternative communication. *Augmentative and Alternative Communication, 30*(1), 83–92.

https://doi.org/10.3109/07434618.2013.87 8751

Stewart, C.A. (2017). *Bilingual AAC intervention: A case study* (Master's thesis, University of Colorado at Boulder). Retreived from https://pdfs.semanticscholar.org/b34e/ aa40793fcca1d184d1cbc2730c680fe50e6e .pdf

Trembath, D., Balandin, S., Togher, L., & Stancliffe, R. J. (2009). Peer-mediated teaching and augmentative and alternative communication for preschool-aged children with autism. *Journal of Intellectual and Developmental Disability, 34*, 173–186. https://doi .org/10.1080/13668250902845210

Wright, P. W. D. (2004). *The Individuals with Disabilities Education Improvment Act of 2004.*(URL link would be helpful to readers) https://www.wrightslaw.com/idea/ index.htm

Yu, B. (2013). Issues in bilingualism and heritage language maintenance: Perspectives of minority-language mothers of children with autism spectrum disorders. *American Journal of Speech-Language Pathology, 22*, 10–24. https://doi.org/10.1044/1058-0360(2012/10-0078)a

Zablotsky, B., Black, L. I., & Blumberg, S. J. (2017). Estimated prevalence of children with diagnosed developmental disabilities in the United States, 2014-2016. *NCHS Data Brief.*

Zangari, C., Lloyd, L. L., & Vicker, B. (1994). Augmentative and alternative communication: An historic perspective. *Augmentative and Alternative Communication, 10*(3), 27–59.

Zangari, C., & Wise, L. (2016). *TELL ME: AAC in the preschool classroom.* Verona, WS: Attainment Company.

Zurawski, L. P. (2014). Speech-language pathologists and inclusive service delivery: What are the first steps? *Perspectives on School-Based Issues, 15*(1), 5. https://doi .org/10.1044/sbi15.1.5

APPENDIX 3–A
Morning Meeting Script

Morning Meeting
Table of Contents

Page 2	Greeting	
Page 3	Calendar Report	
Page 4	Weather Report	
Page 6	Lunch Menu Report	
Page 7	Class Jobs	
Page 9	Current Events	

Material created by Jennifer Lyons, ATS and Lauren Seeley, CCC-SLP, Fulton County School System, 2020
® symbols from WordPower™ © PRC-Saltillo/SymbolStix/Inman Innovations www.prc-saltillo.com

2

Greeting	
I say...	**I touch...**
Hello, class!	
Who do you want to say hello to?	
Hello, _____!	

Material created by Jennifer Lyons, ATS and Lauren Seeley, CCC-SLP, Fulton County School System, 2020
® symbols from WordPower™ © PRC-Saltillo/SymbolStix/Inman Innovations www.prc-saltillo.com

3

Calendar Report

I say...	I touch...
Let's check our calendars. (students have individual calendars out) What are you doing today?	QUESTION ► / what ? / you ► / do
Who will you see today?	QUESTION ► / who ? will / you ► / see (eye)
We will see (people's names from school may be programmed in empty cells of the school people)	I / will / see (eye) PEOPLE ► / SCHOOL PEOPLE
Who has a birthday this month?	QUESTION ► / who has / GROUPS ► / PARTY ► / birthday (cake)
What fun events do we have this month?	QUESTN ► / what ? / DESCRIBE ► / fun (balloon)

4

Weather Report	
I say...	**I touch...**
What's the weather like today?	
It is rainy.	
It is cloudy.	
It is sunny.	
It is windy.	
It is cold.	
What do we need? (Use visuals or objects in a box/bag: sunglasses, scarf, jacket, umbrella, etc. Use photos of people dressed for various weather conditions).	

Material created by Jennifer Lyons, ATS and Lauren Seeley, CCC-SLP, Fulton County School System, 2020
® symbols from WordPower™ © PRC-Saltillo/SymbolStix/Inman Innovations www.prc-saltillo.com

5

Lunch Report	
I say...	**I touch...**
What's for lunch today? (Use your school lunch menu- add pictures or read it and point to items using Chat Editor)	QUESTN ▶ — what — 's — GROUPS ▶ — FOOD ▶ — lunch
What do you want to eat?	QUESTN ▶ — what — you ▶ — eat ▶
I want to eat _____ (model what you might choose from the menu, or have a student model)	I — want — to eat ▶ — MEALS ▶

Material created by Jennifer Lyons, ATS and Lauren Seeley, CCC-SLP, Fulton County School System, 2020
® symbols from WordPower™ © PRC-Saltillo/SymbolStix/Inman Innovations www.prc-saltillo.com

6

Class Jobs	
I say...	**I touch...**
What is your job this week?	QUESTION ? / what ? / -'s / your — HOME / GROUPS / JOBS / job
Who will say hello and goodbye?	QUESTION ? / who / will — ACTIONS / say / SOCIAL / hello
Who will sweep the floor?	QUESTION ? / who / will — ACTIONS / ACTIONS A-Z / s / → / sweep
Who will clean the tables?	QUESTION ? / who / will / ACTIONS / clean
Who will collect the trash?	QUESTION ? / who / will / get / GROUPS / CONTAINERS / trash bag

Material created by Jennifer Lyons, ATS and Lauren Seeley, CCC-SLP, Fulton County School System, 2020
® symbols from WordPower™ © PRC-Saltillo/SymbolStix/Inman Innovations www.prc-saltillo.com

7

Current Events	
I say...	**I touch...**
Let's get our Last Night sheets out.	get out
What did you do last night?	QUESTN what you do TIME last nite
Who do you want to ask?	QUESTN who do you → → ask

Material created by Jennifer Lyons, ATS and Lauren Seeley, CCC-SLP, Fulton County School System, 2020
® symbols from WordPower™ © PRC-Saltillo/SymbolStix/Inman Innovations www.prc-saltillo.com

APPENDIX 3–B
Door Script

Door Script
When you leave/return to the classroom
*Depending on your students' current needs, model 1+ words on the AAC system. Use this script as a guide, modify the number of words modeled as appropriate.

When you leave the classroom	
I say...	**I touch...**
Where are you going?	
I'm going to P.E.	*If your student is using WordPower below 108, add the word "P.E." to your student's device on the Places page. Use the search term "gym class" for an appropriate symbol.
I'm going to the lunchroom.	
I'm going to the playground.	
I'm going to music.	
I'm going to OT.	

Material created by Jennifer Lyons, ATS and Lauren Seeley, CCC-SLP, Fulton County School System, 2020
® symbols from WordPower™ © PRC-Saltillo/SymbolStix/Inman Innovations www.prc-saltillo.com

I'm going to speech therapy.	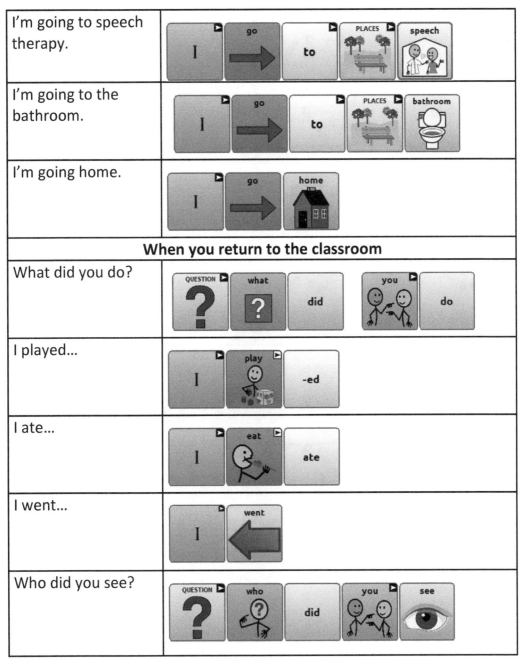
I'm going to the bathroom.	
I'm going home.	
When you return to the classroom	
What did you do?	
I played...	
I ate...	
I went...	
Who did you see?	

Material created by Jennifer Lyons, ATS and Lauren Seeley, CCC-SLP, Fulton County School System, 2020
® symbols from WordPower™ © PRC-Saltillo/SymbolStix/Inman Innovations www.prc-saltillo.com

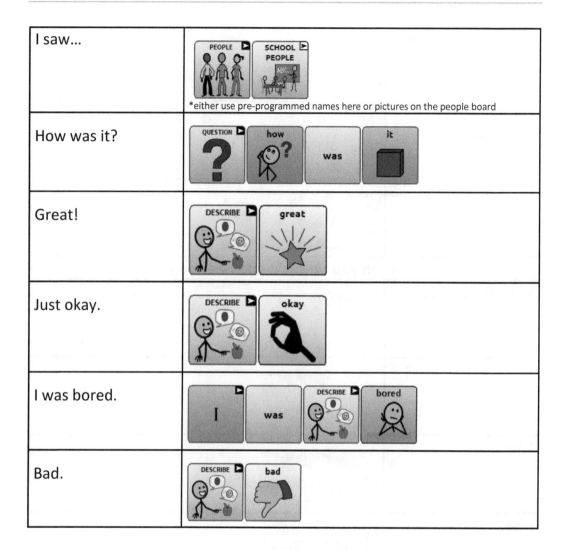

I saw...	PEOPLE ▶ SCHOOL PEOPLE ▶
	*either use pre-programmed names here or pictures on the people board
How was it?	QUESTION ▶ how was it
Great!	DESCRIBE ▶ great
Just okay.	DESCRIBE ▶ okay
I was bored.	▶ I was DESCRIBE ▶ bored
Bad.	DESCRIBE ▶ bad

4

AAC in Schools: Mastering the Art and Science of Inclusion

Nancy B. Robinson and Gloria Soto

■ Introduction

Although significant advances in inclusive education for ALL students are evident in policy and practice in school programs for students with disabilities, students with complex communication needs (CCN) often remain on the margins, spending most of the school day in self-contained classrooms or in separate schools (Kleinert et al., 2015; NCD, 2018; Thurlow, Ghere, Lazarus, & Liu, 2020). This may be partly due to the specialized support that students with CCN need to use their AAC systems effectively in the classroom and across all school environments. In addition, increasing cultural and linguistic diversity of the student population impacts AAC services in schools, creating the need for AAC systems that are individualized to include each student's language and cultural background. We are in a time of great challenges, change, and progress in education. We have better tools to support students to have access to AAC through computers, touch screen tablets, such as iPads, interactive displays and more. Yet, educators, including Speech-Language

Pathologists (SLPs), who are prepared to provide AAC services that are both inclusive and culturally responsive, are in short supply (Andzik, Schaefer, Nichols, & Chung, 2018; Kulkarni & Parmar, 2017). Students with CCN often do not get the support they need to participate with their peers throughout the school day, potentially leading to exclusion from full participation in society beyond the school years.

In this chapter, we will examine the issues, challenges, and solutions to achieve the goal of inclusion for students with CCN who represent the diversity of our schools to access academic, social interaction and cultural learning in all settings. There are several developments in U.S. public education that support this goal, including Multi-Tiered System of Supports (MTSS), Universal Design for Learning (UDL), culturally responsive practices (CRP), Interprofessional Education (IPE), and Interprofessional Practice (IPP). UDL is a foundational concept and set of principles that provides the basis for access to learning through careful planning of each educational environment. MTSS offers a comprehensive framework that brings best practice in inclusive education together, building on a Response to Intervention (RtI) model in successive tiers of student support and whole school collaboration. CRP is integral to service delivery to include students who rely on AAC from all language and cultural backgrounds. IPE and IPP, originated in health care, integrate decades of learning about the importance of collaboration into a comprehensive framework with identified competencies for professional teams to create seamless systems of care. Although we face many challenges to fully include students who rely on AAC to learn and to communicate with peers without disabilities, the resources to achieve inclusion are available. We will first identify the issues and challenges and then provide solutions for equitable access to learning for students who rely on AAC and represent diverse cultural and language backgrounds.

■ Identifying Issues and Challenges Impacting Inclusion in Education for Students With Disabilities

The Education for All Handicapped Children Act (EAHCA, 94-142), now the Individuals with Disabilities Education Act (IDEA) of 2004, was passed in 1975 to provide a free appropriate public education to all students with disabilities. Since that time, understanding and implementation of inclusion in schools has evolved. From the initial legislative requirement in the United States that all students are to be educated in the Least Restrictive Environment (LRE), terminology has changed from "LRE" and "mainstreaming" to "inclusion." Recent reauthorizations of the IDEA do not use the word "inclusion" as

a requirement, yet the concept and practice of inclusive education for all students is clearly the mandate of U.S. educational policy and a goal for public school systems. The concept of inclusion is operationalized differently depending on the specific policies and practices in states, districts, and schools. In some inclusive settings, special education professionals assume the majority of responsibility for teaching students with disabilities in a general education classroom. For the purpose of this chapter, inclusive education refers to situations where students with disabilities are rightful and integral members of general education classrooms and receive instruction by general education teachers in collaboration with special education professionals in the same settings as their peers without disabilities. Inclusion transforms general education classrooms into settings where differences of any kind are treated as "ordinary" (McLeskey & Waldron, 2000). In a comprehensive historical review of U.S. special education legislation, policy and practice, Hossain (2012) traced the development of inclusion in education as a result of parental activism followed by research that documents the benefits of including students with disabilities in general education settings with non-disabled peers. As Hossain stated, "Moving from the goal of a free and appropriate education to meaningful inclusion has taken decades to achieve and is still a work in progress" (Hossain, p. 3).

Given the LRE requirement and the development of inclusion in school systems in the U.S. since 1975, it is surprising that many students with significant disabilities, particularly those with CCN, remain in separate educational settings for much of the school day. Researchers in the field have voiced their concerns that after more than four decades since the passage of legislation to require LRE, students with CNN are often excluded from inclusive learning with their peers (Kleinert, Kearns, Liu, Thurlow, & Lazarus, 2019; Vandercook, Kleinert, Jorgenson, Sabia, & Lazarus, 2019).

In order to gain perspective on the extent of inclusion in U.S. schools, federal data on inclusion is reported in terms of educational placement. The U.S. Department of Education reported in 2015, 95% of students with disabilities, ages 6 to 21 years of age were served in public school programs. Of these students, their percentage of participation in the general education classroom was as follows: 62.5% participated 80% or more; 19% participated from 40% to 79%; and 17% participated less than 40% (Institute of Education Science, National Center on Education Statistics (IES/NES), 2019a). Yet the concept of "participation" is very vague and broad, ranging from sharing school lunch with peers in the school cafeteria to being a full member of a general education classroom.

Status of Inclusion of Students With CCN Who Rely on AAC

There are no conclusive data as to the prevalence of inclusive placements, (i.e., participation in general education classrooms), for students with CCN who use AAC. This could be due to the heterogeneity of students who use AAC and the fact that in large placement studies, students with CCN could be "classified" according to their disability rather than according to whether they use AAC to communicate. Qualitative research provides further insight to better understand the experiences of students with CCN

in general educational settings. Several researchers, in the United States and internationally, have conducted observational and interview studies that show patterns of inclusion, exclusion, and restricted participation by students with CCN in schools (Bourke-Taylor, Cotter, Johnson, & Lalor, 2018; Mehr, 2017; Østvik, Balandin, & Ytterhus, 2017; Raghavendra, Olsson, Sampson, Mcinerney, & Connell, 2012).

Rather than looking only at the educational placement setting, inclusion was measured as "participation" in the same activities with peers and opportunities for communication interaction. Existing research indicates students who use AAC have few communication partners who understand their systems and limited opportunities to interact in peer groups and to develop conversational skills (Biggs, Carter, & Gustafson, 2017; Lilienfeld & Alant, 2005; Smith, 2005).

Researchers have explored the impact of limited opportunities for students who rely on AAC to communicate with peers without disabilities from several perspectives, including the views of students with CCN. In the context of this research, the voices of students who rely on AAC demonstrate their own preferences and perceptions. A key finding by Wickenden (2011a, 2011b) is that students who rely on AAC are reported to see themselves with the same interests and challenges as their peers without disabilities.

Some of the key findings from observational studies have shown students with CCN infrequently use their AAC devices to communicate with peers, even when in close proximity (Chung, Carter, & Sisco, 2012). Raghavendra et al. (2012) compared the social participation of students between 10 to 15 years of age in three groups: those without disabilities, those with physical disabilities and those with

CCN. They found the students who used AAC experienced limited opportunities for interaction; rarely used their AAC devices for peer directed social interaction; and had fewer acquaintances and friends.

Interview studies with parents, teachers, and students with CCN have corroborated the findings of observational studies. Bourke-Taylor et al. (2018) interviewed 47 participants that included students with disabilities, their parents, and teachers. Although only 4 of 7 students interviewed included those with CCN, the overall finding was that students with physical disabilities participate less with peers. In Norway, Østvik et al. (2017) interviewed students from grades 1 to 4, their peers, teachers, and parents and found students using AAC spent less time engaged in activities with peers without disabilities.

Clearly, the impact of limited social participation with communication partners without disabilities has significant implications for inclusion of students with CCN in general education classrooms. The models of service delivery in schools, while intended to advance the language development of students with CCN to use their AAC devices effectively with communication partners in many settings, may have the opposite effect. Nearly two decades ago, Clarke, McConachie, Price, and Wood (2001a, 2001b) investigated perspectives of both SLPs and their students who used AAC systems regarding varying models of speech therapy in the United Kingdom. SLPs reported a range of therapy models were implemented that included AAC services within and outside the classroom. Their students reported a preference for one-to-one speech therapy outside of the classroom, perhaps indicating their peers and classroom teachers were not effective communication partners. More recently, Erikson and Geist (2016) suggested more communication

with adults, compared to interaction with peers without disabilities, may actually pose a barrier for students with CCN to interact with peers without disabilities. In addition to the pattern of limited frequency and quality of interaction, there is also the phenomenon of restricted social networks for students with CCN, mentioned earlier (Raghavendra et al., 2012). These findings are profound with implications that students with CCN experience progressively restricted social networks, with limited opportunities for interactions outside of classroom environments. The long-term effects of limited social networks are linked to increased social isolation and exclusion for students with CCN (Ballin & Balandin, 2008).

Another aspect of communication interaction is the need for language intervention so that students with CCN can effectively express themselves with AAC tools. Despite years of intervention and advances in language and communication skills, many students who use aided AAC continue to struggle to communicate effectively (see Smith, 2005; McNaughton & Nelson Bryen, 2007). It is well documented that individuals who use AAC have limited expressive language abilities that include difficulties building and using novel vocabulary; and forming appropriate and grammatically complete utterances. The expressive language of individuals who use AAC is often characterized by the predominant use of single word utterances (commonly nouns), or brief utterances that are morphologically and syntactically incorrect or immature (Binger & Light, 2008; Soto & Hartmann, 2006; Sutton, Soto, & Blockberger, 2002). Equally, their communication systems are often insufficient to meet the increasing demands for peer socialization and conversation associated with classroom participation (Smith, 2005).

The picture painted in recent research broadens the meaning of inclusion in education beyond only looking at educational placement. Although the amount of time that students with CCN spend in the general education is one glimpse of inclusion, there are multiple dimensions to consider. A student may be placed in a general education classroom and still experience exclusion from meaningful participation. The degree of access and participation in the general education curriculum, communicative interactions with peers, access to linguistically robust AAC systems, comprehensive language intervention, and social interaction across the school day are all dimensions of inclusive education that impact educational outcomes for each student. In order to design inclusive education, each of the above dimensions needs to be addressed with intentionality. An additional dimension is that of students' cultural and linguistic diversity. Students with disabilities who are dual language learners are reported to experience "double" exclusion, both from general education classroom where instruction is in English, and from bilingual education programs where students without disabilities received instruction both in home language and in English (Cioé-Peña, 2017). In the next section, we consider the impact of cultural and linguistic diversity on the inclusion/exclusion of students who rely on AAC.

Status of Inclusion of Students of Culturally and Linguistically Diverse Backgrounds

The changing demographics of U.S. schools reveal that groups perceived as "minorities" with respect with cultural and language background are becoming the "majority" of the student population in public schools. For example, ethnic, racial and language statistics reported in federal education data (IES/NCES, 2019b) show percentages of students in public elementary and secondary schools in the United States identified as Hispanic increased from 16% to 26% from 2000 to 2015, while the percentages of White students decreased from 61% to 49% in the same time period. At the state level, demographic changes have clearly reversed the measure of minority compared to majority of the student population. For example, in California in the 2018 to 2019 school year, 55% of public-school students were identified as Hispanic or Latino while 23 percent were White. Other groups including Asian, African-American, Pacific Islander, American Indian and Filipino are much smaller percentages. With the increasing diversity of cultural backgrounds comes a diversity of languages.

In 2017, 23% of public-school students in the U.S. were reported to speak a language other than English at home (Ziegler & Camarota, 2018). Liu et al. (2013) found that the IDEA child count data for the 2009 to 2010 school year reported 518,088 students with disabilities in U.S. public schools were also classified as limited English proficient (LEP), representing approximately 8.5% of all students with disabilities. Further, of these students, the highest percentage, 39%, were in California. In California, there are 2.6 million public school students who speak a language other than English at home, representing about 42% of school enrollment (California Department of Education, 2019). Among these students are those enrolled in programs to improve English proficiency, variously referred to as students with Limited English Proficient (LEP), English Language Learners (ELL), and English

Learners (EL). There are 5 million English Learners (identified as LEP students in federal reporting) in U.S. public schools and one-third of these students (1.2 million) are in California schools (California Department of Education (CDE), 2019a; Langdon, Saenz, Dominquez, Clark, & McCollum, 2017). In California's public schools, EL students make up 19.3 percent of the total enrollments and data is reported on a total number of 67 primary languages including Spanish, Vietnamese, Mandarin, Arabic, Filipino, Cantonese, Korean, Punjabi, Russian, and Hmong in the top ten.

It is difficult to determine the prevalence of disabilities within the population of EL students, due to potential overlap of the students who may be identified in more than one category and challenges in differentiating between language learning difference or disability in young children. Although the extent of EL students with CCN is not delineated in state reporting data, the high representation of language diversity reported clearly reinforces the need to attend to cultural and language backgrounds in AAC services. These findings provide a very general picture of the status of inclusion in general education classrooms for students with disabilities and indications of disparities for particular groups, including those with CCN and those who are members of culturally and linguistically diverse communities.

The importance of becoming attuned to each individual student's cultural and language background in the provision of AAC services was identified over two decades ago (Soto, Huer, & Taylor, 1997). Kulkarni and Parmar (2017) reviewed a series of studies from 2000 to 2017 that focused on the need for including cultural and linguistic considerations in the design and delivery of AAC services in school set-tings. Their review of 11 studies revealed five major themes in each of these areas: (a) Device Limitations and Lack of support, (b) Family and Professional Dynamics, (c) Cultural Perceptions, (d) Language Supports, and (e) Home-Based Communication Supports and Interventions. In each of these areas, the authors discussed areas of concern identified by families and professionals that need to be addressed for effective AAC services that include the cultural and linguistic diversity of students and their families; in particular, the positive contributions of the child's first language as a bridge to learning English and partnering more effectively with families (Soto & Yu, 2014). Further, research in bilingualism and the student's heritage language strengthens our understanding of the efficacy of including first language foundations as a means to support students, even those with disabilities, to access language learning in a second language (Soto & Yu, 2014; Wagner, 2018; Yu, 2013).

When considering the cultural and language diversity of student populations in U.S. schools and increased globalization of society in general, it is imperative that inclusion takes on the dimension of culturally responsive practices (CRP) to address each of the areas identified by Kulkarni and Parmar (2017). Considering the multiple variables that impact inclusion in general education for students with CCN, the complexity of achieving inclusive education is clear. Figure 4–1 shows the multidimensional relationships of key variables in creating meaningful participation and inclusion of students with CCN, discussed thus far.

In the following sections of the chapter, evidence-based approaches will be presented as solutions to address the challenges discussed and to achieve inclusion

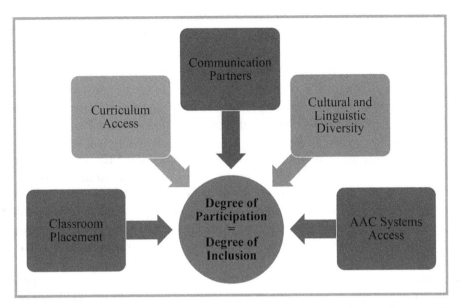

Figure 4–1. Variables that impact classroom inclusion for students with CCN. This figure was created by the authors to illustrate the multiple variables that are documented in research to impact to create inclusive education for all students, including those students with CCN who rely on AAC.

for students with CCN in school settings, both at the systems level and classroom-based intervention.

■ Systems-Level Solutions for Inclusion

For each of the dimensions of inclusion of students with disabilities discussed thus far and shown in Figure 4–1, there are systems-level solutions needed to create effective support for students to participate in all aspects of the school day with their peers (Kleinert et al., 2019). The challenges and conditions in public education in the United Sates impact all students including shortages of teachers and specialist personnel, inequities in technology resources, building infrastructure, state funding, safety, absenteeism,

discipline, and student diversity (Litinov, Alvarez, Long, & Walker, 2018). Several national and state initiatives respond to the challenges for inclusion of students with disabilities. At the systems level, professional development that includes CRP, MTSS and UDL offer promise to benefit all students. Each of these areas is discussed as a solution to advance inclusive education for students with CCN.

Professional Preparation

The need for professional preparation to provide AAC services in schools is widely identified for both speech-language pathologists and teachers. Ratcliff, Koul, and Lloyd (2008) surveyed speech-language pathology programs (both undergraduate and graduate level) and found varied results with 73% of the responding programs offering at least one stand-alone AAC course, 10% offering more than one course, and 80% infusing AAC content in other courses. Only about half of the programs required completion of an AAC course and only about one-third of program graduates reported being prepared to provide AAC services upon graduation. Given the increase in the school population of students with CCN who can benefit from AAC services, Ratcliff et al. concluded there is a critical shortage of AAC training and recommended speech-language pathology programs expand courses, clinical work, research and faculty expertise in AAC. Since the Ratcliff et al. (2008) study, the American Speech Hearing Association included AAC in the Standards of Clinical Practice. This change appears to have had a positive influence on preservice training for Speech-Language Pathology.

In a follow-up survey, Johnson and Prebor (2019) reported 86% of programs in Speech Language Pathology offered at least one course with primary content in AAC. This is a 13% increase since the last survey by Ratcliffe et al. in 2008. Johnson and Prebor also found 91% of the programs reported AAC instruction was included in other content courses. Still lacking are clinical experiences in AAC service provision for their graduate students. Most programs indicated they did not require students to demonstrate specific operational competency in the use of AAC technologies and supports, or professional competency working with individuals who use AAC. This is alarming considering 75% of SLPs feel inadequately prepared to provide AAC services to their clients (Costigan & Light, 2010).

The same patterns apply to teacher preparation in AAC. Andzik et al. (2018) conducted a nationwide survey with over 9,500 teachers who reported they were not well prepared to support students using AAC in their classrooms. Further, teachers reported students often did not use their AAC systems effectively, limiting their communicative interactions to basic requests rather than using their AAC systems to engage in academic content in the classroom. Teachers surveyed also reported they had limited access to SLPs with specialized skills in AAC who were available to provide training and support in the classroom setting. Recommended strategies to address the needs for teachers' proficiency in AAC included greater collaboration with SLPs, special educators, and professional development at the school level.

The role of classroom teachers to optimize students' use of their AAC systems is critical as they are the people most often with their students. In order to effectively support students with CCN to succeed and to participate fully in the classroom, teachers need specialized support (Andzik et al., 2018). Collaboration among the school team in all aspects of assessment, decision-making, goal setting, intervention and progress evaluation is also essential. As Light (1989) pointed out over two decades ago, and other researchers have subsequently reinforced, AAC services require an entire team for students to be successful. Soto, Müller, Hunt, and Goetz (2001a, 2001b) identified a host of supports and resources needed for effective inclusion of students with AAC that included administrative support, professional development, professional expertise, support for teachers, and team collaboration. Forbes (2018) advocated for the implementation of the conjoint behavioral consultation (CBC) model of collaboration as a means to engage the school team in a four-stage process that includes:

(a) needs identification, (b) needs analysis, (c) plan implementation, and (d) plan evaluation. The challenges to apply collaboration include limited preparation for many professionals to practice the skills needed for effective teamwork.

Models of Interprofessional Education (IPE) and Interprofessional Practice (IPP) that originated in health care have applications to education (Nunez, 2015). ASHA adapted the World Health Organization (2010) definition of IPE and IPE as follows:

> IPE is an activity that occurs when two or more professions learn about, from, and with each other to enable effective collaboration and improve outcomes for individuals and families whom we serve. Similarly, IPP occurs when multiple service providers from different professional backgrounds provide comprehensive healthcare or educational services by working with individuals and their families, caregivers, and communities- to deliver the highest quality of care across settings. (ASHA, n.d.)

Interprofessional Education (IPE) and Interprofessional Practice (IPP) are now required in professional preparation for SLPs and Audiologists, both in certification standards and program accreditation (ASHA, 2020; CAA, 2017). To apply IPE and IPP in practice, the Interprofessional Education Collaborative (IPEC, 2020) identified the following four core competency areas:

- Competency 1: Work with individuals of other professions to maintain a climate of mutual respect and shared values. (Values/Ethics for Interprofessional Practice)
- Competency 2: Use the knowledge of one's own role and those of other professions to appropriately assess and address the health care needs of patients and to promote and advance the health of populations. (Roles/Responsibilities)
- Competency 3: Communicate with patients, families, communities, and professionals in health and other fields in a responsive and responsible manner that supports a team approach to the promotion and maintenance of health and the prevention and treatment of disease. (Interprofessional Communication)
- Competency 4: Apply relationship-building values and the principles of team dynamics effectively in different team roles to plan, deliver, and evaluate patient/population- centered care and population health programs and policies that are safe, timely, efficient, effective, and equitable. (Teams and Teamwork)

Given the increasing cultural and linguistic diversity of students in U.S. public schools, researchers identified needs for professionals to be prepared to provide culturally responsive services. CRP in AAC include building partnerships with families to reflect cultural diversity and primary languages in the development and implementation of AAC services in schools (ASHA, 2013, 2014; Kulkarni & Parmar, 2017; Solomon-Rice, Soto, & Robinson, 2018). In response to personnel preparation needs in AAC that include interprofessional collaboration and CRP, about 10% of universities in the United States have developed specialized training in AAC through competitive personnel preparation grants awarded by the United States Department of Education/Office of Special Education Programs (USDOE/OSEP) (Johnson & Prebor, 2019). The peer-reviewed grant application and award process assures programs are designed to advance inclusive practices, aligned with research discussed in this chapter. Table 4–1 highlights six USDOE/OSEP Personnel Preparation grants, awarded since 2015, that have enabled the development of AAC specialization at their respective universities.

Through personnel preparation grants such as those highlighted, universities have opportunities to build capacity to prepare qualified personnel to expand AAC services in school settings. One of these programs, Project Building Bridges, focused on culturally responsive AAC services in schools and developed a competency guide, *Augmentative and Alternative Communication With Focus on Culturally Responsive Practice: Assessment of Knowledge and Skills Acquisition*. Table 4–2 includes the five core domains and infusion of those competencies that target culturally responsive AAC practices. Students and their faculty complete formative and summative assessment using the guide at entry, during internships, and at exit from the program. Data collection is ongoing and results collected to date demonstrate positive changes in knowledge and skills from both the student and faculty perspectives. The complete guide is available in publication by Solomon-Rice, Soto, and Robinson (2018).

In addition to professional preparation at the university level, teachers and the school team require professional development resources to effectively support students with CCN to participate fully in school settings. Several national and state initiatives in education, discussed in the following section, provide resources for practicing professionals to advance inclusive practice.

Multi-Tiered System of Supports for Inclusive Education

Multi-Tiered System of Supports (MTSS) is broad term to describe a process for integration of state, district, and school resources to create comprehensive school improvement so that all students' needs are met in coordinated and inclusive education. In California, MTSS is defined as,

"an integrated, comprehensive framework that focuses on Common Core State Standards, core instruction, differentiated learning, student-centered learning, individualized student needs, and the alignment of systems necessary for all students' academic, behavioral, and social success . . . MTSS offers the potential to create needed systematic change through intentional design and redesign of services and supports that quickly identify and match the needs of all students." (CDE, 2019b)

MTSS incorporates and moves beyond Response to Intervention (RtI) and Positive Behavioral Instructional Supports (PBIS), classroom-based intervention models to support students with academic and behavioral needs from pre-referral to identification and intervention. The RtI approach, designed in multiple tiers of support to meet the needs of students at-risk for learning disabilities, starts at Tier 1 with universal screening

Table 4–1. USDOE/OSEP Discretionary Personnel Preparation Grants in AAC, Funded Since 2015

Grant Name	University	Principal Investigator	Focus
Augmentative and Alternative Communication, Language, and Literacy Initiative to Prepare Speech-Language Pathologists	University of Tennessee	Jillian McCarthy Ilsa Schwartz	Prepare SLPs to improve the language and literacy outcomes of children who use or could benefit from augmentative-alternative communication strategies or equipment (AAC).
Project Building Bridges	San Francisco State University	Gloria Soto	Prepare SLPs to work effectively with culturally and linguistically diverse children with significant disabilities and augmentative communication needs, ages birth to 21.
Penn State AAC Collaboration Project	Pennsylvania State University	Jessica Caron	Provide interdisciplinary training for SLPs and Special Educators to enhance the quality of services and results for children with high-intensity needs who require augmentative and alternative communication (AAC) and assistive technology.
Special Education and Communication-Interdisciplinary Training	University of Kentucky	Judith Page	Provide interdisciplinary training for SLPs and Special Educators for communication programming for students with severe disabilities and complex communication needs.
Penn State AAC Doctoral Leadership Project	Pennsylvania State University	Janice Light	Prepare doctoral training for faculty to conduct research and provide preservice training for speech language pathologists in augmentative and alternative communication (AAC)/assistive technology.
Project GROW (Guiding Responsive Communication Within Inclusive Early Childhood Settings)	San Francisco State University	Amber Friesen	Provide interdisciplinary preparation of Early Childhood Special Educators and SLPs to deliver family-centered, culturally and linguistically responsive services for young children from minority and low-income backgrounds through collaborative and inclusive services that include Augmentative and Alternative Communication (AAC).

Source: Office of Special Education Programs. (n.d.). *Discretionary Grants Database.* Available at: https://publicddb.osepideasthatwork.org

Table 4–2. Augmentative and Alternative Communication With Focus on Culturally Responsive Practice: Assessment of Knowledge and Skills Acquisition: Core and Culturally Responsive Competencies

Core Competency Area	Culturally Responsive AAC Competencies
AAC Systems in Language and Literacy: Assessment	1.2 Demonstrate culturally responsive skills to involve families in the AAC assessment process. 1.3 Demonstrate skills to conduct AAC assessment with interpreters 1.4 Identify cultural views of disability and individual family preferences for communication support related to AAC. 1.5 Determine level of bilingual development regarding first and second language acquisition stage for individual children. 1.6 Conduct ethnographic assessment to include perspectives of family members in consideration of AAC and determination of language mastery for child in first and second language.
AAC Systems in General Education: Programming and Intervention	2.1 Demonstrate knowledge of the cultural background, traditions and history of families and students represented in the SF Bay Area including families of Latino, Chinese, Pacific Islander, Filipino, Eastern European and other backgrounds. 2.2 Incorporate first and second language exposure in the design of AAC systems with individual children. 2.3 Demonstrate culturally responsive skills to determine individual and family preferences for language and communication modality in AAC systems. 2.5 Incorporate cultural and language background of client in design of AAC system. 2.6 Develop culturally and linguistically relevant low and high-tech AAC systems for children and families.
AAC Systems: Collaboration	3.2 Demonstrate self-awareness of cultural competence to include families of CLD backgrounds in AAC teams through completion of ASHA's Self-Assessment of Cultural Competence (ASHA, n.d.) 3.3 Demonstrate culturally responsive skills to involve families in the language, literacy, and AAC team process. 3.4 Demonstrate skills to access and include interpreter services, as needed, to ensure family participation in team meetings and communication.
AAC Systems in Schools: Literacy Development	4.4 Demonstrate knowledge and skills to ensure representation of individual cultural and linguistic diversity in literacy and language curriculum materials. 4.9 Determine level of bilingual development regarding first and second language acquisition stage for individual children in the design of language and literacy goals to meet academic standards.

Table 4–2. *continued*

Core Competency Area	Culturally Responsive AAC Competencies
AAC Systems in Schools: Professional Development	5.2 Demonstrate continued professional development to provide culturally responsive practice to involve families in the language, literacy, and AAC assessment and intervention process.

Source: Solomon-Rice, P., Soto, G., & Robinson, N. (2018). Project Building Bridges: Training speech-language pathologists to provide culturally and linguistically responsive Augmentative and Alternative Communication Services to school-age children with diverse backgrounds. *Perspectives of the ASHA Special Interest Groups*, SIG 12, 3. American Speech-Language-Hearing Association. (Part 4). 136–137. Retrieved from https://pubs.asha.org/doi/pdf/10.1044/persp3.SIG12.186

then moves to progress monitoring at Tier 2 and to identification of students in need of more intensified support in Tier 3 (Freeman, Miller, & Newcomer, 2015; Grether, 2009). Also, in a tiered model, PBIS approaches are designed to support students considered at risk of social, emotional and behavioral support needs in successively intensive interventions (Horner, Sugai, & Anderson, 2010). MTSS has been described as the merging of RtI and PBIS and is also much more. MTSS builds districtwide leadership with involvement at all levels including administrators, teachers, specialists, family members, consultants, staff, other relevant personnel, and community members (Freeman, Miller, & Newcomer, 2015).

The implications of the MTSS movement nationally, and in many states, are significant for SLPs supporting students with CCN, who may find traditional service delivery approaches are challenged with more emphasis on working within the general education classroom. As Sylvan (2018) points out, MTSS offers new opportunities for SLPs to collaborate with teachers to create conditions that support students with CCN to interact with their peers. Key premises of MTSS include UDL and CRP at all levels of support, which

have specific applications for students with CCN and AAC needs.

Three national centers, funded by the U.S. Department of Education, Office of Special Education Programs, provide ongoing comprehensive resources to assist school systems and educators to design and implement MTSS initiatives. Notably, each of the centers described below have recently updated their Web-based resources to include materials for educators to provide online education, when needed.

Schoolwide Integrated Framework for Transformation (SWIFT)

SWIFT is a national technical assistance center, a part of the University of Kansas Lifespan Institute, has developed resources to support states to implement MTSS through building capacity of school districts and communities to provide academic and behavioral support to improve outcomes for all students (Schoolwide Integrated Framework for Transformation [SWIFT], 2020). The following quote from the IDEA website describes the scope of the SWIFT Education Center:

> "SWIFT Education Center provides executive leadership coaching, professional learning, and differentiated technical assistance (TA) to education entities through contractual agreements. These services are based on a framework for inclusive schoolwide transformation in which Multi-Tiered System of Supports (MTSS) is the mechanism that drives improved student outcomes and is scaffolded by four domains of evidence-based practices for successfully installing and sustaining MTSS: Administrative Leadership, Integrated Educational Framework, Family and Community Engagement, and Inclusive Policy Structure and Practice." (IDEA, n.d.)

SWIFT's system-level focus demonstrates the emphasis on leadership involvement in the implementation MTSS at the state and district level. SWIFT Education Center has partnered with states to support Lead Education Agencies (LEAs) to create district leadership teams and professional development for district personnel across the United States On the SWIFT Education Center website, educators, family members, administrators, and state leaders will find comprehensive professional development guides and demonstrations of MTSS implementation in classrooms and districts.

Collaboration for Effective Educator Development, Accountability, and Reform (CEEDAR)

CEEDAR, based at the University of South Florida with national partners, the Ameri-

can Institutes for Research and Council of Chief State School Officers, states their mission as follows:

> "Our mission is to support students with disabilities in achieving college- and career-ready standards by building the capacity of state personnel preparation systems to prepare teachers and leaders to implement evidence-based practices within multi-tiered systems of support" (CEEDAR, 2020).

To accomplish this mission, CEEDAR partners with state departments, universities, school districts and other stakeholders to assist in developing inclusive education at the levels of teacher preparation, credentialing and licensing, evaluation and policy development. Educators, administrators, state policy makers, and university faculty will find extensive resources for planning and implementing inclusive education that include course enhancement modules, research reports, and policy tools.

WestEd National Center for Systemic Improvement (NCSI)

As described on their website, the NCSI is designed to assist states in the development of "Results Driven Accountability" to ensure access to education services for all students with disabilities and that programs focus on meaningful and measurable outcomes (WestEd NCSI, n.d.). NCSI technical assistance services are primarily aimed at the state level with a tiered approach that includes universal, targeted, and intensive technical assistance with differentiated levels of support. Resources available on their website include an extensive library of topics primarily relevant for state and district leaders in addition some that are more relevant to practitioners and families such as Interprofessional Practice (IPP), evidence-based practice and tele-practice.

Universal Design for Learning and Students with CCN

Universal Design for Learning (UDL) is defined as "the design of instructional materials and activities that allow the learning goals to be achievable by individuals with wide differences in their abilities to see, hear, speak, move, read, write, understand English, attend, organize, engage, and remember" (Orkwis & McLane, 1998, p. 9). Three essential qualities of UDL include: (a) multiple representations of content, (b) multiple options for expression, and (c) multiple options for engagement (Rose, Meyer & Hitchcock, 2005). The application of UDL principles and practices has become increasingly relevant to support students with CNN to effectively use AAC in general education classrooms, at all tiers of support. Robinson and Soto (2013) provided strategies for SLPs and the educator team to apply UDL in AAC services and these are adapted in Table 4–3.

Table 4–3. Application of UDL for Students With CCN Through All MTSS Tiers

- Provide alternatives to print materials with simultaneous use of print, icons, photos, and other visual images to convey key concepts.

- Consult with teachers to determine flexible methods to engage all students through increased use of visual supports throughout the classroom such as core vocabulary charts and posters, visual schedules, and photos of recent class/school events.

- Procure assistive technologies to assure access for students who require alternative methods for reading such as text-to-speech formats.

- Design classrooms to accommodate students with CVI or related visual needs to provide high contrast, enlarged images, and controlled sensory input.

- Conduct regular progress monitoring with students who rely on AAC to determine ongoing adaptations for expression using a range of no, mid-, and high-tech systems.

- Evaluate core curriculum to determine goals, adaptations and differentiated instructional methods for students using AAC systems to comprehend, express, and interact with content.

- Promote a classroom culture to accept diverse learning styles and modalities of communication such as enabling each student to respond in group activities using his/her AAC system.

- Anticipate barriers for inclusion in the general education curriculum and problem-solve with teachers to provide multiple modes of expression and communication that include a full range of no, mid- and high-tech AAC. See the National Center for UDL Educator Checklist for additional resources (CAST, 2018).

Source: Adapted from Robinson, N., & Soto, G. (2013). *AAC in Schools: Best Practices for Intervention.* Verona, WI: Attainment Company, Inc.

Culturally Responsive AAC Practices

As discussed earlier in the chapter, the cultural and linguistic diversity (CLD) of the student population in U.S. schools requires inclusion of individual students' backgrounds and home languages in the curriculum. Approaches to support students with diverse cultures and languages in schools are referred to as culturally responsive teaching, culturally responsive pedagogy, culturally relevant teaching, and culturally responsive practices. In their review of 45 classroom-based studies that included any of the above terms, Morrison, Robbins, and Rose (2008) synthesized recommended multiple culturally relevant practices that included: modeling, scaffolding, and clarification of challenging curriculum; using student strengths as starting points and building on their funds of knowledge; investing and taking personal responsibility for students' success; creating and nurturing cooperative environments; having high behavioral expectations; reshaping the prescribed curriculum; encouraging relationships among schools and communities; critical literacy; engaging students in social justice work; making explicit the power dynamics of mainstream society; and sharing power in the classroom. Morrison, Robbins, and Rose (2008) acknowledged implementation of culturally relevant pedagogy is challenging to traditional teaching and requires a "constructivist" approach to respond to the cultures and languages of the learners.

When applied to students from CLD backgrounds who rely on AAC, researchers emphasize the need for culturally responsive methods to engage students and families for effective access to language development and learning

(Kulkarni & Parmar, 2017; Soto, 2018; Wagner, 2018). As Soto stated:

> "Culturally responsive practice [in AAC] requires a different type of clinician. It is impossible for clinicians to know all the languages/cultures of the clients they serve. But it is possible for clinicians to collaborate with families and other professionals to build a clinical practice where different language practices are included and legitimized; where there are materials not only in multiple modalities, but also in different languages; where clients are allowed to use whatever communication resources they have and not wait until they have the "legitimate" ones to develop their own voice." (Soto, 2018, p.137)

From their review of 11 studies related to AAC use in culturally and linguistically diverse populations internationally, Kulkarni and Parmar (2017) identified the need for continued research to understand the impact of cultural and language diversity on effective and culturally responsive practices in AAC. Implications for promising practices and recommendations were identified and are summarized from Kulkarni and Parmar (2017) as follows:

- Provide communication partner instructions within a storybook context to increase turn-taking and multisymbol messaging (Binger, Kent-Walsh, Berens, Del Campo, & Rivera, 2008; Rosa-Lugo & Kent-Walsh 2008; Soto, 2012).
- Intentionally consider socioeconomic factors, increase knowledge

about the intricacies of the home communication environment, provide ongoing support to both the child and caregivers, conduct home-based interventions and individualized AAC materials and build on existing communication (Bunning, Gona, Newton, & Hartley, 2014; McCord & Soto, 2004).

- Recognize family members as the most significant communication partners for students and acknowledge the importance of cultural sensitivity (Parette & Huer, 2002a; Parette, Huer, & Wyatt, 2002b; Stuart & Parette, 2002).
- Collaborate with families in making assistive technology decisions regarding overlays, language options, and training for AAC applications and devices to support families in implementation and access to AAC devices in different contexts outside of school and with a variety of communication partners (Hue, Parette, & Saenz, 2001; Joginder Singh, Hussein, Mustaffa, & Hassan, 2017).
- Work as team to consider and include child's home language in communication and AAC intervention (Pickl, 2011).
- Introduce communication technology to underserved populations to demonstrate increased desire and ability to communicate, improved socialization and safe online communication (Rasid & Nonis, 2015).

Implementation of UDL and CPR are powerful tools that SLPs and educators can employ to design access and inclu-

sion for students using AAC, throughout all MTSS tiers and degrees of support needed for each student.

■ Classroom-Based Solutions for Inclusion

Thus far, in this chapter, we have discussed inclusive education practices that can support students with CCN at the systems level. In this final section, practical solutions for classroom and clinical practice are highlighted that are evidence-based and relevant for increasing meaningful participation and access to communication and learning for students using AAC. Established strategies to promote professional teamwork, curriculum access and communication interaction will be discussed and demonstrated in sample intervention scenarios at each tier of the MTSS framework.

Collaboration and Teamwork

Some years ago, Soto, Müller, Hunt, and Goetz (2001a, 2001b) identified the need for collaborative teamwork and shared professional skills for all members of the educational team to effectively support students with CNN in inclusive classrooms. Now, nearly two decades later, models of service delivery to support inclusion of students with CCN are still evolving. In a qualitative study, McLaren, Bausch, and Ault (2007) interviewed 96 general and special education teachers including, resource teachers and itinerant specialists in ten different states. Teachers responded to questions regarding the strategies they used to collaborate and provide assistive technology AAC services to students with disabilities. Forty-seven percent of teachers reported serving students with mild disabilities in inclusive settings, while only 24 percent of teachers of students with significant disabilities served these students in inclusive settings. Most teachers reported their teams relied on the expert model, in which one professional with expertise "directs" another professional rather than engaging in a process of shared goal setting and joint decision making. Further, most special education teachers and specialists reported being the only person who bore responsibility for the students with disabilities and integrating AT into their instruction. Special education teachers reported they did not feel adequately prepared to collaborate with their general education professional peers. Opportunities for joint professional preparation and professional development can help break rigid professional barriers and provide a shared knowledge and language that will be needed to collaborate on issues they have learned together as described below.

Interprofessional Practice

As introduced earlier in the chapter, Interprofessional Education (IPE) and Interprofessional Practice (IPP) are now included in the professional preparation for future SLPs. However, among practicing educators, IPP in a comprehensive culture of working together throughout a school may not be prevalent. Collaborative teamwork has long been advocated as a means to create cohesive programs for students with disabilities, particularly students with CCN to effectively use AAC. IPP offers the potential to prioritize teamwork in school systems, particularly due to the emphasis on MTSS by school

leadership. The importance of working across disciplines, bringing the expertise of special educators, general education teachers, SLPs, school psychologist, physical therapists, occupational therapists, school nurses, counselors, English language specialists, reading specialists, principals, staff, and all relevant members together around the supporting students is now prominent and represents shift in school culture.

Marks (2018) identified strategies for SLPs to apply IPE and IPP competencies to build collaboration in school settings that include: (a) establishing agreement that teamwork is important for the best interests of the student; (b) recognizing contributions of each profession; (c) sharing knowledge in understandable terms, and (d) encouraging ideas from other team members. For the SLP and educator who embark on planning support for students with CCN to participate in general education, the opportunity to launch IPP at the school level is timely. Kerins (2018), an 18-year veteran SLP in the schools, found applying the IPEC Competencies provided an effective framework to improve collaboration in a special education setting. She reported, "key elements of valuing other professionals, communicating clearly, and establishing and appreciating one another's strengths improved efficiency and aided student success" (Kerins, p. 33). For more guidelines and resources on implementing IPP to build the school team and support students with CCN, see Bruce and Bashinski (2017).

Peer Mentoring: Moving From the AAC Expert to the Coaching Model

In many schools and districts, AAC specialists (often an SLP) are in short supply and have responsibility for students who rely on AAC systems through a given district. In other settings, the SLP with AAC specialization develops a mentorship and consultant role, providing professional development for other SLPs and educators to support students to use AAC in classroom settings. Increasingly, AAC specialists are finding that moving toward a professional development model is more effective and far-reaching to support the multitude of students on their caseloads. As other SLPs, teachers, and family members gain skills to support students with CCN and to implement AAC services, the AAC specialist becomes a mentor and less of a direct service provider. Croft, Coggshall, Dolan, Powers, and Killion (2010) reported on the development of Job Embedded Professional Development (JEPD) model that provides applications for SLPs to provide ongoing training and job-embedded coaching to move from an AAC expert to a collaborative model to support implementation and build sustainability in AAC services by teachers and related services professionals on school teams.

Communication Interaction

A key aspect of inclusion is the ability of students who rely on AAC to communicate effectively with all members of their communities, including peers, adults, and family members. As reported earlier, observational and interview research showed students using AAC systems generally communicated less with their peers, and more often with adults when compared to other students. This finding creates concern, as the social circles were more restricted for students with CCN. Communication partner interven-

tion with peers has demonstrated positive approaches to support extended and more extended communication between students with CCN and their peers.

Communication Partner and Peer-Mediated Instruction

Several approaches to peer-mediated interventions to increase social interaction and communication between students using AAC and peers without disabilities have shown positive results (Biggs et al., 2017; Therrien & Light, 2018; Trottier, Kamp, & Mirenda, 2011). In each setting, researchers reported increased communicative turns, sustained interactions between peers, and increased use of AAC systems by students with CCN. Biggs, Carter, and Gustafson (2017) coached peers and found they were able to use the following strategies with fidelity: (a) providing communication opportunities, (b) using expectant delay, (c) prompting communication and (d) responding appropriately. The efficacy of these approaches is promising to increase sustained communication between peers both in and beyond the classroom setting.

Language and Literacy Development for Curriculum Access

Research-based approaches to adapting curriculum for students with different learning needs include differentiated instruction and contextualized intervention. For students who rely on AAC, language and literacy development are particularly challenging, as discussed earlier in the chapter. Evidence shows through explicit instruction and systematic language intervention, students who use AAC can improve their expressive vocabulary and learn to generate grammatically correct utterances (e.g., Binger, Kent-Walsh, King, Webb, & Buenviaje, 2016; Binger, Maguire-Marshall, & Kent-Walsh, 2011; Kent-Walsh, Murza, Malani, & Binger, 2015). Two of these language intervention methods, AAC include Augmented Language Input and Conversation Based Intervention, provide tools for including students who rely on AAC in the general education classroom and are further described in following sections.

Contextualized Intervention

Ukrainetz (2007) described contextualized intervention with specific application to language and literacy development as an approach that combines elements of naturalistic intervention in contexts such as the classroom with purposeful, explicit, and systematic instruction. Key elements of contextualized intervention include the following:

- Language and literacy interventions in school settings that are relevant to the classroom curriculum
- Intervention goals based on state standards and developed in collaboration with the classroom teacher
- The focus of intervention is on the underlying language skills that enable the student to learn and apply knowledge
- Explicit skill instruction is implemented in context of the curriculum with a variety of content and methods
- Meaning and purpose for the student are keys to maintaining student engagement in the curriculum goals

The above elements provide guidelines for the SLP to work within the curriculum for students to learn using their AAC systems. Through "backward mapping," the SLP and educator can collaboratively determine the curriculum goal and analysis of the skills needed for the student to access the content. Through design of contextualized intervention, goals and activities are embedded in meaningful activities for the student, such as creating an e-mail message for a family member or friend using targeted vocabulary in a sentence, rather than a general sentence that is not embedded in context.

Differentiated Instruction

Adaptations of curriculum to meet the individualized learning needs for students are referred to as differentiated instruction (Hall, Vue, Strangman, & Meyer, 2003). SLPs and special educators are very familiar with adapting curriculum so that students who rely on AAC systems can engage with the same curriculum content as peers without disabilities. The process of differentiated instruction involves task analysis to identify steps in reaching the defined goal of the curriculum, such as identifying the main characters in a story that is read aloud. The applications of prompt hierarchies and scaffolding for students to respond to teacher's question are often needed to aid in comprehension and identification of the key elements in a narrative. Hall et al. (2003) identified guidelines to assist educators design differentiated instruction to engage students in learning through providing the appropriate level of scaffolding as follows:

- Clarify key concepts and generalizations.

- Use assessment as a teaching tool to extend instruction, rather than to only measure skills.
- Emphasize critical and creative thinking to expand on student responses and apply to personal experience.
- Engage all learners with differentiated prompting.
- Provide a balance between teacher-assigned and student-selected task, offering frequent choices.

Augmented Language Input Strategies for Students Using AAC

A number of techniques to support students with CCN to associate symbols with language in their AAC systems fall under the description of "augmented language input." Depending on the language development target for a given student, SLPs and educators can employ a variety of methods to model and scaffold the student's use of AAC to understand and express language. The approaches and terminology vary somewhat and are employed by modeling specific location of symbols in the students' AAC system in a naturalistic manner. Terms used include Aided Language Stimulation (Beukelman & Mirenda, 2013; Goosens', 1989; Romski & Sevcik, 1996), System for Augmenting Language (Romski, Sevcik, Cheslock, & Barton, 2006), Natural Aided Language (Cafiero, 2001), Aided Language Modeling (Drager et. al., 2006), and Aided AAC Modeling (Binger & Light, 2007). Implementations of these methods are largely similar with minor differences depending on the population and student's language target. Each approach has been shown to be effective to increase specific use of language targets and serve as effective tools for SLPs to extend modeling and the student's language use in a naturalistic manner (Sennott, Light, & McNaughton, 2016).

Conversation-Based Language Interventions

Conversation-Based Interventions (CBIs) implement verbal scaffolding procedures (e.g., clarifications, reformulations, explicit corrections), during student-centered conversations where the adult presents the student with implicit or explicit corrective feedback immediately following a student's incomplete, immature or ungrammatical utterance (Eisenberg, 2013, 2014). In CBIs, the adult uses verbal scaffolding, within the context of personally motivating conversations for the student, to make linguistic targets more salient at the specific moment at which the student has something to say, and with minimal disruption to the flow of the conversation. Such scaffolding techniques afford the student opportunities to hear the target form being used in a meaningful way, and to contrast their own utterance with a more complex or grammatically correct one.

CBIs have shown to be effective with students with autism (Scherer & Olswang, 1989), specific language impairment (Camarata & Nelson, 2006; Nelson, Camarata, Welsh, Butkovsky, & Camarata, 1996; Plante et al., 2014), language learning disabilities (Stiegler & Hoffman, 2001), language delay (Ruston & Schwanenflugel, 2010), and motor speech disorders who use aided AAC (Soto & Clarke, 2017). Soto and Clarke (2017) used a conversation-based intervention (CBI) to teach eight students aged 8 to 13 with motor speech disorders who used speech-generating devices (SGDs) to form more complex and grammatically correct utterances. Improvements seen in intervention were generalized to conversations with familiar adults. In the Soto and Clarke study, clinicians used recasting of students' AAC-mediated utterances and direct prompting for the repair of incomplete or ungrammatical utterances in conversations around personal events chosen by the child.

■ Classroom-Based Profiles for Inclusion

In this final section of the chapter, three profiles of students who rely on AAC demonstrate the application of solutions for inclusion discussed thus far. These solutions include evidence-based practices both at the systems level and in the classroom for each student and their education team. Each case profile represents an example of differing levels of intervention needed for each student, at each of three tiers of intervention, in an MTSS framework. Highlights of each student's profile and inclusion practices are summarized in Table 4–4, followed by more detailed explanation.

Tier 1: Universal Support

Alejandro, an 8-year-old boy who lives with his extended family, including his

Table 4–4. Classroom-based AAC Inclusion Solutions in MTSS Framework

Tier	Focus Student	AAC Strategies
Tier 1: Universal Support	Alejandro, age 8 years	SLP, EL, Teachers, Team consult to design UDL access with visual display of words and icons for all students.
	First language is Spanish, both English and Spanish spoken at home	
	Limited verbal speech, shows age-level comprehension of Spanish	Application of CRP with dual language representation
	Recognizes extensive sounds and sight word vocabulary in Spanish	Small group shared story time in with visual icons of key story elements.
	Recently received an AAC device with touch screen tablet with dynamic symbols	Peer-Mediated Conversations to retell stories from small group story time
	Quickly learned to access vocabulary symbols with both English and Spanish printed label	IPP to collaborate in adapting curriculum with EL & Classroom Teacher input using Differentiated Instruction
	Responds to visual communication symbols to answer questions in English	SLP coaches EL Teacher to implement Aided AAC Modeling to expand vocabulary and CBI to target complex sentence development.
	Highly social and greets peers and adults in classroom	
	Takes turns in conversations when prompted by peer or adult	Create "daily news" to take home in English and Spanish on AAC device.

Table 4–4. *continued*

Tier	Focus Student	AAC Strategies
Tier 2: Supplemental Support	Jasmine, age 10 years Family speaks Cantonese and English at home Vocalizes and gestures to demonstrate yes/no Understands basic Cantonese phrases, songs, stories Responds to English vocabulary Accesses AAC system on tablet with communication APP with direct selection Generates one and two-word responses to questions with minimal help on her device Shows limited initiation to others unless prompted Shows difficulty in early literacy and reading skills to blend sounds	SLP, Teachers, Team members apply IPP to consult weekly re: supplemental support for Jasmine and all focus students. Design language-rich classroom with application of UDL to create multiple modes of representation in visual displays, tablet access, and communication books. Peer-Mediated instruction to retell language/literacy stories in context of grade level curriculum, using her AAC system SLP demonstrates and coaches teaching staff to implement Aided AAC Language Modeling and CBI in small group language activity aligned with curriculum. SLP assists teaching staff to construct personal narratives with Jasmine about family events with text-to-speech application and photos with Chinese characters and English vocabulary (applying CRP and CBI).
Tier 3: Intensive Interventions	Sara, age 12 years Family speaks Punjabi and English. Sari responds to Punjabi and English at basic level to include familiar nouns, function words, actions, with core of approximately 50 words. Diagnosed with cerebral palsy and Cortical Visual Impairment Responds to choices with facial expression for yes/no Uses 2-step scanning with SDG, with verbal coaching Indicates choices to navigate to multiple screens on SDG in response to partner assisted scanning	SLP, Teachers, Team members apply IPP to consult weekly re: intensive interventions for Sara and all focus students. Peer mentoring with team by Vision Specialist to design low-sensory and high contrast learning areas to accommodate CVI learning needs Design low-sensory and high contrast areas in classroom using UDL principles. SLP conducts peer mentoring with teachers to apply Aided AAC Modeling, CBI, and Differentiated Instruction to adapt core curriculum. SLP applies CRP and coaches personal assistant to conduct individual sessions to build family narrative in AAC device using photos provided by parents, in both English and Punjabi vocabulary.

mother, older sister, brother, and grandparents. He was diagnosed in his early life with a form of cerebral palsy that primarily affects his speech with some muscle weakness on his right side. He is very active and plays soccer with his siblings and friends to the best of his ability. His family recently emigrated from Guatemala, where his father continues to work and plans to join his family in the next year. His grandparents speak primarily Spanish and his siblings are rapidly learning English. His mother works many hours outside of the home, leaving most of the family care to the grandparents. His family has always been concerned about Alejandro's speech. Although he tries to speak often and shows understanding of everything that is said to him, only his family can understand him with limited success. As a result, his mother and his early educators in Guatemala developed a gesture and picture-based system that included print in Spanish. He has also developed the ability to spell many words and phrases with an alphabet board. He entered public school in the United States as a kindergartner one year ago, at age 7 years. For most of his previous school year, his teacher found it difficult to engage him in classroom activities due to lack of verbal speech.

Based on assessment in both Spanish and English by the SLP, Special Education Teacher, and English Language Teacher, Alejandro showed near age-appropriate language and concept development in Spanish. For this reason, it was determined learning English was his primary need and focus of his education program. Following an AAC assessment, his SLP also introduced an AAC device to Alejandro (tablet with dynamic communication symbols). Since he began using the tablet in the classroom, Alejandro has shown significant gains in English language development through the use of his device, both orally and in sight words. His teacher has observed Alejandro responds to questions in English when she points to corresponding visual symbols on his device.

Alejandro's education team includes his general education teacher, English language (EL) teacher, instructional aide, and his mother with consultation from the SLP. In their initial planning meeting, the team considered Alejandro's rapid acquisition of English vocabulary since obtaining his AAC device. They applied CRP (Kulkarni & Parmar, 2017) and found dual language representation in both Spanish and English further aided his learning and response to questions. This information and recent assessment results helped to inform the team's application of UDL (CAST, 2018) to plan the classroom environment and activities with visual tools for all students, including Alejandro. For example, to implement UDL within shared reading, the SLP consulted with the classroom and EL teacher to provide visual icons projected on an interactive screen for each student to point to characters and events in the story in a large group. The SLP also consulted with classroom and EL teacher to conduct small groups to include Alejandro to facilitate peer-mediated conversations (Biggs et al., 2017), structured around the story between communication partners to review, feelings, reactions and share favorite parts of the story.

In order to support Alejandro to access the first-grade curriculum, the EL teacher, SLP and general education teacher applied Interprofessional Practice (IPP; Bruce & Bashinski, 2017) and collaborated to adapt materials using differentiated instruction (Hall et al., 2003) so that Alejandro and other students with

EL needs would have different levels of prompting and be able to answer questions using visual communication tools. Further, the SLP coached the EL teacher to implement Aided AAC Modeling (Binger & Light, 2007) with Alejandro to expand and locate vocabulary in both Spanish and English and respond in-group activities. As a means to expand his expressive language, the SLP collaborated with the EL teacher to implement a form of CBI (Soto & Clarke, 2017) to build upon Alejandro's brief sentences in English by modeling and recasting his phrases with language targets that included adjectives and verbs in his AAC device. Following individual sessions with Alejandro, the EL teacher coached his instructional aide to assist Alejandro to generalize language targets conversations with a peer. To further incorporate CRP (Kulkarni & Parmar, 2017), Alejandro participated in small group and individual literacy activities with his instructional aid to build sentences using his AAC device and create a "school news" report to share with his family, both in English and Spanish.

Tier 2: Supplemental Support

Jasmine, a 10-year-old girl, lives with her parents and grandparents and two older brothers. She is particularly fond of animals and helps to care for several cats with her grandparents. Although both English and Cantonese are spoken at home, her family often communicates in Cantonese, her grandparents' primary language. Since birth, Jasmine and her family have participated in early intervention and special education programs with her, due to her continued developmental and learning needs. Jasmine's speech remains a primary concern for her parents, as she vocalizes and gestures to demonstrate "yes" and "no" with a limited expressive vocabulary that only her family and those who are familiar with her can understand. Her family reported Jasmine shows her understanding of basic Cantonese phrase, songs, and stories through her responses and many English words. She has used AAC tools since first grade and currently uses a tablet device, which she accesses using with minimal assistance with direct selection of many English vocabulary words. Her special education teacher observed Jasmine recently began to use her AAC device more independently, answering questions with single words and word combinations. She often responds to her peers and teachers but shows limited initiation in her communication with others. Her education and speech therapy services to date have been in a separate classroom with individualized therapy. In addition to her progress in speech and language development through AAC, her teachers found Jasmine showed strengths in emerging literacy development through sound-letter correspondence but experienced difficulty in early reading skills. The school psychologist completed his assessment and recommended support strategies for early literacy and reading activities. Given this information, her family and education team decided in her IEP meeting that a general education classroom placement with supplemental supports would be the most appropriate to meet her educational goals. Supplemental supports in the general education classroom, in small group and individual activities, were designed to meet Jasmine's educational goals by her team, including the SLP, general education teacher, special education teacher, instructional aide, her parents, and school psychologist.

Through weekly consultation, both in person and through online formats, Jasmine's team applied IPP (Bruce & Bashinski, 2017) to share perspectives of her success and additional support needs relative to her goals, based on each professional's input. As a result, the team continually evaluated the level of support needed for Jasmine's participation and success. In addition, the team applied UDL (CAST, 2018) to support Jasmine's inclusion in language and literacy curriculum through designing a language-rich classroom with visual displays of weekly vocabulary in printed and icon formats in large posters for all students to view. Tablet technology was also utilized to highlight specific vocabulary activities in small groups for Jasmine and other students with English learning needs. A further supplement for improved access to vocabulary, communication books were developed with core vocabulary and specific vocabulary introduced in the reading curriculum. These were placed at learning stations throughout the classroom and provided as learning tools for all learners. Through language and literacy rich displays for the classroom as a whole and representation of vocabulary and literacy concepts with alternative formats in small groups, Jasmine and other students received supplemental support in multiple formats with repeated opportunities for participation and learning.

Following the small group literacy activities, Jasmine communicated, using her AAC device in peer-mediated instruction (Biggs et al., 2017), with another student and teacher's assistant to construct narratives based on the selected reading for the class. This activity is also incorporated with contextualized intervention (Ukrainetz, 2007) to embed goals for Jasmine to build vocabulary in the context of the core curriculum expected in her classroom.

In order to supplement language learning with Jasmine, the SLP also provided consultation and peer mentoring (Croft et al., 2010) with her teacher and instructional aide, focusing on language intervention strategies. The SLP first demonstrated Aided AAC Language Modeling (Binger & Light, 2007) to support Jasmine to effectively construct sentences using her AAC device. After several sessions, the SLP coached the teacher and instructional aide to implement CBI (Soto & Clarke, 2017) to assist Jasmine to respond in conversations and expand on her sentences in brief narratives. Further, through narrative construction about school news and family events, the SLP applied culturally responsive practice (Kulkarni & Parmar, 2017) to assist teaching staff to support Jasmine in building short 3-sequence stories to share with her family and peers, using both English vocabulary and Chinese characters available in her AAC device.

Tier 3: Intensive Intervention

In an MTSS model, at the Tier 3 level, students with more significant needs receive more intensive interventions within the general education classroom environment as the primary educational placement. Although there may be variations in the location for individualized services, inclusive education remains the goal. Sara is a 12-year-old girl with complex communication needs in addition to physical and sensory disabilities. Her profile illustrates how the SLP and education team provide intensive interventions in the general education classroom. Sara lives with her family that includes her parents, live-in personal assistant, two younger brothers, and her grandmother, where both English and Punjabi are spoken. Although Sara was born in the United States, her grandmother and mother emigrated from the Punjab State of India nearly 20 years earlier. Sara's family reports she responds to both Punjabi and English at a basic level, showing her understanding of familiar nouns, function words, and actions up to a total of 50 words in both languages. She is particularly fond of music of all kinds, particularly listening to traditional Punjab music with her grandmother. Sara was diagnosed with cerebral palsy that limits her motor abilities, overall, and her speech in particular. In addition, cortical visual impairment (CVI) significantly affects her vision. She often vocalizes her feelings and reactions to others, with no identifiable words. Her primary modes of communication include gestures and facial expression to indicate "yes" and "no" in response to partner-assisted scanning methods. With her AAC device, Sara activates a two-step scanning switch to select choices when coached directly by her communication partner.

Sara's education team includes the SLP, general education teacher, special education teacher, vision specialist, physical therapist, personal assistant, and her parents. Her school-based team meets weekly to review progress, to coordinate services and to complement each member's intervention programs, using IPP (Bruce & Bashinski, 2017) to share perspectives with Sara's overall IEP goals in mind. Sara's team identified an area for their own professional development related to accommodations for students with cortical visual impairment. Through mentoring by the vision specialist (Croft

et al., 2010), the team designed low-sensory areas in the classroom with tools for displaying enlarged and high contrast materials for individualized support for Sara and other students with CVI, applying UDL principles (CAST, 2018). In addition, Sara's parents meet periodically with the team for updates and input about Sara's responsiveness at home. In order to provide curriculum access for Sara and other students with complex communication needs, the SLP created a professional peer-mentoring group (Croft et al., 2010) for teachers at the school who meet monthly. In the peer mentoring meetings, the SLP coaches school team members in applying Aided AAC Language Modeling (Binger & Light, 2007), CBI (Soto & Clarke, 2017) and differentiated instruction (Hall et al., 2003) strategies in the classroom, focused on adapting core curriculum to input into students' AAC devices throughout the school. Additionally, the SLP applies peer mentoring and culturally responsive practice (Kulkarni & Parmar, 2017) through weekly consultation and coaching with Sara's personal assistant in the classroom to build family narratives in her AAC device that she can retell at home in Punjabi and with peers in the classroom in English.

Discussion of Student Profiles

In each of the above student profiles, the application of solutions for inclusion for students who rely on AAC to communicate and to learn with communication partners and peers without disabilities require systems-level policy, infrastructure and leadership by school administrators. As described earlier, MTSS is a framework that brings together all levels of the education system and stakeholders in schools and districts to align resources to build comprehensive and cohesive school-wide services to meet the needs of all students in a tiered instructional continuum. MTSS holds the promise and potential for education teams to create inclusive educational environments for all students, particularly those who rely on AAC, through implementing evidence-based practices that have demonstrated positive educational outcomes described in this chapter. Although a majority of states report implementation of MTSS initiatives, diverse goals and varying degrees of success are reported (Bailey, 2018). Often, students with significant disabilities and the professionals who serve them are not included in MTSS initiatives (Thurlow et al., 2020). Yet, MTSS increasingly shows positive outcomes for those districts who implement comprehensive planning and resource allocation (Bailey, 2018). Thurlow et al. advocate for MTSS to advance inclusion of all students by adhering to the premise and practice that students receiving special education services are general education students first, and that special education services are supplementary services. The focus on educating all students together with a continuum of supports in the general education setting is a significant shift in practice for many SLPs and educators, yet necessary to achieve inclusion for students with complex communication needs.

■ Summary

We have examined the development of inclusive education for students with disabilities and all learners, with specific focus on students with CCN who benefit from and rely on AAC systems. As Vandercook et al. (2019) conclude, for inclusion to succeed in the classroom for all students with disabilities, change must occur at the systems level. Although progress has been made, the inclusive education of students who rely on AAC requires concerted initiatives at all levels of the system and include leadership, preparation of future professionals, and support for practicing professionals. With the many resources now available, the challenge ahead is to work together in comprehensive ways to apply the accumulated knowledge and research that is within our reach.

The implementation of solutions for inclusion is based on both art and science. The science of inclusion relies on the application of evidence-based educational practices that can be applied at different levels, or tiers, of intervention to meet the individual needs of each student. Most students can benefit from universal support, some require supplemental support, and a few need intensive support to learn and participate with their peers without disabilities. Continued evaluation by the education team determines the level of support needed to create equity for all students. For students who rely on AAC, the SLP with AAC specialization is a critical member of the team with language intervention expertise. The art of inclusion is achieved by the application of evidence-based practice (science) so that each student has equitable access to the curriculum. In order to achieve inclusion for students with CNN who rely on AAC, the SLP and the whole school team need to continually evaluate and adjust intervention, combining art and science, in the context of the general education classroom.

"There are many places with incredible inclusion programs, yet we have a lot of work to do to get to a level where MTSS is truly a well-oiled system with a universally designed foundation that serves most kids well. Then, our 'ninja' people come in to do their super-powers. That is the vision."

Kristin Wright, Director, Special Education Division, California Department of Education (Robinson, 2020)

■ References

American Speech-Language-Hearing Association. (n.d). *Interprofessional Education/Interprofessional Practice (IPE/IPP)*. Retrieved from https://www.asha.org/Practice/Interprofessional-Education-Practice/

American Speech-Language-Hearing Association. (2013). *Issues in ethics: Cultural and linguistic competence*. Retrieved from www.asha.org/Practice/ethics/Cultural-and-Linguistic-Competence/.

American Speech-Language-Hearing Association. (2014). *Cultural competence*. Retrieved from http://www.asha.org/Practice-Portal/Professional-Issues/Cultural-Competence/

American Speech-Language-Hearing Association. (2020). *2020 Standards and implementation procedures for the Certificate of Clinical Competence in speech-language pathology*. Retrieved from https://www.asha.org/Certification/2020-SLP-Certification-Standards/

Andzik, N .R., Schaefer, J. M., Nichols R. T, & Chung, Y-C. (2018). National survey describing and quantifying students with communication needs. *Developmental Neurorehabilitation, 21*(1) 40–47. https://doi.org/10.1080/17518423.2017.1339133

Bailey, T. R. (2018). Is MTSS/RTI here to stay? All signs point to yes! *American Institutes for Research*. Retrieved from https://www.rti4success.org/blog/mtssrti-here-stay-all-signs-point-yes

Ballin, L., & Balandin, S. (2008). An exploration of loneliness: Communication and the social networks of older people with cerebral palsy. *Journal of Intellectual & Developmental Disability, 32*(1), 315–326. https://doi.org/10.1080/13668250701689256

Beukelman, D., & Mirenda, P. (2013). *Augmentative and alternative communication: supporting children and adults with complex communication needs* (4th ed.). Brookes.

Biggs, E. E., Carter, E. W., & Gustafson, J. (2017). Efficacy of peer support arrangements to increase peer interaction and AAC use. *American Journal on Intellectual and Developmental Disabilities, 122(*1), 25–48, 93–95. https://doi.org/10.1352/1944-7558-122.1.25

Binger, C., Kent-Walsh, J., Berens, J., Del Campo, S., & Rivera, D. (2008). Teaching Latino parents to support the multi-symbol message productions of their children who require AAC. *Augmentative and Alternative Communication, 24*, 323–338. https://doi.org/10.1080/07434610802130978

Binger, C., Kent-Walsh, J., King, M., Webb, E., & Buenviaje, E. (2016). Early sentence productions of 5-year-old children who use augmentative and alternative communication. *Communication Disorders Quarterly, 38(*3), https://doi.org/10.1177/1525740116655804

Binger, C., & Light, J. (2007). The effect of aided AAC modeling on the expression of multisymbol messages by preschoolers who rely on AAC. *Augmentative and Alternative Communication, 23*, 30–43. https://doi.org/10.1080/07434610600807470

Binger, C. & Light, J. (2008). The morphology and syntax of individuals who use AAC: Research review and implications for effective practice. *Augmentative and Alternative Communication, 24*, 123–138. https://doi.org/10.1080/07434610701830587.

Binger, C., Maguire-Marshall, M. & Kent-Walsh, J. (2011). Using aided AAC models, recasts, and contrastive targets to teach grammatical morphemes to children who use AAC. *Journal of Speech, Language, and Hearing Research, 54*, 160–176. https://doi.org/10.1044/1092-4388

Bourke-Taylor, H., Cotter, C., Johnson, L., & Lalor, A. (2018). Belonging, school support and communication: Essential aspects of school success for students with cerebral palsy in mainstream schools. *Teaching and Teacher Education, 70*, 153–164. https://doi.org/10.1016/j.tate.2017.11.016

Bruce, S. M., & Bashinski, S. M. (2017). The trifocus framework and interprofessional collaborative practice in severe disabilities. *American Journal of Speech-Language Pathology, 26*(2), 162–180. https://doi.org/10.1044/2016_AJSLP-15-0063

Bunning, K., Gona, J. K., Newton, C. R., & Hartley, S. (2014). Caregiver perceptions of children who have complex communication needs following a home-based intervention using augmentative and alternative communication in rural Kenya: An intervention note. *Augmentative and Alternative Communication, 30*, 344–356. https://doi.org/10.3109/07434618.2014.970294

Caifero, J. (2001). The effect of an augmentative communication intervention on the communication, behavior and academic program of an adolescent with autism. *Focus on Autism and Other Developmental Disabilities, 16*, 179–193.

California Department of Education. (2019a). *Basic facts—California Language Census: Fall 2018. Facts about English Language Learners in California, CalEd Facts.* Retrieved from http://www.cde.ca.gov/ds/sd/cb/cefelfacts.asp

California Department of Education. (2019b). *Definition of MTSS.* Retrieved from https://www.cde.ca.gov/ci/cr/ri/mtsscomprti2.asp

Camarata, S., & Nelson, K. E. (2006). Conversational recast intervention with preschool and older children. In R. McCaule & M. Fey (Eds.), *Treatment of language disorders in children* (pp. 237–264). Brookes.

CAST. (2018). *Universal design for learning guidelines version 2.2.* Retrieved from http://udlguidelines.cast.org

Chung, Y., Carter, E. W., & Sisco, L. G. (2012). Social interactions of students with disabilities who use augmentative and alternative communication in inclusive classrooms. *American Journal on Intellectual and Developmental Disabilities, 117*(5), 349–367. Retrieved from https://search-proquest-com.jpllnet.sfsu.edu/docview/1074762720?accountid=13802

Cioè-Peña, M. (2017). Who is excluded from inclusion?: Points of union and division in bilingual and special education. *Theory, Research, and Action in Urban Education: Special Issue on #BlackLivesMatter, 5*(1). Retrieved from https://blmtraue.commons.gc.cuny.edu/2017/02/24/who-is-excluded-from-inclusion-points-of-union-and-division-in-bilingual-and-special-education/

Clarke, M., McConachie, H., Price, K., & Wood, P. (2001a). Speech and language therapy provision for children using augmentative and alternative communication systems. *European Journal of Special Needs Education, 16*(1), 41–54. https://doi.org/10.1080/08856250150501798.

Clarke, M., McConachie H., Price, K., & Wood, P. (2001b). Views of young people using augmentative and alternative communication systems. *International Journal of Language and Communication Disorders, 36*(1), 107–115. https://doi.org/10.1080/13682820119446

Collaboration for Effective Educator Development, Accountability, and Reform (CEEDAR). (2020). *CEEDAR Center.* University of Florida. Retrieved from https://ceedar.education.ufl.edu/

Costigan, F. A. & Light, J. (2010). A review of preservice training in augmentative and alternative communication for speech-language pathologists, special education teachers, and occupational therapists. *Assistive Technology, 22*(4), 200–212. https://doi.org/10.1080/10400435.2010.492774.

Council on Academic Accreditation in Audiology and Speech-Language Pathology. (2017). *Standards for accreditation*. Retrieved from https://caa.asha.org/wp-content/uploads/Accreditation-Standards-for-Graduate-Programs.pdf

Croft, A., Coggshall, J. G., Dolan, M., Powers, E., & Killion, J. (2010). Job-embedded professional development: What it is, who's responsible, and how to get it done well. *Issue Brief. Washington, DC: National Comprehensive Center for Teacher Quality*. Retrieved from https://files.eric.ed.gov/fulltext/ED520830.pdf

Drager, K. D. R., Postal, V. J., Carrolus, L., Castellano, M., Gagliano, C., & Glynn, J. (2006). The effect of aided language modeling on symbol comprehension and production in two preschoolers with autism. *American Journal of Speech-Language Pathology, 15*, 112–125. https://doi.org/10.1044/1058-0360(2006/012)

Eisenberg, S. L. (2013). Grammar intervention: Content and procedures for facilitating children's language development. *Topics in Language Disorders, 33*, 165–178.

Eisenberg, S. (2014). What works in therapy: further thoughts on improving clinical practice for children with language disorders. *Language, Speech and Hearing Services in the Schools, 45*(2), 117–126. https://doi.org/10.1044/2014_LSHSS-14-0021

Erickson, K. A., & Geist, L. A. (2016). The profiles of students with significant cognitive disabilities and complex communication needs. *Augmentative and Alternative Communication, 32*(3), 187–197. https://doi.org/10.1080/07434618.2016.1213312

Forbes, H. J. (2018). Augmentative and alternative communication intervention in public schools: Achieving meaningful outcomes through collaboration. *Perspectives of the ASHA Special Interest Groups, SIG 12, 3*(12), 55–69. https://doi.org/10.1044/persp3.SIG12.55

Freeman, R., Miller, D., & Newcomer, L. (2015). Integration of academic and behavioral MTSS at the district level using implementation science. *Learning Disabilities—A Contemporary Journal, 13*(1), 59–72. Retrieved from https://eric.ed.gov/?id=EJ1080597

Goosens, C. (1989). Aided communication intervention before assessment: A case study. *Augmentative and Alternative Communication, 5*, 14–26. https://doi.org/10.1080/07434618912331274926.

Grether, S. M. (2009). Response to intervention: Applications for AAC in preschool settings. *Perspectives on Augmentative and Alternative Communication, 18*(1), 4–10. https://doi.org/10.1044/aac18.1.4

Hall, T., Vue, G., Strangman, N., & Meyer, A. (2003). *Differentiated instruction and implications for UDL implementation*. Wakefield, MA: National Center on Accessing the General Curriculum. Retrieved from http://aem.cast.org/about/publications/2003/ncac-differentiated-instruction-udl.html

Horner, R., Sugai, G. & Anderson, C.M. (2010). Examining the evidence base for schoolwide positive behavior support. *Focus on Exceptional Children, 42*, 1-14. https://doi.org/10.17161/fec.v42i8.6906.

Hossain, M. (2012). An overview of inclusive education in the United States. In J.E Aitken, J. Pedego Fairley, & J. K. Carlson (Eds.), *Communication technology for students in special education and gifted programs* (pp. 1–25). IGI Global. Retrieved from https://ici.umn.edu/products/impact/261/261.pdf

Huer, M. B., Parette, H. P., Jr., & Saenz, T. I. (2001). Conversations with Mexican Americans regarding children with disabilities and augmentative and alternative communication. *Communication Disorders Quarterly, 22*, 197–206. https://doi.org/10.1177/152574010102200405

IDEAs that work. (n.d.). *SWIFT Education Center*. Retrieved from https://osepideasthatwork.org/swift-education-center

Institute of Education Science, National Center on Education Statistics. (2019a). *Fast facts: Inclusion of students with disabilities*. Retrieved from https://nces.ed.gov/fastfacts/display.asp?id=59

Institute of Education Science, National Center on Education Statistics. (2019b). *Status and trends in the education of racial and ethnic groups*. Retrieved from https://nces.ed.gov/programs/raceindicators/indicator_rbb.asp

Interprofessional Education Collaborative. (2020). *Core competencies for interprofessional collaborative practice: 2016 update*. Retrieved from https://www.ipecollaborative.org/core-competencies.html

Joginder Singh, S., Hussein, N.H., Mustaffa Kamal, R., & Hassan, F. H. (2017). Reflections of Malaysian parents of children with developmental disabilities on their experiences with AAC. *Augmentative and Alternative Communication, 33*, 110–120. https://doi.org/10.1080/07434618.2017. 1309457

Johnson, R. K., & Prebor, J. (2019). Update on preservice training in augmentative and alternative communication for speech-language pathologists. *American Journal of Speech-Language Pathology, 28*(2), 536–549. Retrieved from https://www.ncbi.nlm.nih.gov/pubmed/31136246

Kent-Walsh, J., Murza, K. A., Malani, M. D., & Binger, C. (2015). Effects of communication partner instruction on the communication of individuals using AAC: A meta-analysis. *Augmentative and Alternative Communication, 31*(4), 271–284. https://doi.org/10.3109/07434618.2015.1052153

Kerins, M. (2018). Promoting interprofessional practice in schools. How can school-based SLPs get more deliberate about working across disciplinary boundaries to bolster student learning? *The ASHA Leader, 23*(12) 32–33. https://doi.org/10.1044/leader.SCM.23122018.32

Kleinert, H., Towles-Reeves, E., Quenemoen, R., Thurlow, M., Fluegge, L., Weseman, L., & Kerbel, A. (2015). Where students with the most significant cognitive disabilities are taught: Implications for general curriculum access. *Exceptional Children, 81*, 312–329.

Kleinert, J., Kearns, J., Liu, K. K., Thurlow, M. L. & Lazarus, S. S. (2019). *Communication competence in the inclusive setting: A review of the literature (TIES Center Report 103)*. University of Minnesota, The TIES Center.

Kulkarni, S. S. & Parmar, J. (2017). Culturally and linguistically diverse student and family perspectives of AAC. *Augmentative and Alternative Communication, 33*(3), 170–180.

Langdon, H. W., Saenz, T. I., Dominquez, G., Clark, S. & McCollum, M. (2017). Collaborating with interpreters and translators. CSHA task force on collaborating with interpreters. Position Paper. *California Speech, Language, and Hearing Association*. Retrieved from https://www.csha.org/collaborating-with-interpreters-and-translators-2017/

Light, J. (1989). Toward a definition of communicative competence for individuals using augmentative and alternative communication systems. *Augmentative and Alternative Communication, 5*, 137–144. https://doi.org/10.1080/07434618912331275126.

Lilienfeld, M. & Alant, E. (2005) The social interaction of an adolescent who uses AAC: The evaluation of a peer-training program. *Augmentative and Alternative Communication, 21*(4), 278–294, https://doi.org/10.1080/07434610500103467.

Litinov, A., Alvarez, B., Long, C., & Walker, T. (2018). 10 challenges facing public education today. *NEA Today*. Retrieved from http://neatoday.org/2018/08/03/10-challenges-facing-public-education-today/

Liu, K., Watkins, E., Pompa, D., McLeod, P., Elliott, J., & Gaylord, V. (Eds). (Winter/Spring 2013). *Impact: Feature Issue on Educating K-12 English Language Learners with Disabilities, 26*(1), 1–2, 33. University of Minnesota, Institute on Community Integration and Research and Training Center on Community Living. Retrieved from https://ici.umn.edu/products/impact/261/

Marks, A. K. (2018) Interprofessionalism on the augmentative and alternative communication team: Mending the divide. *Perspectives of the ASHA Special Interest Groups, SIG 12, 3*(12), 70–79. https://doi.org/10.1044/persp3.SIG12.70

McCord, M. S., & Soto, G. (2004). Perceptions of AAC: An ethnographic investigation of Mexican-American families. *Augmentative and Alternative Communication, 20*,

209–227. https://doi.org/10.1080/07434610 400005648

McLaren, E. M., Bausch, M. E., & Ault, M. J. (2007). Collaboration strategies reported by teachers providing assistive technology services. *Journal of Special Education Technology, 22*(4), 16–29. https://doi.org/10 .1177/016264340702200402

McLeskey, J., & Waldron, N. (2000). *Inclusive education in action: Making differences ordinary.* ASCD.

McNaughton, D., & Nelson Bryen, D. (2007). AAC technologies to enhance participation and access to meaningful societal roles for adolescents and adults with developmental disabilities who require AAC. *Augmentative and Alternative Communication, 23*(3), 217–229. https://doi.org/10.1080/ 07434610701573856

Mehr, D. L. (2017). Supporting the communication needs of students with severe disabilities in inclusive settings: Practices and perspectives. *Culminating Projects in Special Education. 32.* Retrieved from https:// repository.stcloudstate.edu/sped_etds/32

Messinger-Willman, J., & Marino, M. T. (2010). Universal design for learning and assistive technology: Leadership considerations for promoting inclusive education in today's secondary schools. *NASSP Bulletin, 94*(1), 5–16. https://doi.org/10.1177/0192636510 371977

Morrison, C. A., Robbins, H. H., & Rose, D. G. (2008). Operationalizing culturally relevant pedagogy: A synthesis of classroom-based research. *Equity & Excellence in Education, 41,* 433–452. https://doi.org/10.1080/1066 5680802400006

National Council on Disability. (2018, February). *IDEA series: The segregation of students with disabilities.* Retrieved from https://ncd.gov/sites/default/files/NCD_ Segregation-SWD_508.pdf

Nelson, K. E., Camarata, S. M., Welsh, J., Butkovsky, L., & Camarata, M. (1996). Effects of imitative and conversational recasting treatment on the acquisition of grammar in children with specific language impairment and younger language-normal children. *Journal of Speech, Language, and Hearing Research, 39*(4), 850–859. https:// doi.org/10.1044/jshr.3904.850

Nunez, L. (2015). Achieving quality and improved outcomes through interprofessional collaboration. *American Speech-Language and Hearing Association.* https:// www.asha.org/Articles/Achieving-Quality- and-Improved-Outcomes-Through-Inter- professional-Collaboration/

Office of Special Education Programs. (n.d.). *Discretionary Grants Database.* Retrieved from https://publicddb.osepideasthatwork .org

Orkwis, R., & McLane, K. (1998). A curriculum every student can use: Design principles for student access. *ERIC/OSEP Topical Brief.* Council for Exceptional Children. Retrieved from https://eric.ed.gov/?id=ED423654

Østvik, J., Balandin, S., & Ytterhus, B. (2017). A "Visitor in the class": Marginalization of students using AAC in mainstream education classes. *Journal of Developmental and Physical Disabilities, 29*(3), 419–441. https:// doi.org/10.1007/s10882-017-9533-5.

Parette, Jr. H. P., & Huer, M. B. (2002a). Working with Asian American families whose children have augmentative and alternative communication needs. *Journal of Special Education Technology, 17,* 5–13. https://doi .org/10.1177/016264340201700401

Parette, Jr. H. P., Huer, M. B., & Wyatt, T. A. (2002b). Young African American children with disabilities and augmentative and alternative communication issues. *Early Childhood Education Journal, 29,* 201–207. https://doi.org/1082-3301/02/0300-0201/0

Pickl, G. (2011). Communication intervention in children with severe disabilities and multilingual backgrounds: Perceptions of pedagogues and parents. *Augmentative and Alternative Communication, 27,* 229–244. https://doi.org/10.3109/07434618.2011.63 0021

Plante, E., Ogilvie, T., Vance, R., Aguilar, J. M., Dailey, N. S., Meyers, . . . Burton, R. (2014). Variability in the language input to children enhances learning in a treatment context. *American Journal of Speech-Language*

Pathology, 23, 530–545. https://doi.org/10.1044/2014_AJSLP-13-0038

Raghavendra, P., Olsson, C., Sampson, J., Mcinerney, R., & Connell, T. (2012). School participation and social networks of children with complex communication needs, physical disabilities, and typically developing peers. *Augmentative and Alternative Communication, 28*(1), 33–43, https://doi.org/10.3109/07434618.2011.653604

Rasid, N. N. B. M., & Nonis, K. P. (2015). Exploring communication technology behavior of adolescents with cerebral palsy in Singapore. *International Journal of Special Education, 30*, 17–38. Retrieved from http://www.internationaljournalofspecialed.com/articles.php?y.2015&v.30&n.3

Ratcliff, A., Koul, R., & Lloyd, L. (2008). Preparation in augmentative and alternative communication: An update for speech-language pathology training. *American Journal of Speech Language Pathology, 17*(1), 48–59. https://doi.org/10.1044/1058-0360(2008/005)

Robinson, N. (2020). MTSS in California: A conversation with Kristin Wright, Director Special Education Division, California Department of Education. *CSHA Magazine*, Fall/Winter Issue (2019/2020), 52–56. Retrieved from http://digital.apogee-mg.com/publication/?i=642100&p=&pn=52

Robinson, N., & Soto, G. (2013). *AAC in schools: Best practices for intervention*. Attainment Company.

Romski, M. A., & Sevcik, R. A. (1996). *Breaking the speech barrier: Language development through augmented means*. Brookes.

Romski, M. A., Sevcik, R. A., Cheslock, M., & Barton, A. (2006). The system for augmenting language: AAC and emerging language intervention. In R. J. McCauley & M. E. Fey (Eds.), *Treatment of language disorders in children*. Brookes.

Rosa-Lugo, L. I., & Kent-Walsh, J. (2008). Effects of parent instruction on communicative turns of Latino children using augmentative and alternative communication during storybook reading. *Communication Disorders Quarterly, 30*, 49–61. https://doi.org/10.1177/1525740108320353

Rose, D. H., Meyer, A., & Hitchcock, C. (2005). *The universally designed classroom: Accessible curriculum and digital technologies*. Harvard Education Press.

Ruston, H. P., & Schwanenflugel, P. J. (2010). Effects of a conversation intervention on the expressive vocabulary development of pre-kindergarten children. *Language, Speech, and Hearing Services in Schools, 41*, 303–313. https://doi.org/10.1044/0161-1461(2009/08-0100)

Scherer, N. J., & Olswang, L. B. (1989). Using structured discourse as a language intervention technique with autistic children. *Journal of Speech and Hearing Disorders, 54*, 383–394. https://doi.org/10.1044/jshd.5403.383

Schoolwide Integrated Framework for Transformation (SWIFT). (2020). *SWIFT Education Center*. Retrieved from http://www.swiftschools.org

Sennott, C. S., Light, J. C., & McNaughton, D. (2016). AAC modeling intervention research review. *Research and Practice for Persons with Severe Disabilities, 14*(12), 101–115. https://doi.org/10.1177/1540796916638822

Smith, M. (2005). The dual challenges of aided communication and adolescence. *Augmentative and Alternative Communication, 21*, 67–69. https://doi.org/10.1080/10428190400006625

Solomon-Rice, P., Soto, G., & Robinson, N. (2018). Project Building Bridges: Training speech-language pathologists to provide culturally and linguistically responsive augmentative and alternative communication services to school-age children with diverse backgrounds. *Perspectives of the ASHA Special Interest Groups, SIG 12, 3*(12), 136–137. https://doi.org/10.1044/persp3.SIG12.186

Soto, G. (2012). Training partners in AAC in culturally diverse families. *Perspectives on Augmentative and Alternative Communication, 21*(4), 144–150. https://doi.org/10.1044/aac21.4.144

Soto, G. (2018). Introduction to the special issue on cultural and linguistic diversity and AAC. *Perspectives of the ASHA Special Interest Groups, SIG 12, 3*(12), 136–137. https://doi.org/10.1044/2018_PERS-SIG12-2018-0013

Soto, G., & Clarke, M. T. (2017). Effects of a conversation-based intervention on the linguistic skills of children with motor speech disorders who use augmentative and alternative communication. *Journal of Speech-Language and Hearing Research. 60*(7), 1980–1998. https://doi.org/10.1044/2016_JSLHR-L-15-0246

Soto, G., & Hartmann, E. (2006). Analysis of narratives produced by four children who use augmentative and alternative communication. *Journal of Communication Disorders, 39*, 456–480. https://doi.org/10.1016/j.jcomdis.2006.04.005

Soto, G., Huer, M., & Taylor, O. (1997). Multicultural issues. In L. Lloyd, D. Fuller, & H. Arvidson (Eds.), *Augmentative and alternative communication: A handbook of principles and practices* (pp. 406–413). Allyn & Bacon.

Soto, G., Müller, E., Hunt, P., & Goetz, L. (2001a). Critical issues in the inclusion of students who use augmentative and alternative communication: An educational team perspective. *Augmentative and Alternative Communication, 17*(2), 62–72. https://doi.org/10.1080/aac.17.2.62.72

Soto, G., Müller, E., Hunt, P., & Goetz, L. (2001b). Professional skills for serving students who use AAC in general education classrooms: A team perspective. *Language, Speech, and Hearing Services in Schools, 32*(1), 51–56. https://doi.org/10.1044/0161-1461(2001/005)

Soto, G., & Yu, B. (2014). Considerations for the provision of services to bilingual children who use augmentative and alternative communication. *Augmentative and Alternative Communication, 30*, 83–92. https://doi.org/10.3109/07434618.2013.878751

Stiegler, L. N., & Hoffman, P. R. (2001). Discourse-based intervention for word finding in children. *Journal of Communication Disorders, 34*, 277–303. https://doi.org/10.1016/S0021-9924(01)00051-X

Stuart, S., & Parette, Jr. H. P. (2002). Native Americans and augmentative and alternative communication issues. *Multiple Voices for Ethnically Diverse Exceptional Learners, 5*, 38–53. https://doi.org/10.5555/muvo.5.1.p8006861217m5414

Sutton, A., Soto, G., & Blockberger, S. (2002). Grammatical issues in graphic symbol communication. *Augmentative and Alternative Communication, 18*, 192–204. https://doi.org/10.1044/aac17.2.56

Sylvan, L. (2018). Tiers to communication success: How can SLPs join in the MTSS framework many schools are adopting to catch students' special education needs earlier and provide levels of intervention? *The ASHA Leader, 23*(8) 44–53. https://doi.org/10.1044/leader.FTR1.23082018.44

Therrien, M. C. S., & Light, J. C. (2018). Promoting peer interaction for preschool children with complex communication needs and autism spectrum disorder. *American Journal of Speech-Language Pathology, 27*(1), 207–221. https://doi.org/10.1044/2017_AJSLP-17-0104

Thurlow, M. L., Ghere, G., Lazarus, S. S., & Liu, K. K. (2020). *MTSS for all: Including students with the most significant cognitive disabilities*. University of Minnesota, National Center on Educational Outcomes/TIES Center. Retrieved from https://nceo.umn.edu/docs/OnlinePubs/NCEOBrief MTSS.pdf

Trottier, N., Kamp, L., & Mirenda, P. (2011). Effects of peer-mediated instruction to teach use of speech-generating devices to students with autism in social game routines. *Augmentative & Alternative Communication, 27*(1), 26–39. https://doi.org/10.3109/07434618.2010.546810

Ukrainetz, T. (2007). *Contextualized language intervention: Scaffolding PreK-12 literacy achievement*. Thinking Publications

Vandercook, T., Kleinert, H., Jorgenson, C., Sabia, R., & Lazarus, S. (2019). The hope of lessons learned: Supporting the inclusion of students with the most significant disabilities into general classrooms. *Impact, 31*(2), 1–3. Retrieved from https://ici.umn.edu/products/impact/312/#Cover

Wagner, D. K. (2018). Building augmentative communication skills in homes where English and Spanish are spoken: Perspectives of an evaluator/interventionist. *Perspectives of the ASHA Special Interest Groups, SIG 12, 3*(12), 172–185. https://doi.org/10.1044/persp3.SIG12.172

WestEd National Center for Systemic Improvement. (n.d.). *Transforming state systems to improve outcomes for students with disabilities.* Retrieved from https://ncsi.wested.org/

Wickenden, M. (2011a). Talking to teenagers: Using anthropological methods to explore identity and the life worlds of young people who use AAC. *Communication Disorders Quarterly, 32*, 3. https://doi.org/10.1177/1525740109348792

Wickenden, M. (2011b). Whose voice is that?: Issues of identity, voice and representation arising in an ethnographic study of the lives of disabled teenagers who use augmentative and alternative communication. (AAC). *Disability Studies Quarterly, 31*, 4. https://doi.org/10.18061/dsq.v31i4.1724

World Health Organization. (2010). *Framework for action on interprofessional education & collaborative practice.* Health Professions Networks Nursing & Midwifery Human Resources for Health. WHO. Retrieved from https://apps.who.int/iris/bitstream/handle/10665/70185/WHO_HRH_HPN_10.3_eng.pdf?sequence=1

Yu, B. (2013). Issues in bilingualism and heritage language maintenance: Perspectives of minority-language mothers of children with autism spectrum disorders. *American Journal of Speech-Language Pathology, 22*, 10–24. https://doi.org/10.1044/1058-0360

Zeigler, K., & Camarota, S. (2018). Almost half speak a foreign language in America's largest cities. *Center for Immigration Studies.* Retrieved from https://cis.org/Report/Almost-Half-Speak-Foreign-Language-Americas-Largest-Cities

5

Supporting Participation and Communication in Employment and Volunteer Activities for Adolescents With Complex Communication Needs

David McNaughton and Salena Babb

■ Introduction

The special education team at Central High School[1] meets each month to develop transition plans for the adolescents with disabilities at the school, including the students with complex communication needs. Their goal is to identify key future environments (e.g., employment/volunteer activities, independent/group home living) for each student, and to implement activities that would prepare that individual for success. Mrs. Stoltz, who has been a speech-language pathologist at the school for seven years, takes the lead in coordinating communication services, and investigating and supporting the use of AAC for the students at the school. In thinking about options for Ivan, a 16-year old with autism spectrum disorder (ASD) and limited speech, she realizes the team faces many of the same challenges they have faced in working with other adolescents with complex communication needs.

---

[1]This story is based on a real student, however, the name of the school, the educational team members, and the student have been changed to protect confidentiality. Additional details are available in Babb et al. (2020)

Ivan had been a student in the school district for over 10 years, and was well-liked by school staff. He liked popular movies with superheroes, and participated appropriately when given short, clear directions in familiar routines. Communication was a challenge, however. Ivan had difficulty participating in interactions with other people, and would often repeat back what he had been told (i.e., repeat the question or instruction), or turn away. An AAC system (a tablet-based app) had been introduced five years previously, but this approach had been of limited assistance in supporting his comprehension during interactions with others. For expressive communication, Ivan preferred to use his speech and gestures. Even after extensive training, Ivan only made use of the AAC device when explicitly directed to do so.

The school team thought Ivan could learn to work in a setting with a predictable routine (e.g., shelving books in a library, bagging groceries in a store). However, in past efforts to teach new vocational skills (e.g., wiping down gym equipment, routine cleaning tasks at an animal shelter), Ivan had required ongoing prompting from a teacher's aide to complete activities. Ivan also did not initiate communication or seek assistance from others, even when needed. The special education team realized that like many adolescents with complex communication needs, an effective transition plan for Ivan would require supports for learning new skills, and for communicating with others.

■ Participation and Communication

Adolescents with complex communication needs (and their family members) have new expectations for life after high school, including participation in meaningful employment and community-building volunteer activities (McNaughton, Arnold, Sennott, & Serpentine, 2010; Rossetti, Lehr, Pelerin, Huang, & Lederer, 2016). Many parents express sentiments comments like those expressed by the mother of Haylie (a young woman with significant cognitive challenges and complex communication needs):

> Haylie thrives on interaction with people. She likes that what she does has a sense of purpose (helping others). She also likes to be "on the go." She would be miserable idling her time away at home or "killing time" in a segregated setting. (McNaughton et al., 2010, p. 113)

Despite the desire for active participation and interaction, individuals with complex communication needs often are not provided with needed opportunities and supports, and only a small percentage of adults with complex communication needs are employed (McNaughton et al., 2010; McNaughton & Bryen, 2007). Too often, adolescents with complex communication needs are not provided with the needed instruction and vocational experiences, and leave high school without the skills needed to participate in the workplace (Carter et al., 2010; Carter, Austin, & Trainor, 2012).

In addition, communication challenges often create barriers to participation in workplace and volunteer settings. For example, 30% of individuals with ASD do not develop functional speech (Wodka, Mathy, & Kalb, 2013), and over 50% of adolescents with Down syndrome are not intelligible to anyone other than close caregivers (van Gameren-Oosterom et al., 2013).

Without access to appropriate AAC, these individuals are often restricted in their ability to interact with others, resulting in limited participation and social isolation. As Robert Rummel-Hudson (2018) wrote in describing the experiences of his daughter, Schuyler (a young woman with complex communication needs):

> People with disabilities are treated like partial people by our society because our society doesn't know them. Much of our society doesn't even realize they are knowable. And until those relationships become real, until students in school and adults in their workplaces . . . begin to see people like Schuyler existing and working and laughing and cursing and living messy lives right next to them, there will always be a divide.

Clearly, the transition to the adult world poses many challenges for adolescents and young adults with complex communication needs, and their families. As the parent of an adult with Down syndrome commented, "The biggest challenge was after high school . . . that was the scariest point and because her birthdate is October, she actually went to the transition program until she was 22. BUT THEN IT ALL JUST ENDS." (Hanson, 2003, p. 359) To support successful transition to adult roles, school intervention teams must ensure that both *participation supports* (e.g., assistance in learning to perform new skills), and *communication supports* (e.g., AAC systems for communicating with others) are well established before the individual leaves school (Hunt-Berg, 2005). Successful intervention will require attention both to general principles of effective AAC intervention (Beukelman & Light, 2020), as well as issues specific to successful outcomes in employment and volunteer settings (McNaughton et al., 2010). To promote engagement in workplace and volunteer settings in adult life, the individual with complex communication needs must have opportunities to practice the use of appropriate participation and communication supports in these key future environments while the individual is still in school.

In this chapter, we will address three main topics. First, we will review what is known about the workplace and volunteer participation of adolescents and young adults with complex communication needs. Second, we will examine the role of assistive technology and AAC systems in supporting participation and communication for individual with complex communication needs in these settings.

Finally, we will describe an innovative support to participation and communication, the use of *video visual scene displays*, and provide a case example of its use with an adolescent with ASD who required AAC.

Employment and Community-Building Volunteer Activities

There is growing evidence that participation in employment and community-building volunteer activities are realistic goals for individuals with disabilities who make use of AAC (Light, Stoltz, & McNaughton, 1996; McNaughton, Symons, Light, & Parsons, 2006; Richardson, McCoy, & McNaughton, 2019). To date, however, the most promising outcomes have been observed for individuals who are highly educated, highly literate, and expert users of sophisticated AAC systems (Isakson, Burghsthahler, & Arnold, 2006; McNaughton, Light, & Arnold, 2002; McNaughton, Light, & Groszyk, 2001; Trembath, Balandin, Stancliffe, & Togher, 2010). Too often individuals with intellectual and developmental disabilities (IDD) and complex communication needs are unemployed or underemployed. Based on the results of the National Longitudinal Transition Study (NLTS-2), Newman et al. (2011) reported that young adults with ID had an employment rate of 46%, whereas young adults with ASD had an employment rate of 45%. The additional challenge of complex communication needs results in even lower levels of employment and volunteer activity (McNaughton & Bryen, 2007).

Supporting Participation

Success in the workplace (and volunteer settings) requires attention to the knowledge and skills that are valued in the community, including the performance of work or volunteer activities (McNaughton et al., 2010). Although some skills can be learned in classroom settings, often the best place to learn most skills is in the actual setting in which the skills will be used, where the individual learns to deal with the wide range of work requirements and supports that exist in the real world (Mirenda, 1996; Wehman, 2006). To "bridge" the gap from the classroom to the workplace, many schools now provide vocational placements (with educational staff support) while students are still in school. These activities can help alert educational staff, and the student, to skills that will be important in future employment and volunteer settings.

Traditional approaches to teaching often involved instruction in which a trained partner would provide one-to-one instruction in new skills in a workplace setting. Although effective, this type of training requires a trained instructor, and can result in prompt-dependency (i.e., a reliance on cues from another individual) for the learner with disabilities (Hume, Boyd, Hamm, & Kucharczyk, 2014).

A variety of visual supports has been investigated to teach new skills and promote more independent completion of a task. *Visual activity schedules*—the presentation of an organized sequence of photographs, line drawings, or symbols that serve as cues for the independent performance of the steps in a task—have been demonstrated to be of benefit for a wide variety of activities for a wide variety of learners (Spriggs, Mims, van Dijk, & Knight, 2017; van Dijk & Gage, 2019). For example, Carson, Gast and Ayres (2008) described the positive impact of the use of a visual activity schedule on transitions between vocational tasks (i.e., moving on to the next task when one task was completed) for three young adults with intellectual disabilities. All three participants demonstrated higher levels of successful transitions when the visual activity schedule (i.e., a book with a series of photos depicting target behaviors) was provided.

The introduction of portable tablet devices has made *video prompting* a viable instructional approach for many individuals with IDD (Collins & Collet-Klingenberg, 2018; Park, Bouck, & Duenas, 2019). In this approach, the learner is shown a video that depicts a series of steps in a task (e.g., preparing a meal, completing a work activity). After viewing a step in the video, the learner performs the behavior that they observed, and then views (and performs) the next step in the video, until the activity is completed. Early research provides evidence that video prompting is an effective and efficient method for teaching new skills to adolescents and young adults in vocational settings. For example, Kellems and Morningstar (2012) used video models provided via a small tablet device to improve task performance for four young adults with ASD. Following the introduction of the video clips, all four learners demonstrated performance at or above mastery levels for the targeted tasks (taking inventory, recycling cardboard). More recently, Gilson and Carter (2018) described the positive impact of a video-modelling intervention on the employment-related social behaviors of young adults with ID. All five participants learned to complete both targeted employment activities (e.g., delivering supplies to a classroom, operating a snack cart) as well as engage in appropriate social behaviors (e.g., initiating conversation, asking for help when needed).

In summary, there is growing evidence that video modeling can serve as a powerful instructional technique for individuals with IDD for a wide range of skills, including skills related to employment and volunteer settings (Hong et al., 2016; Park et al., 2019). To date, however, there is only limited information on how video modelling might address the communication needs of individuals who would benefit from the use of AAC.

Supporting Communication

In addition to demonstrating the necessary job skills, it is essential that individuals demonstrate the ability to interact in the workplace. As Bryen, Potts, and Carey (2007) reported, employers identify the ability to communicate successfully as an essential skill for employment. Communication in workplace and volunteer settings, however, may pose special challenges for many individuals with IDD. Communication in the workplace serves a wide variety of functions, including giving and receiving instructions, requesting assistance, and participating in social interactions. Frequently, there is an expectation that an individual will be able to convey a message effectively and efficiently (McNaughton, Light, & Gulla, 2003; McNaughton & Chapple, 2013). Difficulties in communication can lead to breakdowns in workplace interactions, and the failure to meet the social expectations of employers is one of the primary reasons why employees with IDD lose their jobs (Chadsey, 2007).

At present, there is only limited information on providing appropriate communication supports for the large number of individuals with IDD who will not develop functional speech, and will need AAC (National Association of State Directors of Developmental Disabilities Services and Human Services Research Institute, 2017). Early research to address communication in the workplace for persons with complex communication needs has recognized the importance of access to individualized AAC supports. For example, Storey and Provost (1996) described the positive impact of the introduction of communication skills instruction and communication books featuring personalized vocabulary on the workplace interactions of three workers with complex communication needs. More recently, Richardson, McCoy, and McNaughton (2019) described the benefits of AAC for seven young adults with ASD who were employed in community settings. The individuals with ASD were employed in a variety of community businesses, including both customer service (e.g., grocery store, bookstore, butcher shop) and cleaning service (i.e., commercial cleaning company) businesses. The use of a variety of AAC approaches, including picture communication books and tablets with AAC apps, supported successful interaction in the workplace.

Although there is clear evidence that persons with IDD and complex communication needs can successfully participate in employment and volunteer activities, both employers and family members have noted the challenge of learning to participate in these settings. In order to address the dual challenges of learning both new participation and communication skills, Light and colleagues (2014) proposed the use of videos with embedded visual scene displays (i.e., video VSDs). A *visual scene display* (VSD) is a photograph of a meaningful event that has been programmed on a tablet computer (using an app) to support communication (Beukelman & Light,

2020). Using the VSD app, *hotspots* (i.e., highlighted areas within the image) can be added to the VSD to support expressive communication (Light, McNaughton, & Caron, 2019). When touched, the hot spot produces speech output for a recorded word or phrase. For example, an adolescent with complex communication working at a grocery store might have a VSD showing the individual and a coworker at the check-out counter. When the programmed hotspot is activated, the phrase, "Do you need any paper or plastic bags for your check-out station?" is spoken.

A *Video VSD* approach combines the participation supports of video prompting with the communication supports of VSDs (Light et al., 2019). Using a specialized app, VSDs can be placed within an ongoing video—that is, the video plays, and then pauses to show a VSD. The appearance of the VSD serves as a cue to perform the behavior depicted in the video, and the VSD can also be programmed with hotspots to support communication. Figure 5–1 provides an example of the video VSD application with a hotspot. The hotspots in the VSDs can be used in two ways: some persons with complex communication needs use the speech output of the AAC device to communicate with others, whereas others use the speech output to cue use of their own speech in the interaction (O'Neill, Light, & McNaughton, 2017). (See https://tinyurl.com/rerc-on-aac-vVSD for an example of video VSDs).

The use of video VSDs is an important enhancement of video modeling and provides integrated supports not only for learning new skills, but also for communication (Light, McNaughton, & Jakobs, 2014). The VSDs are programmed to appear at key moments in the video;

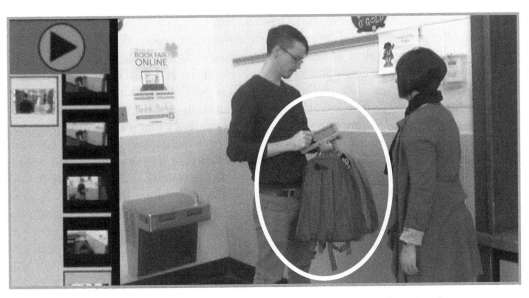

Figure 5–1. A screenshot of the video VSD app with a VSD containing a hotspot (*white circle*). When the hot spot is activated by the student, the following spoken message is produced by the tablet, "I am going to put the backpacks in the storage room."

these pauses at key junctures mark the appropriate opportunity for participation and communication, and the hotspots in the VSD provide the necessary vocabulary for the learner with complex communication needs to fulfill the communication demands at that point in time.

A growing body of research provides evidence of the benefits of a video VSD approach to support both participation and communication. O'Neill et al. (2017) investigated the use of video VSDs for a 16-year-old female ("Lena") with ASD. Lena's transition plan included learning both prevocational tasks (e.g., working in the school office) and community participation skills (e.g., riding public transportation). Prior to the introduction of the video VSD, Lena had been dependent on step-by-step prompts from a teacher to initiate and complete work activities. Lena also was described as a "passive communicator"—she rarely initiated interaction, and typically repeated the speech of her

communication partner or made use of ritualized phrases in response to others.

Once the video VSD was introduced, Lena quickly learned to independently complete the steps as displayed in the video for three activities: completing die cuts in a print shop, shredding paper in the school office, and riding public transportation. In addition, Lena used the hotspots to "cue" her natural speech, and participated appropriately in social exchanges with others (e.g., greeting the school secretaries on entering the office, thanking the bus driver when leaving the bus).

Babb, Gormley, McNaughton, and Light (2019) utilized video VSDs to support participation and communication for "James," an 18-year-old male with ASD, during a prevocational experience. James' transition plan targeted learning four tasks (i.e., checking in books, putting books away, making die cut prints, and paper shredding) in a school library. Prior to the introduction of the video VSD,

James required multiple prompts (e.g., modeling of expected behavior, repetition of oral instructions, physical guidance) in order to complete new tasks and skills. He typically communicated through "yes/no" responses (e.g., signaling "yes" with a thumbs up gesture) to familiar spoken questions from communication partners (e.g., "Do you want a sandwich?"). He also pointed to communicate choices among preferred items. Although an AAC device (iPad with AAC app) had been recommended for James six years prior to the study, he did not use any form of assistive technology to support communication at the time of the study.

Following the introduction of the video VSD, James successfully completed both the task requirements and communication opportunities within each of the four tasks, requiring only a small number of intervention sessions to reach high levels of independence (i.e., greater than 90% accuracy). The four targeted tasks for James each included 11 to 16 steps, and were a combination of motor (e.g., put books in their proper place on the shelves) and communication acts (e.g., tell a staff member "I am finished putting the books away").

More recently, Jung et al. (2020) described the use of a video VSD to assist a young adult with Down syndrome in independent completion of a shopping activity in a large grocery store. Prior to the introduction of the video VSD, the participant was unable to locate shopping list items in the store, and his speech was less than 10% intelligible during interactions with others. After the video VSD was intro-

duced, the participant quickly learned to navigate the store, select desired items, communicate with store staff (e.g., order sliced meats at the Deli counter), and pay for his purchases with a debit card.

In summary, the research to date provides evidence that the use of video VSDs can provide effective supports in key contexts (including employment and volunteer settings) for individuals with IDD and complex communication needs. The integrated support both for learning new skills, and for communicating in new settings with new communication partners, represents a promising approach for this population.[2]

Making a Decision: Video VSDs

Video VSDs are just one approach to meeting the participation and communication needs of adolescents with complex communication needs. There is evidence that the use of both visual activity schedules (Spriggs et al., 2017; van Dijk & Gage, 2019) and video modeling (Gardner & Wolfe, 2013; Hong et al., 2016; Park et al., 2019) can be of benefit in teaching the steps of an activity. A video VSD approach, however, provides the dual benefits of supports for both participation and communication. The research to date provides evidence that it is an effective solution for individuals with no speech, and individuals with limited speech, and may be especially helpful in situations in which there is the goal that the individual both perform a task independently (i.e.,

---

[2]Additional information on the commercial availability of apps to support a video VSD approach is available at https://aac-learning-center.psu.edu/educational-resources/learner-profiles-and-communication-supports/video-visual-scene-displays/

without prompting from a professional) and communicate with new (i.e., unfamiliar) communication partners.

■ Making a Video VSD

Video VSDs can be made to support participation in and communication in a wide variety of activities in the community, including employment settings. The following six-step process is used to create a video VSD.

S— Select a key activity and create a task analysis

T—Take video

A—Add visual scene displays

R—Record communication on hotspots

S—Support use of the video VSD by providing models, guided practice, and independent practice

! — Celebrate success

S—Select a Key Activity and Create a Task Analysis

The first step is to select a key activity for the learner. This may be an activity which is new to the learner, or one in which the learner currently participates but is dependent upon prompting from an instructor to complete the task. It is ideal to select an activity which will be a regular part of the individual's day (or week) so that they will have multiple opportunities to practice the new skill.

Next, create a task analysis for the activity. A *task analysis* supports instruction by breaking a skill down into an ordered series of smaller, more manageable steps (Cooper, Heron, & Heward, 2007). To create a task analysis, first create a "draft" list of the steps that will be needed to complete the task. Next, perform the task yourself (using the draft list as a guide) in order to identify any missing steps, and the appropriate sequence of steps (Snell & Brown, 2006). It may be helpful to perform the task more than once to refine the steps, and ensure that all needed steps have been identified for the learner (Cooper et al., 2007). Table 5–1 provides an example of a task analysis.

One common question in creating a task analysis is the "size" of each step (i.e., how much should a person "do" in each step). This is an individualized decision, dependent on the skills and learning ability

Table 5–1. Task Analysis for Riding the Bus

Step
1. Walk to the bus stop.
2. Wait for the bus.
3. Get on the bus.
4. Say **"Hi, I am going to Mall"** to the bus driver.
5. Show bus pass to the driver.
6. Walk to seat, sit down, and wait.
7. Pull cord when stop is next.
8. Get up and walk to exit.
9. Say **"Thank you"** to the bus driver.
10. Get off the bus.

Note. Steps that are in **bold** are programmed as hot spots to fulfill communication opportunities.

of the learner. For example, consider your own experience in travel instructions: if you are new to a city, you may find it helpful to have each step broken down into smaller steps (e.g., walk to the corner of Main Street and Park Avenue, get on the Downtown bus, get off after three stops at 3rd Street). If you are familiar with the city, one big "chunked" instruction ("take the bus downtown and get off at the State Theater") may be sufficient. When creating the steps of a task analysis, consider the level of support the learner will need so that instruction is both effective and efficient.

One key benefit of video VSDs is the ability to support communication. During the task analysis, identify opportunities for interaction with others. Some of these communication opportunities may be related to task completion (e.g., asking for a key to open a room, asking a supervisor to inspect a completed task), but others may be purely social (e.g., greeting co-workers), a critical part of making an activity enjoyable!

T—Take Video

Once the task analysis is complete, take a video recording of someone performing the steps in the task analysis. Video VSD apps support either creating a new video using the tablet's video camera, or importing an existing video (from the tablet's video library) into the app. The video should clearly show an individual performing each step in the activity (as outlined in the task analysis), and allow the learner to both see and hear the information relevant to their expected participation.

It is not necessary for the model to be the same age or gender as the learner.

Past research provides evidence that individuals with disabilities can effectively learn from models who are markedly different from them (Domire & Wolfe, 2014; Gardner & Wolfe, 2013; Park et al., 2019). There may also be situations in which the individual themselves can perform the skills, but is dependent upon step-by-step prompting. In these situations, the learner can serve as the "model"—the individual can be recorded as they perform the skill, and then the prompting can be edited out, so that all that is seen in the video is the "unprompted" performance of the skill.

A—Add Visual Scene Displays (VSDs)

After the video is recorded, use the video VSD app to create VSDs. The VSDs will appear as still images in the video, and provide a "pause" in the playing of the video. The appearance of the VSD within the video is a cue to the learner that a key step needs to be completed. Although there may be some minor differences among video VSD apps, the creation of a VSD typically includes the following steps:

- Switch to "edit" mode.
- Pause the video at the end of the step outlined in the task analysis (automatically creating a VSD).

When viewed in "play" mode by the learner, the video will pause automatically wherever a VSD has been created.

R—Record Communication by Adding Hotspots

When the step requires communication, add hotspots to provide the needed words and phrases vocabulary. Hotspots can be added to previously created VSDs, or new VSDs can be added and programmed with hotspots:

- Switch to "edit" mode.
- Pause the video at the opportunity for communication (automatically creating a VSD).
- Draw a hot spot on the VSD.
- Record the needed word or phrase using digitized speech.
- Return to "play" mode.

When viewed by the learner, the video will pause automatically wherever a VSD as been created. When the VSD appears, the outline of the hot spot will be displayed momentarily in order to mark a communication opportunity. A video VSD can contain multiple VSDs, and each VSD can contain multiple hotspots, with each hotspot providing appropriate words and phrases.

S—Support Use of the Video VSD by Providing Models, Guided Practice, and Independent Practice

Like any new skill, learners will benefit from instruction in the use of video VSDs. First, *model* the use of the video VSD: watch the video with the learner, and act out the steps shown in the video, ideally in the same situation in which the video VSD will ultimately be used. Encourage the learner to attend to the video, and comment on how you are imitating the behaviors in the video.

Next, provide *guided practice*: assist the learner in gradually becoming more independent in the use of the video VSD. This is a gradual process over time. For example, in an early guided practice session you may press the 'play' button for the first two video clips, but then encourage the learner (e.g., point to the play button, say "your turn") to become more independent for subsequent video clips. You can also verbally encourage the learner to imitate the behavior seen in the video, so that the learner will better understand the expectation that they imitate the video model.

Finally, provide *independent practice*. When you see evidence that the learner is reliably imitating the skills observed in the video VSD and making use of the hotspots, withdraw cues and prompting. Take data on the learner's performance to identify what steps have been mastered (i.e., completed with the assistance of the video VSD), and what steps may need additional instruction (e.g., guided practice with prompting or reinforcement).

■ Case Illustration: Video VSDs to Support Participation and Communication

As part of an ongoing collaboration with a local school district, we investigated the use of video VSDs as a support to communication and participation for four young men (ages 14 to 20) with intellectual and developmental disabilities, all of whom required AAC (Babb et al., 2020). All four individuals—Ivan, Jerry, Keith, and Martin—participated in their school district's transition program for students with disabilities. The program provided employment experiences for the students during their time in middle/high school, with the goal of increasing opportunities for employment after graduation.

Traditionally, employment experiences had focused on easily-learned routines with limited communication demands (e.g., wiping down cafeteria tables, collecting towels in the fitness center). The AAC team wanted to explore more challenging activities for the students at the school, with increased expectations for participation and communication.

The students were recommended by their classroom teachers, who reported that all four were dependent on prompts to complete tasks within the classroom, and all four had difficulty communicating with both familiar and unfamiliar communication partners. Each student had an IEP transition goal that included work experience. Additional information on the background and performance of all four individuals is available in Babb et al. (2020). In this section we focus on the performance of one participant, Ivan (introduced at the beginning of this chapter).

Ivan was a 16-year-old student with a diagnosis of moderate autism spectrum disorder (ASD). He spent most of his day in a special education classroom, with the exception of an elective class (i.e., cooking) with his tenth-grade general education peers. Educational staff described Ivan as very prompt-dependent, and reluctant to participate in tasks without high levels of prompting and reinforcement. Ivan typically communicated with gestures and spoken 2 to 4 word phrases (when prompted by a staff member). He was provided with visual schedules to support his transitions throughout the day. Ivan did not use an AAC system—in past efforts at trialing devices, Ivan had demonstrated a strong preference for his natural speech, even though his use of speech was limited and frequently resulted in communication breakdowns.

It was determined that in order for Ivan to participate appropriately in a vocational activity, he would require supports both for completing the task, and for communicating with others in the work environment.

Implementing the Video VSD Process

Select a Key Activity and Create a Task Analysis

As part of their prevocational transition plans, all participants were expected to participate in school or community-based work experiences for approximately 90 minutes, two days per week. For the past three years, the school district had partnered with the local food bank and YMCA to send food home each weekend for students who participated in the free or reduced-cost lunch programs. Each week, staff members in the school would meet for a few hours after school at a local elementary school and pack the backpacks with food. Based on a discussion between the researchers and the classroom team prior to the start of the study, it was decided that packing food backpacks for students who participated in the food-bank programs would serve as the target activity for the intervention.

Next, a task analysis was created by identifying each of the necessary steps in the activity. As needed, each step was broken down into further, smaller steps, and placed in the most natural ordered sequence (Snell & Brown, 2006). Then, a member of the AAC team performed the task analysis for the activity in order to be sure that the steps made practical sense and produced the desired outcomes. The activity comprised 25 steps. Each step included an action to be completed related to task completion (i.e., motor acts) or communication opportunities (i.e., communication acts). Table 5–2 provides a Task Analysis for Packing Backpacks.

Table 5–2. Task Analysis for Packing Backpacks

Step
1. Walk to and enter the office
2. Greet secretary: "**Hi, how are you?**"
3. Respond to secretary: "**I'm okay.**"
4. Tell her why you are there: "**I'm here to fill the backpacks.**"
5. Ask to be let in to the storage room: "**Can you let me in the storage room?**"
6. Thank secretary: "**Thank you.**"
7. Leave office, walk to storage room and pick up two backpacks
8. Carry the backpacks out of the storage to the cafeteria
9. Put the backpacks at the end of the table
10. Look at the menu
11. Pick up a backpack from the table
12. Fill the backpack with the items
13. Carry the backpacks from the table and put them against the wall
14. Fill the remaining backpacks
15. Ask the supervisor to check your work: **"Can you check my work?"**
16. Zip up the backpacks
17. Tell the supervisor you are going to put the backpacks away: **"I am going to put the backpacks in the storage room."**
18. Carry the backpacks from the cafeteria to the storage room.
19. Put the backpacks in the completed bin.
20. Exit the storage room and close the door.
21. Enter the office
22. Tell the secretary you are finished in the storage room: "**I am finished with the backpacks.**"
23. Let the secretary know you have closed the door: **"I closed the storage room door."**
24. Say goodbye to the secretary: **"Bye! Have a great day!"**
25. Exit the office

Note. Steps that are in **bold** are programmed as hot spots to fulfill communication opportunities.

Take Video

Using the onboard camera of a tablet computer, each step in the task analysis was video recorded. A male graduate student (approximately 27 years of age) served as the model for the demonstration of the target behaviors in the video. As noted above, past research provides evidence that individuals with disabilities can learn from a wide variety of video types, and that the age and gender of the "model" is of limited importance. More importantly, the video clearly demonstrates the target behavior, especially the expected behavior of the participant.

Add Visual Scene Displays (VSDs)

Next, the video was uploaded to the video VSD app. The video was paused at the end of each of the keys step in the task analysis. Pausing the video (while using the video VSD app), automatically created a still VSD at these junctures in the video. These videos served both as a cue for the individual to perform as the next step in the task, and could also be programmed with hotspots for those steps requiring communication.

Record Communication

For those steps in the task analysis which required communication, relevant vocabulary was added to the VSDs with hotspots. In these cases, the AAC team member identified the needed word or phrase (e.g., "I'm here to fill the backpacks"), and identified an appropriate portion of the VSD that could be programmed with a hotspot (e.g., the model speaking to the secretary). The AAC team member then created a hotspot on that portion

of the image using the edit function of the VSD app, and recorded the needed phrase.

Support Use of the Video VSD App Using a Model/Guided Practice/Independent Practice Instructional Sequence

The AAC team taught Ivan a five-step procedure to use the video VSD app and participate in the activity:

A. Press the play button (the arrow located at the top left).
B. Watch the video segment depicting the step from the task analysis (shown in the large area on the right side of the screen).
C. Complete the step by performing the motor act and/or fulfilling the communication act portrayed in the segment (i.e., by selecting the hot spot from the VSD).
D. Press the play button again to watch the video model of the next step, or select the thumbnail of the video of the next step from the menu on the left-hand side.
E. Repeat steps A through D for each step to complete the entire task.

The AAC team used a model, guided practice, independent practice instructional sequence to teach Ivan the five-step procedure. In the *model* step, the instructor first viewed the video VSDs with Ivan, activating each hotspot and providing a short narration of each step in the task analysis (e.g., "First you walk to the office to get the key"). Next, Ivan navigated the tablet to view each video and activate each hotspot. Following this introduction to the app, the instructor provided guided practice in the use of the app.

During *guided practice*, the instructor provided Ivan with the tablet and encouraged him to use the video VSDs to complete the activity. At this stage, the instructor stood close to Ivan and provided prompting and supports as needed. For example, initially Ivan was hesitant to use the app, and simply held the tablet without pressing the 'play' button to watch the first video clip. At this point, the instructor would gesture to the play button as a prompt to support Ivan in starting the task. Similarly, if Ivan watched a step in the task analysis but then did not begin to complete that step, the instructor may have gestured in the direction of the next step (e.g., toward the storage room) or the instructor may have provided a verbal cue such as, "Enter the office." As Ivan became more confident with the technology and with the task, the instructor was able to distance herself and fade the support she was providing. Figure 5–2 provides an image of a student using the video VSD app to greet the secretary.

Once Ivan was consistently demonstrating high levels of performance during the guided practice sessions, he began *independent practice*. During these sessions, the instructor did not provide cues or prompts for Ivan (as was provided in guided practice), but did provide assistance if Ivan made an error or omitted a necessary step. The goal in independent practice is to prepare the learner to perform the needed skills without the support of the instructor.

The model/guided practice/independent practice instructional sequence quickly resulted in positive outcomes for Ivan. Before Ivan had access to the video VSD app, he typically completed only 1 of the 25 steps (5%) correctly. Immediately after the introduction of the video VSD support (and a modelling session), he performed 11 of the steps (45%) correctly. Ivan then performed 21 steps (84%) correctly after only his second guided practice session. At the end of five sessions with the video VSD app, Ivan was

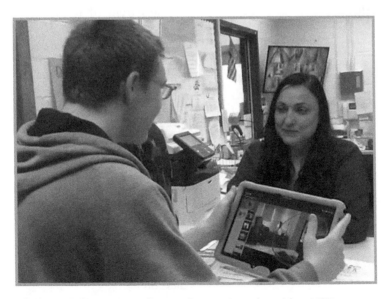

Figure 5–2. Image of a student using the video VSD app to greet the secretary.

completing 23 or more (90% or better) of the 25 steps correctly (and independently). Ivan continued to demonstrate mastery levels of performance 2 and 4 weeks after the last intervention session had been provided. Figure 5–3 provides a "Graph of Percentage of Steps Performed Correctly for Ivan."

The intervention resulted not only in increases in participation and communication using the video VSD app, but also in Ivan's use of speech. During the baseline sessions, Ivan did not make use of any speech at all. Following the introduction of the video VSD, Ivan touched the hotspots to obtain models of the needed words and phrases and used these as models (i.e., for the needed vocabulary) for his speech during the interaction. Although his speech was difficult to understand, the combined use of his natural speech and the speech from the tablet resulted in successful communication. As he gained confidence in the activity, he also smiled and made use of short phrases (e.g., "Did it!") to communicate his pride in his completion of activities.

!—Celebrate Success!

Ivan was just one of four adolescents with complex communication needs who successfully used video VSDs to complete both targeted tasks and communication acts during the volunteer activity (Babb et al., 2020). The increases from baseline to intervention were observed for all four participants, with each demonstrating an immediate change in performance following the introduction of the app. Figure 5–4 provides an image of student with backpacks.

The success of the four participants was recognized both by the members of the AAC team, as well as other school staff who observed the work and interactions of the students as they completed the backpack activity. As one staff member described:

A lot of teachers stopped by to check it out, not just special education teachers, there were other teachers that came by that were interested. . . . Even the parents that were coming in the

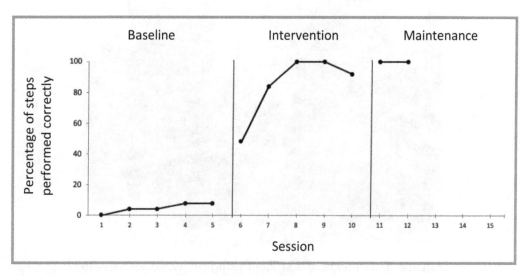

Baseline   Intervention   Maintenance

Figure 5–3. Graph of percentage of steps performed correctly by Ivan.

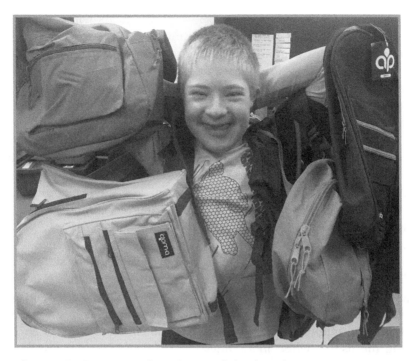

Figure 5–4. Image of student with backpacks.

door were checking it out. We got a lot of people; it's like a little community all involved in it. It wasn't just us, it was other people cheering them on and wanting them to do well.

Comments from staff members and others made clear that changed perceptions not only for this particular task, but for expectations more broadly:

- "I thought it was great that other people got to see how well they could do. They (the other people) asked questions and wanted to know what was going on . . . that bar got so high for them."
- "They were able to accomplish what they set out to do. It was amazing to start with them needing one-on-one attention and then to see them independently be able,

with very little help, to pack the backpacks."
- " . . . those kids were able to feel success. I think they felt like they were a productive adult within this building. I think it built a whole lot of self-esteem with those kids. It exceeded our expectations."

The intervention was widely regarded as a success. In fact, the school district viewed the program so positively that it was continued the following school year, and expanded it to include additional students and additional workdays.

■ Conclusions

AAC intervention must address socially meaningful outcomes (Light & McNaughton, 2015; Ogletrec, 2007). A Video VSD approach can provide powerful participation and communication supports for individuals with complex communication needs in desired activities—in this case, participating in a community-building volunteer activity. For the four individuals who participated in this study, only limited AAC supports were being used prior to the video VSD intervention. Like many individuals who make some limited use of speech, it had been seen as difficult to provide AAC approaches that supported and complemented their use of speech, and did not add complexity to learning a new skill. For these individuals, the use of one "integrated" support reduced the challenge of learning how to both complete a new task and interact with new communication partners at the same time. In addition, the use of video modelling may have better supported the learning of complicated tasks than would have been possible with the use of static images (i.e., photos) as traditionally used in a visual schedule approach.

Additional research is needed to better understand the contexts in which a video VSD approach can provide appropriate participation and communication supports—for example, situations in which a majority of the participation and communication demands can be reasonably anticipated. Future research should also address strategies to easily integrate video VSDs into the communication systems of individuals who are already making use of an AAC technique (e.g., an AAC app on a tablet device). For example, individuals could be taught to navigate between a video VSD app (for access to integrated support for participation and communication) and a previously learned AAC technique (for the generation of novel utterances, as appropriate).

Individuals with complex communication needs have new expectations for engagement in society (Rossetti et al., 2016; Williams, Krezman, & McNaughton, 2008); however, they often experience significant challenges at these times (Light & McNaughton, 2015). Intervention must address not only the provision of vocabulary for communication, but address the supports needed to maximize participation in key environments. As noted by Light and McNaughton (2015),

> . . . Individuals who require AAC must develop sufficient skills to meet the functional communicative demands within real-world interactions with various partners in their natural environment. Communication is not an end goal in and of itself; rather, it is a tool to allow individuals to participate effectively and attain their goals at home, at school, at work, or in the community. (p. 88)

A growing body of research provides evidence that video VSD is an effective technique for supporting interaction for individuals with complex communication needs (Babb et al., 2019, 2020; Jung et al., 2020; Laubscher, Light, & McNaughton, 2019; O'Neill et al., 2017). The integrated provision of support for both participation and communication is a promising approach to creating new employment and volunteer opportunities for persons who benefit from the use of AAC.

Note. The contents of this chapter were developed, in part, under a grant to the Rehabilitation Engineering Research Center on Augmentative and Alternative Communication (The RERC on AAC) from the US Department of Health and Human

Services, National Institute on Disability, Independent Living, and Rehabilitation Research (NIDILRR grant #90RE5017). Salena Babb was supported by the Penn State AAC Doctoral Leadership Project, a doctoral training grant funded by U.S. Department of Education grant #H325D170024. The contents do not necessarily represent the policy of the funding agency, and you should not assume endorsement by the federal government.

■ References

Babb, S., Gormley, J., McNaughton, D., & Light, J. (2019). Enhancing independent participation within vocational activities for an adolescent with ASD using AAC video visual scene displays. *Journal of Special Education Technology, 34*, 120–132. https://doi.org/10.1177/0162643418795842

Babb, S., McNaughton, D., Light, J., Caron, J., Wydner, K., & Jung, S. (2020). Using AAC video visual scene displays to increase participation and communication within a volunteer activity for adolescents with complex communication needs. *Augmentative and Alternative Communication*, 1–12.

Beukelman, D. R. & Light, J. C. (2020). *Augmentative and alternative communication: Supporting children and adults with complex communication needs* (5th ed.). Brookes.

Bryen, D. N., Potts, B. B., & Carey, A. C. (2007). So you want to work? What employers say about job skills, recruitment and hiring employees who rely on AAC. *Augmentative and Alternative Communication, 23*, 126–139. https://doi.org/10.1080/07434610600991175

Carson, K. D., Gast, D. L., & Ayres, K. M. (2008). Effects of a photo activity schedule book on independent task changes by students with intellectual disabilities in community and school job sites. *European Journal of Special Needs Education, 23*, 269–279. https://doi.org/10.1080/08856250802130475

Carter, E. W., Austin, D., & Trainor, A. A. (2012). Predictors of postschool employment outcomes for young adults with severe disabilities. *Journal of Disability Policy Studies, 23*, 50–63. https://doi.org/10.1177/1044207311414680

Carter, E. W., Ditchman, N., Sun, Y., Trainor, A. A., Swedeen, B., & Owens, L. (2010). Summer employment and community experiences of transition-age youth with severe disabilities. *Exceptional Children, 76*, 194–212. https://doi.org/10.1177/001440291007600204

Chadsey, J. G. (2007). Vocational skills and performance. In J. W. Jacobson, J. A. Mulick, & J. Rojahn (Eds.) *Handbook of intellectual and developmental disabilities: Issues in clinical child psychology* (pp. 619–634). Springer.

Collins, J. C., & Collet-Klingenberg, L. (2018). Portable electronic assistive technology to improve vocational task completion in young adults with an intellectual disability: A review of the literature. *Journal of Intellectual Disabilities, 22*, 213–232. https://doi.org/10.1177/1744629516689336

Cooper, J. O., Heron, T. E., & Heward, W. L. (2007). *Applied behavior analysis*. Pearson.

Domire, S. C., & Wolfe, P. (2014). Effects of video prompting techniques on teaching daily living skills to children with autism spectrum disorders: A review. *Research and Practice for Persons with Severe Disabilities, 39*, 211–226. https://doi.org/10.1177/1540796914555555

Gardner, S., & Wolfe, P. (2013). Use of video modeling and video prompting interventions for teaching daily living skills to individuals with autism spectrum disorders: A review. *Research and Practice for Persons with Severe Disabilities, 38*, 73–87. https://doi.org/10.2511/027494813807714555

Gilson, C. B., & Carter, E. W. (2018). Video-based instruction to promote employment-related social behaviors for high school students with intellectual disability. *Inclusion, 6*, 175–193. https://doi.org/10.1352/2326-6988-6.3.175

Hong, E. R., Ganz, J. B., Mason, R., Morin, K., Davis, J. L., Ninci, J., . . . Gilliland, W. D. (2016). The effects of video modeling in teaching functional living skills to persons with ASD: A meta-analysis of single-case studies. *Research in Developmental Disabilities, 57,* 158–169. https://doi.org/10.1016/j.ridd.2016.07.001

Hume, K., Boyd, B. A., Hamm, J. V., & Kucharczyk, S. (2014). Supporting independence in adolescents on the autism spectrum. *Remedial and Special Education, 35,* 102–113. https://doi.org/10.1177/07419325135 14617

Hunt-Berg, M. (2005). The Bridge School: Educational inclusion outcomes over 15 years. *Augmentative and Alternative Communication, 21,* 116–131. https://doi.org/10.10 80/07434610500103509

Isakson, C. L., Burghstahler, S., & Arnold, A. (2006). AAC, employment, and independent living: A success story. *Assistive Technology Outcomes and Benefits, 3*(1), 67–79.

Jung, S., Ousley, C., McNaughton, D., & Light, J. (2020, January 30). *Supporting participation and communication in community shopping using video VSDs.* Poster session presented at the Annual Conference of the Assistive Technology Industry Association, Orlando, FL.

Kellems, R. O., & Morningstar, M. E. (2012). Using video modeling delivered through iPods to teach vocational tasks to young adults with autism spectrum disorders. *Career Development and Transition for Exceptional Individuals, 35,* 155–167. https://doi.org/10.1177/0885728812443082

Laubscher, E., Light, J., & McNaughton, D. (2019). Effect of an application with video visual scene displays on communication during play: Pilot study of a child with autism spectrum disorder and a peer. *Augmentative and Alternative Communication, 35,* 299–308. https://doi.org/10.1080/0743 4618.2019.1699160

Light, J., & McNaughton, D. (2015). Designing AAC research and intervention to improve outcomes for individuals with complex communication needs. *Augmentative and Alternative Communication, 31,* 85–96. https://doi.org/10.3109/07434618.2015.10 36458

Light, J., McNaughton, D., & Caron, J. (2019). New and emerging AAC technology supports for children with complex communication needs and their communication partners: State of the science and future research directions. *Augmentative and Alternative Communication, 35,* 26-41. https://doi.org/ 10.1080/07434618.2018.1557251

Light, J., McNaughton, D., & Jakobs, T. (2014). Developing AAC technology to support interactive video visual scene displays. *RERC on AAC: Rehabilitation Engineering Research Center on Augmentative and Alternative Communication.* Retrieved from https://rerc-aac.psu.edu/development/ d2-developing-aac-technology-to-support-interactive-video-visual-scene-displays/

Light, J., Stoltz, B., & McNaughton, D. (1996). Community-based employment: Experiences of adults who use AAC. *Augmentative and Alternative Communication, 12,* 215–229. https://doi.org/10.1080/0743461 9612331277688

McNaughton, D. B., Arnold, A., Sennott, S., & Serpentine, E. (2010). Developing skills, "Making a match," and obtaining needed supports: Successful employment for individuals who use AAC. In D. McNaughton & D. R. Beukelman (Eds.) *Transition strategies for adolescents and young adults who use AAC* (pp. 111–127). Brookes.

McNaughton, D., & Bryen, D. N. (2007). AAC technologies to enhance participation and access to meaningful societal roles for adolescents and adults with developmental disabilities who require AAC. *Augmentative and Alternative Communication, 23,* 217–229. https://doi.org/10.1080/07434610701 573856

McNaughton, D., & Chapple, D. (2013). AAC and communication in the workplace. *Perspectives on Augmentative and Alternative Communication, 22*(1), 30–36. https://doi.org/10.1044/aac22.1.30

McNaughton, D., Light, J., & Arnold, K. (2002). "Getting your wheel in the door": Successful full-time employment experiences of individuals with cerebral palsy who use Augmentative and Alternative Communication. *Augmentative and Alternative Communication, 18*, 59–76. https://doi.org/10.1080/07434610212331281171

McNaughton, D., Light, J., & Groszyk, L. (2001). "Don't give up": Employment experiences of individuals with amyotrophic lateral sclerosis who use augmentative and alternative communication. *Augmentative and Alternative Communication, 17*, 179–195. https://doi.org/10.1080/aac.17.3.179.195

McNaughton, D., Light, J., & Gulla, S. (2003). Opening up a 'whole new world': Employer and co-worker perspectives on working with individuals who use augmentative and alternative communication. *Augmentative and Alternative Communication, 19*, 235–253. https://doi.org/10.1080/0743461031000 01595669

McNaughton, D., Symons, G., Light, J., & Parsons, A. (2006). "My dream was to pay taxes": The self-employment experiences of individuals who use augmentative and alternative communication. *Journal of Vocational Rehabilitation, 25*, 181–196.

Mirenda, P. (1996). Sheltered employment and augmentative communication: An oxymoron? *Augmentative and Alternative Communication, 12*, 193–197.

National Association of State Directors of Developmental Disabilities Services and Human Services Research Institute. (2017). *National core indicators: Adult consumer survey 2016–2017*. Retrieved from https://www.nationalcoreindicators.org/upload/core-indicators/NCI_2016-17_ACS_NATIONAL_REPORT_PART_I_%286_29%29.pdf

Newman, L., Wagner, M., Knokey, A.-M., Marder, C., Nagle, K., Shaver, D., & Wei, X. (2011). *The post-high school outcomes of young adults with disabilities up to 8 years after high school: A report from the National Longitudinal Transition Study-2 (NLTS2). NCSER 2011-3005*. National Center for Special Education Research. Retrieved from https://eric.ed.gov/?id=ED524044

Ogletree, B. T. (2007). What makes communication intervention successful with children with autism spectrum disorders? *Focus on Autism and Other Developmental Disabilities, 22*, 190–192.

O'Neill, T., Light, J., & McNaughton, D. (2017). Videos with integrated AAC Visual Scene Displays to enhance participation in community and vocational activities: Pilot case study with an adolescent with autism spectrum disorder. *Perspectives of the ASHA Special Interest Groups, 2*(12), 55–69. https://doi.org/10.1044/persp2.SIG12.55

Park, J., Bouck, E., & Duenas, A. (2019). The effect of video modeling and video prompting interventions on individuals with intellectual disability: A systematic literature review. *Journal of Special Education Technology, 34*, 3–16. https://doi.org/10.1177/0162643418780464

Richardson, L., McCoy, A., & McNaughton, D. (2019). "He's worth the extra work": The employment experiences of adults with ASD who use augmentative and alternative communication (AAC) as reported by adults with ASD, family members, and employers. *Work, 62*, 205–219. https://doi.org/10.3233/WOR-192856

Rossetti, Z., Lehr, D., Pelerin, D., Huang, S., & Lederer, L. (2016). Parent involvement in meaningful post-school experiences for young adults with IDD and pervasive support needs. *Intellectual and Developmental Disabilities, 54*, 260–272. https://doi.org/10.1352/1934-9556-54.4.260

Rummel-Hudson, R. (2018). *The care and feeding of monsters*. Retrieved from http://belovedmonsterandme.blogspot.com/2018/05/the-care-and-feeding-of-monsters.html

Snell, M. E., & Brown, F. (2006). Designing and implementing instructional programs. In M. E. Snell, & F. Brown (Eds.), *Instruction of students with severe disabilities* (6th ed). pp. 111–169. Pearson.

Spriggs, A. D., Mims, P. J., van Dijk, W., & Knight, V. F. (2017). Examination of the evidence base for using visual activity schedules with students with intellectual disability. *The Journal of Special Education, 51,* 14–26. http:// doi:10.1177/0022466916658483

Storey, K., & Provost, O. (1996). The effect of communication skills instruction on the integration of workers with severe disabilities in supported employment settings. *Education and Training in Mental Retardation and Developmental Disabilities, 31,* 123–141.

Trembath, D., Balandin, S., Stancliffe, R. J., & Togher, L. (2010). "Communication is everything": The experiences of volunteers who use AAC. *Augmentative and Alternative Communication, 26,* 75–86. https://doi.org/10.3109/07434618.2010.481561

van Dijk, W., & Gage, N. A. (2019). The effectiveness of visual activity schedules for individuals with intellectual disabilities: A meta-analysis. *Journal of Intellectual & Developmental Disability, 44,* 384–395. https://doi.org/10.3109/13668250.2018.1431761

Van Gameren-Oosterom, H. B., Fekkes, M., Reijneveld, S. A., Oudesluys-Murphy, A. M., Verkerk, P. H., Van Wouwe, J. P., & Buitendijk, S. E. (2013). Practical and social skills of 16–19-year-olds with Down syndrome: Independence still far away. *Research in Developmental Disabilities, 34,* 4599–4607. https://doi.org/1016/j.ridd.2013.09.041

Wehman, P. (2006). *Life beyond the classroom: Transition strategies for young people with disabilities* (4th ed.). Brookes.

Williams, M. B., Krezman, C., & McNaughton, D. (2008). "Reach for the stars": Five principles for the next 25 years of AAC. *Augmentative and Alternative Communication, 24,* 194–206. https://doi.org/10.1080/08990220802387851

Wodka, E. L., Mathy, P., & Kalb, L. (2013). Predictors of phrase and fluent speech in children with autism and severe language delay. *Pediatrics, 131*(4), e1128–e1134. https://doi.org/10.1542/peds.2012-2221

PART III
AAC Challenges and Solutions: Adult Disorders

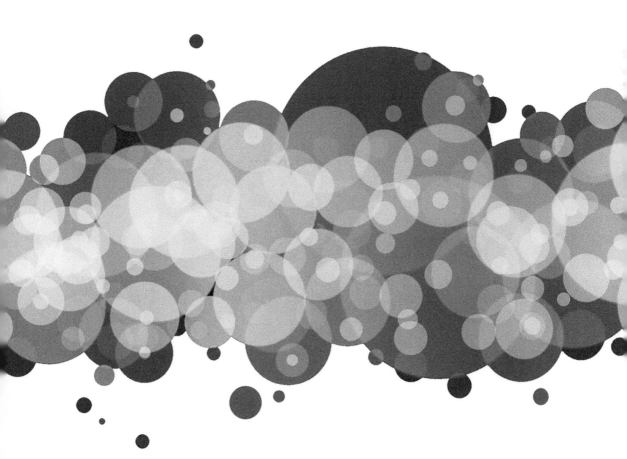

6

AAC Interventions in Persons with Aphasia

Tiffany Chavers, Cissy Cheng, and Rajinder Koul

■ Introduction

Aphasia is a language impairment resulting from damage to areas of the brain that are responsible for the comprehension and formulation of language (Koul, 2011). Persons with aphasia (PWA) tend to experience a wide variability in linguistic and cognitive characteristics based on factors such as the size of the lesion, the damaged brain area's role in processing distinct brain functions, and remote effects of the lesion on distant brain tissue (Brookshire & McNeil, 2014; Goodglass & Kaplan, 1983; Kertesz, 1982; Mountcastle, 1978; Porch, 1981). Variability in linguistic and cognitive characteristics include issues related to attention, working memory, resource allocation, executive function, spontaneous speech, auditory comprehension, reading, writing, and metacognitive, and metalinguistic skills among others (Erickson, Goldinger, & LaPointe, 1996; Garrett & Kimelman, 2000; Petroi, Koul, & Corwin, 2014). These factors in combination with socio-demographic, environmental, and psychological variables (e.g., age, education, partner support, motiva-

tion, depression) play a significant role in the recovery of language function in PWA (Koul, 2011). Thus, aphasia is a complex condition that requires comprehensive intervention targeting both language and cognitive systems.

Whereas some PWA regain speech and language function through restorative therapy approaches, others may continue to have severe communication impairment with little to no functional speech. Such persons may benefit from the use of Augmentative and Alternative communication (AAC) methods, techniques, and strategies. An effective AAC intervention is multifaceted and facilitates expressive and receptive communication, reduces cognitive load, enhances executive function, and promotes independent participation across diverse communicative settings (Beukelman & Mirenda, 2013; Brock, Koul, Corwin, & Schlosser, 2017; Dada, Stockley, Wallace, & Koul, 2019; Garret & Lasker, 2005; Koul, 2011; Koul, Corwin, Nigam, & Oetzel, 2008).

Despite facilitative effects of AAC, it may often be considered a resource of last resort by clinicians, clients, and other stakeholders with PWA (e.g., Frankoff

& Hatfield, 2011). That means AAC may only be considered as an option when restorative therapy fails to meet the goal of facilitating communication primarily through spoken modality. However, AAC strategies must always be considered as an option for patients with severe aphasia to both facilitate the recovery of natural speech and language and/or compensate for severe communication impairment (Garret & Lasker, 2005). The following quote (Corwin, 2011) from a paid caregiver at an assisted living facility describing communication with the resident with aphasia clearly indicates communication challenges in the absence of communication supports such as the use of AAC techniques and strategies.

> Most of the time it is very frustrating because he's trying to tell me something and I don't understand. Sometimes he can get the word out. If he can give me a one-word clue, I can go from there. You know, if you just have an area to start with . . . If you just don't have a clue, then it's . . . you've got the whole world to think about [laugh]. But, most of the time, it's pretty frustrating. And, he's gotten better. At first, it was just horrible [laugh] because it was just so hard. But he's gotten better with, the . . . okay, he can't say it . . . just stop for a minute . . . and you tell him, "Just rest a minute and think about it." And sometimes he'll just come up with a word or two that will give me a clue and I can just kind of go from there, because if he says, "Go," I'll find out if he wants to go somewhere. And I can ask him, "Where?" and he

> can either point in a direction, or sometimes he will say, "Street" . . . down the street, or something. And you just kind of go from there . . .

The purpose of this chapter is to provide practitioners with an overview of AAC intervention approaches for PWA. We will present approaches that use technology such as speech generating devices (SGDs) to facilitate communication and approaches that are primarily low tech or no tech. However, even as experienced clinicians plan and implement AAC intervention for PWA they find significant challenges in addressing factors such as cognitive-linguistic competencies, design of interface displays, partner involvement, and device abandonment (Koul, 2011). It is critical to factor these challenges while implementing a successful AAC intervention for PWA. We will first present the nature of these challenges, followed by each section of the chapter offering evidence-based solutions to these challenges.

The first challenge is related to considering cognitive factors while devising AAC intervention for PWA. Cognitive strategies that are critical to the use of AAC techniques and strategies include perceptual processing, attention, memory, resource allocation, and capacity. Research has indicated that PWA demonstrate reduced working memory capacity and deficits in allocation of attentional resources and executive functioning (e.g., Koul, 2011; McNeil, Odell, & Tsend, 1991; Purdy & Dietz, 2010). Use of AAC strategies and techniques tend to increase the information processing demands for PWA during communicative interactions. For example, to share information with a communication partner using a taxonomic grid display, PWA must rely on their declarative and semantic memory stores while maintaining in working memory the commentary of communication partners and the purpose of the response s/he is producing using the AAC system. Executive functioning deficits are often observed in PWA in situations where they are unable to resolve communication breakdowns by using an alternative strategy that is available to them.

The second challenge is related to the design of message selection and enhancement approaches that reduce cognitive effort and provide greater flexibility in generating novel messages during spontaneous interactions. It is important that display interfaces be designed in a way that builds upon the relatively intact visuospatial skills and episodic memory of PWA, thereby reducing the cognitive demands to successfully use the interface.

Although AAC strategies are intended to facilitate communication in PWA, research has indicated that PWA may abandon high-tech AAC approaches because of cognitive demands related to navigating complex interfaces, inadequate individualization of messages stored on the SGDs, slow rate of communication, and stigmatization associated with using devices (Johnson, Inglebret, Jones, & Ray, 2006). This challenge can be reduced and/or eliminated by integrating communication partner training, evaluating participatory patterns of PWA, and conducting periodic follow up assessments to determine whether the AAC system is meeting the socio-communication and socio-relational needs of PWA.

These challenges are clearly identified in the following communication partner excerpts (Corwin, 2011). In this excerpt, the communication partner focuses

on limited messages available on AAC device, complex navigation required in identifying and selecting messages, and cognitive effort required to sustain interaction using high-tech AAC.

Interviewer: Does he really use it to communicate with somebody else?

Communication Partner: Uh . . . not so much. I think he uses it more for his own information. You know. And I think he likes to put things in it and then, when the computer says what he's put into it, then he can repeat it, you know. So, I think he uses it more for himself than he does for actually communicating. You know, unless there's something he just really can't get over to . . . you know, especially to me . . . if he's trying to tell me something, I'll go get it and I'll say, "Okay. Find something on there. A word. A picture. Anything." And he can do that. And sometimes that helps.

Interviewer: So, it's programmed adequately to be able to do that?

Caregiver: Uh-huh. I think so. As far as just . . . like in a conversation or something . . . I think a lot of the times it may be something that just . . . that he can't say that comes up only that one time, so that's not programmed, you know, into it. I mean, what's programmed into it are specific things. It's not like something that just might accidentally come up in a conversation, you know, and it would be impossible to get everything like that into it. So . . . but it's helpful as far as, just like I say, words and pictures or if he can find something related to what he's trying to say, then it helps. . . . We've got a couple of different little programs in there that kind of simplify a lot of it. But, you know, if you're trying to find something to say, it's . . . you have to go through too many different pages and too many different things trying to find what you're trying to say.

Interviewer: You can lose the thought by the time you found it?

Caregiver: [laugh] Yeah. Yeah. By the time you find it, it's like, I don't remember now! But I think mostly it's just . . . his patience isn't very long anymore. He gets really frustrated really easily if he has to go through too much trouble. He just won't do it. He'll say, "Oh forget it." So, we have simplified it as far as the program . . . just certain programs . . . as far as his basic needs and personal things . . . you know . . . that works out fine, but I don't know that he would ever really use it in a complete conversation.

■ AAC Intervention Using Technology or No Technology Options

This section provides a comprehensive review of technology-based and no-technology AAC intervention approaches for PWA. The salient feature of technology-based intervention approaches is the use of dedicated speech generating devices (SGDs) and/or software applications that turn computers or hand-held multi-purpose electronic devices (e.g., Apple iPad™, iPhone™, and Google Android™) into communication aids that produce synthetic or digitized speech upon selection of a message (Koul, 2011). In contrast, no-tech intervention approaches do not involve production of speech output upon selection of a message. Examples of no-tech approaches include communication boards/books, gestures and signs, and tangible objects. There is a substantial research evidence to support the effectiveness of both technology-based and no-tech AAC intervention approaches in facilitating communication for PWA (e.g. Ball & Lasker, 2013; Koul, Corwin, & Hayes, 2005; Koul & Harding, 1998; Koul & Lloyd, 1998; Koul et al., 2008; Wallace, Dietz, Hux, & Weissling, 2012).

High Tech AAC Intervention Approaches

Due to rapid advances in software development and miniaturization of hardware, AAC aids such as speech generating devices (SGDs) and software programs for hand-held multipurpose devices (e.g., iPad, Surface Pros) have become increasingly accessible for PWA (Koul, 2011; Koul, Petroi, & Schlosser, 2010). Most dedicated devices, software programs, and applications are recommended to persons with severe communication impairment, irrespective of the nature of their medical diagnosis and linguistic, behavioral, and cognitive characteristics. However, one commercially available SGD, Lingraphica, is designed and promoted for use by PWA (Lingraphica: The Aphasia Company, 2009). The currently available SGDs provide access to several different interface displays. These displays are described in the following sections.

Grid Displays

Commercially available SGDs provide people who rely on AAC options to access and retrieve messages using grid displays. Three types of grid displays are taxonomic, semantic-syntactic, and visual-scene displays (Beukelman & Mirenda, 2013). A taxonomic grid display presents symbols across multiple screens in a logical sequence (Figure 6–1). On the first page, people who rely on AAC may select one of the superordinate categories, such as food. This will correspond to a second screen with several subordinate categories (e.g., breakfast, lunch, dinner, etc.). Selecting "breakfast" on the second page will bring up a subordinate category for types of breakfast foods (e.g., cereals, fruits, drinks, etc.). The screens are designed to display each symbol or message on a distinct grid with an option to produce a spoken message upon selection of a symbol.

Previous research indicates that PWA can access, identify, manipulate, and combine symbols across multiple screens to produce simple sentences and phrases using taxonomic grid displays (Koul & Harding, 1998; Koul et al., 2008; Petroi et al., 2014; Weinrich, Boser, McCall, & Bishop, 2001; Weinrich, Shelton, Cox, & McCall, 1997).

Visual Scene Displays

The visual scene display (VSD) is an option for organizing messages that provides personalization and communicative context for both people who rely on AAC and their communication partners. A typical visual scene display presents an activity, place, or a situation using photographs, places, or virtual environments and contains symbols representing vocabulary elements (e.g., people, descriptors, feelings, etc.) that are organized schematically and accompanied by written phrases or

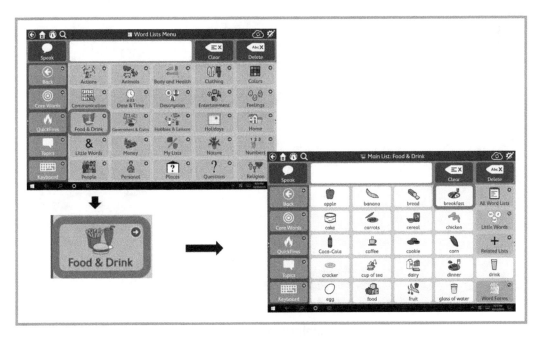

Figure 6–1. An example of a grid display on Tobii Dynavox I-13®.

sentences that support a variety of communicative functions (e.g., comments, questions, labels). PWA can navigate through multiple pages using a navigation ring. A navigation ring is a D-shaped layout where thumbnails of the other possible visual scenes border the currently active VSD. This allows for the PWA to select from a variety of thumbnails to navigate through pages on the SGD rather than sorting through words and icons on SGDs with dynamic displays (Beukelman, Hux, Dietz, McKelvey, & Weissling, 2015; Wallace & Hux, 2014).

When selecting photographs, places, or virtual environments to generate VSDs, data indicates that the combination of con-textualization and personal meaningfulness of photos positively facilitates communication for PWA (Beukelman et al., 2015; Griffith, Dietz, & Weissling, 2014; McKelvey, Hux, Dietz, & Beukelman, 2010). For instance, a picture of a beach does not provide a substantial amount of personal information and is generally decontextualized (Figure 6–2). However, a picture of a beach with a PWA's family sitting on a blanket under an umbrella laughing and playing board games provides both contextual information and personal relevance (Figure 6–3).

The relative effects of grid versus VSDs in facilitating target communicative behaviors in persons with chronic severe

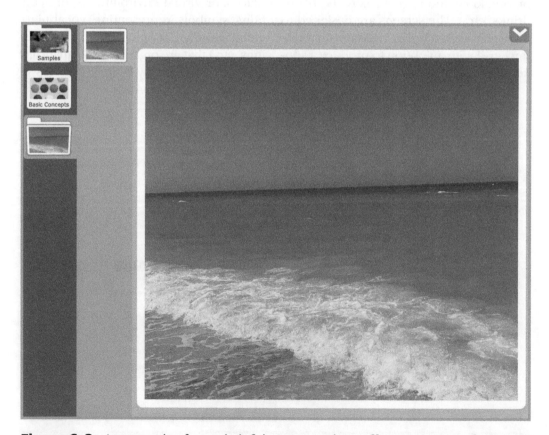

Figure 6–2. An example of an unhelpful picture with insufficient amount of personal information.

aphasia supports the greater potential for VSDs in facilitating communication (Beukelman et al., 2015; Brock et al., 2017). For example, Brock et al. (2017) explored the use of a grid display and a VSD across several communicative tasks during conversational interactions between a PWA and a communication partner. In experiment 1, the PWA watched an episode of *I Love Lucy* and was trained to use both grid and VSDs to engage in communicative interactions about the episode. Following training, the participant engaged in conversations with a communication partner using either the grid display or VSD. For the second experiment, the participant watched a second episode of *I Love Lucy* but did not receive any grid display or VSD training. The investigators examined the number of conversational turns, total conversation time, instances of frustration, navigational errors, complexity of utterances, and response accuracy. Results indicated that the participants' use of VSD resulted in greater number of conversational turns, and fewer instances of navigational errors and frustration. Additionally, the use of VSD resulted in relatively greater response accuracy and production of longer and more complex utterances in contrast to use of grid display. These results suggest that VSD's interface design and photographic content may be less demanding cognitively

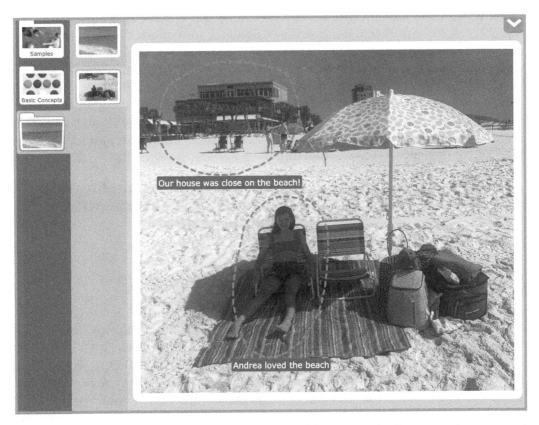

Figure 6–3. An example of a picture with highly personal-relevant and contextual information used in a visual scene display.

compared to the grid displays. Furthermore, graphic symbols in the grid display tend to lack context compared to contextually rich photographs used in VSDs. Thus, it is relatively difficult to combine graphic symbols across screens in a grid display to produce phrases and sentences. To summarize, the relative strengths of VSDs over grid layouts include ease of use, higher navigational accuracy, and greater number of efficient and effective communicative interactions (Beukelman et al., 2015; Brock et al., 2017; Koul, 2011).

Mobile Apps

Mobile tablets with communication apps (e.g., Snap + Core Plus™, SmallTalk™ Proloquo2Go™, Predictable™) will potentially increase accessibility to AAC technology to persons with severe communication impairment. Because mobile tablets support apps for therapy, communication, and entertainment, clinicians must examine models for app selection (e.g., Holland, Weinberg, & Dittelman, 2012; Munoz, Hoffman, & Brimo, 2013). An integral component of the selection and implementation of a communication app is "buy-in" or agreeing how to use the system by both the PWA and their stakeholders. One approach to achieve "buy-in" is to target a communication function valued by the PWA and introduce a communication app that supports that function. For example, hosting a book club may be identified as a meaningful goal. Introducing an app that will aid in specific scenarios or functions important to the PWA may provide the incentive to learn how to operate the tablet and the app. Other factors that affect the adoption of a mobile tablet by a PWA include the commercial availability, durability of a mobile tablet, portability, acceptance, support

from stakeholders, and the ease of finding, selecting, and purchasing apps (Holland, Weinberg, & Dittelman, 2012).

Mobile apps are not as straightforward to operate and maintain as they appear. Successful implementation often includes initial setup, routine updates, troubleshooting, connecting to Wi-Fi or cellular service, and adapting settings to fit the PWA's needs and preferences (Munoz, Hoffman, & Brimo, 2013). To alleviate the inconveniences of using a mobile app, it is crucial that communication partners and other stakeholders are trained and familiar with the PWA's communication app.

Although mobile apps are pervasive in many individuals' lives, it is imperative to remember that the introduction of each mobile app is associated to the introduction of an unfamiliar device (Zimmerman & Vanderheiden, 2008). Many rubrics (e.g., Fonner & Marfilius, 2011; Gosnell, Costello, & Shane, 2011; Lee & Cherner, 2015) are available for clinicians to refer to when selecting communication apps that best fit the PWA's needs and preferences.

Efficacy of Technologically Based AAC Intervention Approaches

Previous research supports the efficacy of technologically based AAC intervention approaches for persons with severe aphasia (Koul & Harding, 1998; Koul et al., 2008; McKelvey, Dietz, Hux, Weissling, & Beukleman, 2007; Nicholas, Sinotte, & Helms-Estabrooks, 2005). Koul (2011) conducted a systematic review of AAC intervention studies with PWA that involved technology as one of the treatment components. A comprehensive search for treatment studies using various databases yielded five single subject design and two group design studies that met the inclusion criteria. Study outcomes were classified as positive, negative, or mixed based on criteria proposed by Rispoli, Machalicek, and Lang (2010). Three single subject design studies reported positive outcomes (Koul & Harding, 1998; Koul et al., 2008; McKelvey et al. 2010; Nicholas et al., 2005) and one single subject design reported mixed outcome (Koul et al., 2005). Both group design studies reported positive outcomes (Beck & Fritz, 1998; van de Sandt-Koenderman, Wiegers, & Hardy, 2005). This systematic review suggested that PWA can use SGDs to identify, select, and combine symbols to produce simple sentences and phrases.

Additionally, Petroi and colleagues (2014) investigated the ability of persons with severe Broca's aphasia to complete a series of experimental tasks involving identification of single symbols and subject-verb-object sentences on an SGD in the absence or presence of competing stimuli. Participants included ten individuals with aphasia due to left hemisphere damage and ten individuals without brain damage who served as matched participants in the control group. Results indicated that both the number of symbols on the display and complexity of the navigation had a significant effect on the accuracy and latency of symbol identification for grid displays. Participants with aphasia demonstrated higher accuracy and identified symbols faster when navigation requirements were minimal. Having fewer number of symbols on the display also enhanced identification accuracy. However, navigation was observed to have a greater impact on identification of symbols than number of symbols on the display. This study indicates that clinicians must design displays for PWA that minimize cognitive effort and are relatively easy to navigate.

Griffith and colleagues (2014) examined the effect of interface design on the communication behaviors of four participants with moderate-severe Broca's aphasia using a narrative retell task. Four narratives were created on an AAC device with combinations of personally relevant photographs, line drawings, and text for each of the participants. The narrative retells were analyzed by expressive modality units used, trouble sources experienced, and trouble sources repaired. Qualitative data were also collected on each participant's perceived helpfulness of the interface features. Results indicated that participants relied more on personal relevant photographs than line drawings. However, participants reported that both picture types were equally helpful. Outcomes measures in trouble sources repaired indicated that visual and linguistic supports do not appear to affect the rate of trouble sources repaired.

Overall, research indicates that PWA are able to use both taxonomic grid and visual scene displays to produce sentences and simple phrases in a variety of settings (Koul et al., 2005; Koul & Harding, 1998; Weinrich et al., 1997; Weinrich et al., 2001). Further, PWA seem to have greater number of conversational turns, and fewer instances of navigational errors and frustration when using VSD compared to a taxonomic grid display (Beukelman et al., 2015; Brock et al., 2017; Koul, 2011). However, efficacy and effectiveness data are primarily based on studies conducted in structured experimental contexts and not in the "real world" settings. Future research should focus on collecting maintenance and generalization data across communicative contexts, settings, and partners.

No Tech AAC Intervention Approaches

Besides high-technology-based AAC strategies, there are several no-technology-based AAC methods that do not involve speech output upon selection of a message (Koul, 2011). No-technology-based AAC strategies include a variety of options for PWA—communication boards (e.g., picture board and spelling board), cue cards, memory books, photo albums, visual scenes, rating scales, signing, gestures, drawing, and so forth. Research indicates that no-technology-based communication strategies are effective to varying degrees in supporting communication for PWA (e.g., Fox, Sohlberg, & Fried-Oken, 2001; Jacobs, Drew, Ogletree, & Pierce, 2004; Lasker, Hux, Garrett, Moncrief, & Eischied, 1997).

Rating Scales

Rating scales are typically used as a strategy to help PWA share feelings, express opinions, and indicate pain. The most commonly used scales are Likert scales. These scales usually consist of numbers, words, or picture symbols. For example, a clinician may use the rating scale depicted in Figure 6–4 to ask a PWA for his food preference. The clinician presents a picture symbol of a type of food and asks the PWA to indicate if he likes it or not on a five-point Likert Scale. Other rating scales, for instance, pain scales are widely used in medical settings to help PWA indicate their level of discomfort.

Talking Mats©

Talking Mats© is a method to help PWA to express their opinions and views. Talking Mats© utilizes a set of pictures and a textured mat to allow PWA to indicate their feelings about various options under a specific topic by placing images below a visual scale (Murphy & Oliver, 2013). For example, PWA can use Talking Mats© to categorize symbols of everyday activities into three groups—things that the PWA is managing well, things that she is not quite sure about, and things that she may require assistance (Figure 6–5). For instance, a PWA is presented with a symbol of "shopping," asked, "how do you feel about going shopping?" Then sym-

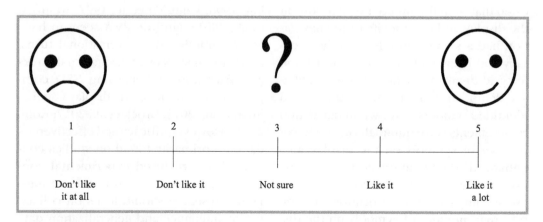

Figure 6–4. A sample rating scale for use with PWA.

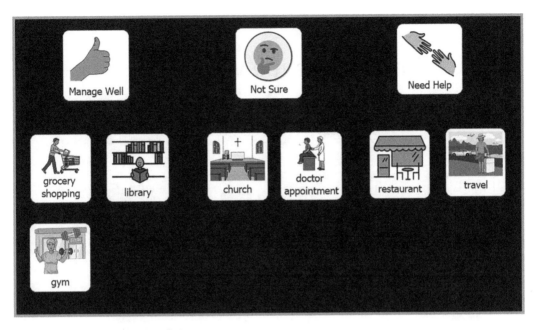

Figure 6–5. Talking Mat© for PWA.

bol is put under the one of the three categories mentioned above according to the PWA's response. By using Talking Mats©, PWA are given opportunities to express opinions and play an active part in the decision-making process.

Communication Board

A PWA may point to the symbols and/or words on a no-technology-based communication board to express his or her wants and needs and transfer information. Clinicians, PWA, and caregivers should work together to organize, and store messages based on PWA's communication needs as well as cognitive-linguistic competencies. Usually, a typical communication board consists of core messages to communicate about frequently occurring activities of daily living and a set of fringe messages to meet PWA's personal needs. Figure 6–6 provides an example of a communication

board for PWA to use in an acute care medical setting.

Spelling Board

Spelling boards are similar to keyboards and are composed of letters, digits, and other operational commands. PWA can point to the letters on a spelling board to convey messages. Sometimes spelling boards include frequently used words or phrases for specific contexts. Figure 6–7 provides an example of a spelling board typically used in a medical setting. One advantage of a spelling board is that it can help PWA communicate whatever they want rather than being limited to pre-stored messages. However, spelling boards can only be used with PWAs who have intact spelling and writing skills. PWAs who have severe reading and writing impairments cannot benefit from spelling boards.

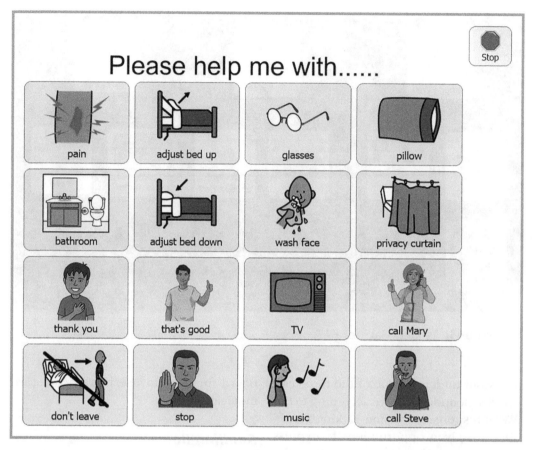

Figure 6–6. A sample communication board for PWA to use in medical settings.

Identification and Communication Card

Identification and communication cards help PWA disclose their communication impairment to unfamiliar speech partners. Figure 6–8 provides an example of an identification card. Identification cards contain information such as the PWA's name, the nature of his or her communication difficulties, and strategies to help facilitate communication. This card, especially the "to help me" section (see Figure 6–8) should be tailored to compensate for PWA's specific communication impairments and to enhance communicative effectiveness. The Aphasia Center's website (http://www.theaphasiacenter .com/pocket-card) provides free customizable options for PWA to create their own identification card.

Summary

No-technology-based AAC strategies can be relatively easy to use and create minimal financial burden for PWA and their family. These AAC strategies must be always individualized to meet PWA's specific needs across various contexts. It is recommended that clinicians provide a variety of no-tech-based AAC options for PWA to facilitate their communication.

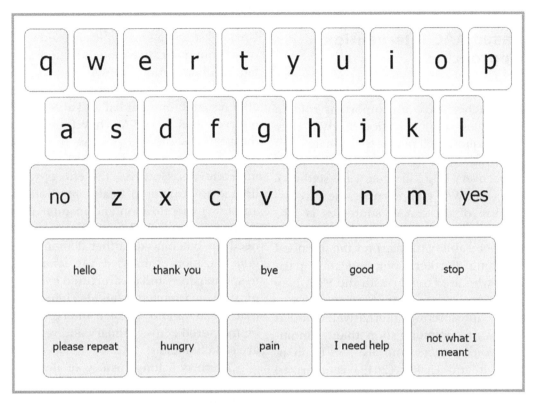

Figure 6–7. A sample of spelling board for PWA.

Please Read This

My name is _____ . I have aphasia from stroke. This means I have trouble understanding you and talking with you. I am intelligent but need some extra support during conversation.

Address: _____
Emergency Contact #: _____

To help me, please:

1. Use simple sentences to speak with me.
2. Ask me a question that I can answer with 'yes' or 'no' if I have trouble answering your open-ended questions.
3. Be patient and allow additional time for me to respond.
4. ......

Figure 6–8. A sample of an identification and communication card.

Efficacy of No-Technology Based AAC Intervention Approaches

No-technology-based AAC intervention approaches have an important role in enhancing communication of PWA. They are uniquely well placed to facilitate communication for PWA in the early stages of recovery (e.g., in acute care settings). Besides PWA's competences, the successful use of these AAC strategies is also dependent upon their communication partner's ability to interpret the intended meaning. Further, communication partners who are familiar with the PWA may experience relatively more success in correctly interpreting alternative, unaided forms of communication than communication partners who are less familiar. Garrett and Lasker (2013) categorized no-technology-based AAC strategies into four categories: unaided strategies, partner-dependent/partner-assisted strategies, use of external stored information, and use of self-formulated/self-generated messages. The descriptions, as well as the efficacy of these four strategies, are discussed below.

Unaided Strategies

Unaided AAC strategies involve the use of a person's own body part for communication purposes (i.e., without external aids or devices). Examples are manual signs, body position, facial expression, pantomiming, stereotypic utterances, and head nods/shakes, and so forth. These types of strategies can help PWA successfully convey messages to familiar communication partners or within familiar contexts. They may be particularly effective when PWA's residual speech is relatively intelligible and the unaided strategies (e.g., manual

sign, pantomiming) are easily discernible. Unaided strategies are typically used with other communicative modalities to facilitate communication in PWA.

Jacob et al. (2004) summarized available research on unaided and aided AAC interventions for PWA. They found that most studies showed positive treatment outcomes for both aided and unaided interventions. However, the effects were limited to structured treatment contexts and few generalization and maintenance data were reported. Thus, there is a critical need for outcome data that demonstrate generalization of unaided AAC strategies to spontaneous and unstructured communicative environments. It is also important that social validity of such interventions be measured across primary and secondary stakeholders.

There is a long history of unaided strategies as part of traditional aphasia intervention. Specifically, the use of symbolic gestures, emblems, and pantomimes has been observed to facilitate communication. Rose and Douglas (2008) and Rose, Raymer, Lanyon, and Attard (2013) observed that gestures were used to compensate as well as to facilitate spoken communication. They found that some PWA benefit from combined gesture and verbal treatment for production of nouns and verbs. They indicated that PWA can acquire symbolic gestures through gesture training that can generate effective treatment outcomes.

Partner-Dependent/ Partner-Assisted Strategies

Partner-dependent or partner-assisted strategies refer to the support provided by communication partners during conversation. The strategies include augmented input, written-choice communication, and other strategies to enhance PWA's auditory comprehension as well as expression.

Augmented input refers to any visual, linguistic, or other modalities of information used by the communication partner to facilitate language comprehension in PWA (Dada et al., 2019). These strategies can help to increase the saliency of the information presented and provide information redundancy that may reduce the cognitive load required to comprehend a message (Garrett & Lasker, 2013; Wallace et al., 2012). One example of augmented input is that the communication partner points to written words or pictures while talking with a PWA. With the same or similar information conveyed through the visual modality, the PWA gains a better understanding of the communication partner's spoken words.

Dada et al. (2019) compared the effectiveness of two augmented input conditions in facilitating auditory comprehension of narratives in PWA. In one condition, the communication partner actively pointed out key content words using visuographic support whereas in the second condition, participant's attention was not purposefully drawn to the visuographic supports. Their results indicated that visuo-graphic support such as high-context images and line drawings may be facilitative of auditory comprehension for some PWA.

Further, Brown, Wallace, Knollman-Porter, and Hux (2018) evaluated change in language comprehension in PWA across the following three conditions: auditory-only, written-only, and combined auditory and written condition. They measured participants' accuracy and preference for each condition. They found that PWA demonstrated significantly higher accuracy for the combined auditory and written condition. One interesting finding was

that compared to persons with mild and moderate aphasia, persons with severe aphasia benefited significantly more from the combined modality condition than the written-only modality. In addition, most participants preferred the information conveyed through both the auditory and written modality than through either one of the two modalities. The authors recommended that clinicians should individualize augmented input strategies based on observed effectiveness, preference, and access to instructional support.

Use of External-Stored Information

The external-stored information strategies refer to a PWA using an alternative mode of communication that has an external source for information. Examples of external-stored information are an album with relevant photographs, a communication book or a high-tech SGD. Research indicates that PWA are able to retrieve external-stored information for transferring information (Garrett & Huth, 2002; Ho, Weiss, Garrett, & Lloyd, 2005).

Fox et al. (2001) investigated the effects of conversational topic choice on the efficacy of AAC intervention in three persons with Broca's aphasia. Participants were assigned to two conditions: choice topic and nonchoice topic. Choice topics were topics of high interest for participants and nonchoice topics were assigned by the investigators. One participant demonstrated greater use of personal photographs, color photographs from magazines, and line drawings with word labels, when discussing choice topics. The other two participants did not demonstrate a difference in the use of type of symbols between the two conditions. The authors summarized that in natural communicative environments, use of AAC was dependent on several other factors (e.g., personal, environmental) besides the features of the symbols themselves. Although topic choice might promote improved use of communication aids for some PWA, other issues must also be considered for successful generalization to natural settings. For instance, PWA's clinical profiles, social network, partners' interests might all exert influence on the use of AAC strategies.

Ho et al. (2005) investigated effects of AAC intervention on several communicative functions in two individuals with global aphasia. These individuals interacted with a speech-language pathologist in three different experimental conditions: no external stored information available, use of Picture Communication Symbols (PCS) displayed in a communication book, and use of remnants (e.g., maps, photographs, magazine covers) displayed in a communication book. Results indicated that the persons with global aphasia had more successful interactions when symbols (either PCS or remnants) were used. They initiated more topics, successfully communicated messages more often, and experienced more positive effects when they had access to a communication book compared to when they did not. Results indicated that the number of unrepaired communication breakdowns were lower when given external communication support (i.e., pictographic book, remnant book). Specifically, remnant book seemed to have a greater effect in facilitating communication than a pictographic book. The authors conducted a follow-up interview with the clinician three years later after completion of data collection. The clinician who previously served as the conversational partner revealed that she and her colleagues continued to develop remnant books instead of pictographic books for persons with global aphasia for use in acute rehabilitation settings. The authors interpreted that the clinician's report provides a degree of social validity of the use of remnant books in the acute care settings. However, the use of remnant books in other settings, and its effectiveness in comparison with the pictographic book, requires further research.

Currently, external-stored information is easily infused with technology (e.g., Pictello™, audio-enhanced paper photos, speech-generating devices) to support PWA's communication and enhance their overall well-being (Griffith et al., 2014; Kurland, Wilkins, & Stokes, 2014; Piper, Weibel, & Hollan, 2014).

Use of Self-Formulated/ Self-Generated Messages

The self-formulated or self-generated messages are used when PWA utilize writing and/or drawing to compensate for their language impairments. With the successful use of self-formulated strategies, PWA can convey messages that may not be stored in their device or communication book. Self-generated drawing or writing are not often the focus of AAC intervention research. Drawing serves more as a component of a multimodality treatment package to boost PWAs' functional communication. Research indicates that drawing, as part of the aphasia intervention, helps PWA with conceptualization (Sacchett & Black, 2011) and naming (Farias, Davis, & Harrington, 2006 Hung & Ostergren, 2019). In contrast, writing was reported to have higher demand on the cognitive and linguistic systems (Harrington, Farias, Davis, & Buonocore, 2007; Hung & Ostergren, 2019). Beeson and Ramage (2000) investigated the benefits of drawing for PWA for the purposes of initiating and maintain communication. They observed that drawing can be successfully used by PWA as a means to augment communication. However, Koul and Corwin (2011) pointed out several challenges for PWA to use self-formulated methods. For example, it is possible that the drawings may be vague, and words might be misspelled. This would exert a burden on the communication partner to correctly interpret the message.

Summary

Based on overall research findings to date, we recommend that AAC intervention that involves multimodalities (e.g., partner-dependent strategies, external-stored information) seems to enhance communicative effectiveness and efficiency of persons with aphasia. Multimodal AAC strategies that increase the level of independence and participation across communicative contexts and settings have potential to enhance communication of PWA (Dada et al., 2019; Pierce, O'Halloran, Togher, & Rose, 2019).

■ AAC Interventions Based on Communication Needs, Competences, and Participation Levels

The previous sections described AAC intervention strategies and techniques based on the use of either dedicated technology or AAC applications used with mobile devices. Lasker, Garrett, and Fox (2007) provide another comprehensive model of AAC intervention based on PWA's communication needs, cognitive-linguistic competencies, and participation patterns. They classified communicative

needs and support required by PWA into two broad categories: partner-dependent and partner-independent communicators.

Partner-Dependent Communicators

Three distinct types of partner-dependent AAC communicators and the importance of partner training are discussed in the next section.

Emerging Communicators

Emerging communicators were previously referred to as basic-choice communicators (Garett & Lasker, 2013). These communicators primarily depict characteristics of persons with global aphasia who demonstrate severe impairment in all aspects of language (e.g., limit comprehension, expression, reading, and writing skills). Their verbal output is typically insufficient to support effective functional communication (Jacobs et al., 2004; Koul & Corwin, 2011). They tend to also have difficulties processing information as well as maintaining attention (Koul, 2011; Petroi et al., 2014).

Garett and Lasker (2013) identified the following intervention goals for emerging communicators: attend to tangible objects (e.g., clothing, food), personal photos or reminiscence items; show acceptance or rejection of a tangible choice using an alternate modality; and follow commands to take and return objects. They highlighted that intervention goals should focus on choice-making and signaling affirmation of preferred items and rejection for nonpreferred items.

They also observed several challenges that may be encountered during the intervention. For instance, PWA may demonstrate attention deficits; they may have poor comprehension without visual or personal contexts; they may have inconsistent signal for meanings (e.g., "yes" or "no"); they may demonstrate emerging awareness of daily routine, but feel confused by changes in new events; and they might not engage in functional speech or gestures. To assist PWA to overcome these challenges, collaboration among patients, familiar communication partners (e.g., family members, caregivers), and clinicians is necessary. Communication partner training is critical for treatment outcomes. Koul and Corwin (2011) suggested allowing an adequate amount of wait time for the PWA to recruit all possible strategies to achieve meaning-

ful communication. Partners should be trained to create choice-making opportunities to manage informational demands and provide multimodal support based on patients' communicative competences. Figure 6–9 provides an example of communication using AAC strategies with emerging communicators.

Contextual-Choice Communicators

The contextual-choice communicators are referred to as controlled-situation communicators. These typically include PWA who may have demonstrated characteristics of following aphasia subtypes: chronic severe Broca's aphasia, severe Wernicke's

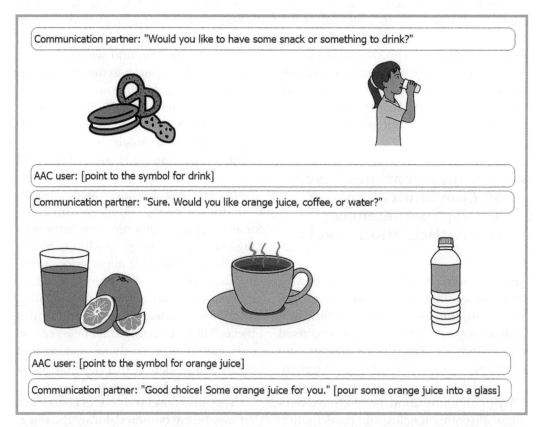

Communication partner: "Would you like to have some snack or something to drink?"

AAC user: [point to the symbol for drink]

Communication partner: "Sure. Would you like orange juice, coffee, or water?"

AAC user: [point to the symbol for orange juice]

Communication partner: "Good choice! Some orange juice for you." [pour some orange juice into a glass]

Figure 6–9. An example of an AAC intervention strategy for the emerging communicator.

aphasia, and transcortical motor aphasia (Koul, 2011). These communicators can answer questions or indicate a preference by pointing to pictures, photos, and line drawings. In addition, they are able to participate in multiturn conversations given partner scaffoldings (e.g., written choice, yes-no questions, augmented input). However, they seldom initiate communication on their own which can lead to social isolation (Koul, 2011).

Garrett and Lasker (2013) suggested the use of a written choice conversation technique to facilitate communication for contextual-choice communicators. During the intervention using the written-choice conversation method, communication partners ask open-ended questions and provide keywords for potential answers in the form of large print words. These choices are usually laid out vertically, which is easier for PWA with visual field deficits to scan and select. However, there is the possibility that none of the anticipated choices offered are appropriate. Thus, the communication partner should offer a standard choice that says, "None of the choices is my answer. Offer some others, please." Garrett and Lasker (2013) also recommended that contextual choice communicators can benefit from using graphic scales or maps to quantifying feelings, events, or locations. Figure 6–10 provides an example of a conversation between a contextual communicator and her communication partner using a written-choice conversation.

For contextual-choice communicators, it is also essential to train their communication partners to provide appropriate scaffolding to facilitate patients' auditory comprehension and expressive communication. If the PWA has a severe deficit in processing auditory information, communication partners should be trained to use augmented input strategies.

Communication partner: What would you like to talk about?
[Writes in large block letters while saying:
{MY DOG "My dog"
MY TRIP TO HAWAII "My trip to Hawaii"
MY FAVORITE FOOD "My favorite food""}]
AAC user: [points to MY TRIP TO HAWAII]
Communication partner: "Sounds interesting! Which islands have you been?"
[Shows a map of Hawaii while saying
AAC user: [Points to Oahu and Maui]
Communication partner: How nice! I have not been to Hawaii yet. I heard it is a beautiful place for a tropical vacation. Which is your favorite part of the trip?
[Writes in large block letters while saying:
SCENERY "Scenery"
FAMILY "Family"
MUSIC "Music"
SHOPPING "Shopping"]
AAC user: [Points to FAMILY, SCENERY, and SHOPPING]

Figure 6–10. An example of the written choice communication strategy for a contextual communicator.

For instance, writing down keywords or presenting photos, pictures, calendars, or maps will compensate for PWA's impaired auditory comprehension. At this stage of intervention, it is crucial to create a supportive environment to encourage PWA to make use of scaffolding to attend to speech partners' questions and maintain conversations.

Transitional Communicators

Transitional communicators are those who have demonstrated improvements over a period of time and are progressing toward being independent communicators with minimal partner support. These communicators can produce stored and novel messages and use various self-generated strategies to facilitate their communication. For example, they can use gestures or refer to photos or location to supplement their verbal expressions (Cress & King, 1999). However, transitional communicators might still rely on their speech partners' cues and prompts to answer questions and maintain conversations. They tend to require constant cueing to access stored messages or switch to an alternative mode of communication. Sometimes they are not able to independently repair communication breakdowns, resulting in frustration and withdrawal.

The AAC intervention goals for transitional communicators are as follows: use no-technology options (e.g., communication boards) or high-technology strategies (e.g., SGDs) to communicate in familiar contexts such as ordering food at a restaurant or answering highly predictable questions; make use of multimodal communication strategies to maximize communication outcomes; and initiate a conversation under familiar occasions or specific contexts with partners' support. Garrett

and Lasker (2013) suggested several strategies that are effective with transitional communicators: scripted interactions and role-playing, asking questions, storytelling, and the use of visual scenes to organize both narrative information and potential comments. The intervention at this stage is aimed at helping PWA to decrease the level of reliance on instructions and cues from clinicians and conversational partners. It is important for communication partners not to provide cues unless they are sure that the PWA is unable to convey messages without further scaffoldings.

The communication partners working with transitional communicators should be trained to provide a supportive communicative environment. For instance, they should provide hints and cues if necessary; allow extra waiting time to pause and expect communication from PWA; provide opportunities for communication about topics highly relevant to PWA's interests; and assist PWA's development of written scripts for role-playing and assist PWA to identify and organize messages on an SGD.

Partner-Independent Communicators

The partner independent communicators are independently able to use AAC strategies to facilitate their communication. Partner-independent communicators require minimal to no contextual support from their partners to initiate or maintain meaningful conversations (Koul, 2011). This category of PWA depict cognitive and linguistic patterns of persons with moderate Broca's aphasia, conduction aphasia, and transcortical motor aphasia. According to Garrett and Lasker (2013), these

PWA have the following characteristics: their auditory comprehension is relatively adequate to support their understanding of speech with little contextual support; they have enough cognitive-linguistic competence to formulate language to convey meaning through both natural communication (e.g., residual speech, gestures) and AAC strategies (e.g., pointing to pictures to compensate for limited speech intelligibility, finding messages stored in an SGD). Some of the main intervention goals for these PWA include using their AAC to repair communication breakdowns and communicate across variety of contexts.

Partner-independent communicators are further subclassified into three categories: stored-message communicators, generative-message communicators, and specific-need communicators.

Stored-Message Communicators

Stored-message communicators can locate messages that have been prestored in their SGDs. They have relatively adequate auditory comprehension to process the spoken language and may independently use AAC strategies to supplement their speech in familiar communicative situations (Garrett & Lasker, 2013; Koul, 2011). However, they might not feel comfortable about generating novel information to discuss unfamiliar topics, as their communicative skills are not adequate to support their independent participation in various communicative scenarios. They need assistance organizing and storing messages in their AAC systems and practicing AAC strategies across communicative settings. The intervention must focus on enhancing their ability to access, identify, and combine symbols and messages across screens to generate meaningful communi-

nication in a timely fashion. For example, an AAC intervention to order food at a restaurant for a stored-message communicator would be to identify and store a menu in an SGD and practice retrieval of the messages that would facilitate ordering food at a given restaurant across communication partners using a script. Garrett and Lasker (2013) recommend evaluating the following related to use of AAC strategies in real life settings: Effectiveness—does the PWA get the message across? Efficiency—what is the frequency of communication breakdowns? Changes—is there anything the PWA could have done to make the interaction go better?

Generative-Message Communicators

Some PWA can independently access messages in their AAC systems to communicate effectively in predictable situations. However, they are not yet capable of generating enough novel information to participate in discussions about unfamiliar topics. Their communication skills are not sufficient to support their participation in free-form conversation (Garrett & Lasker, 2013). Their ability to communicate novel messages is either fragmented or inconsistent resulting in communication breakdowns. For instance, they might experience inefficient communication when encountering highly demanding or unfamiliar communicative contexts; they sometimes require more time or several trials to complete communication attempts. Garrett and Lasker (2013) referred to these persons as comprehensive communicators who wish to participate in variety of communicative settings.

It is recommended to provide these communicators with a sufficient amount of training about different modalities of communications based on their need assessment and participatory patterns. Interventions goals for them include: independently combining various modalities and message components to create new expressions; independently navigating through multiple levels in a communication system to retrieve components and form a single message; mastering the use of prestored message in familiar situations to communicate effectively and efficiently; and being able to recognize communication breakdowns and resolve them with little to no external support. Garrett and Lasker (2013) suggested that intervention strategies for generative-message communicators should involve multimodal communication (e.g., residual speech, writing, gestures, communication board, SGD) to form messages with increased semantic complexity. For example, clinicians can train a PWA to say "that's good" while nodding his head, or pantomime playing golf and after that point to the symbol of golf on his SGD. It is essential for PWA to practice combining messages across modalities to achieve functional communication. They also state that the generative—message communicators should be trained to utilize metacommunicative strategies to repair communication breakdowns such as signaling to communication partners to check if they can understand and deciding about whether to continue or quit.

Koul (2011) suggested that one critical aspect of AAC intervention with generative-message communicators is to provide them with substantial instructions as well as practice opportunities to use their AAC strategies to communicate in real-life settings.

Specific-Need Communicators

Some PWAs who have a mild impairment in expressive language may not need to rely on AAC systems to meet their daily communication needs. They tend to make good use of residual speech, gestures, writing, or other strategies to communicate successfully in most social contexts. However, in some specific situations, they may wish to achieve a higher level of communicative efficiency and clarity. For instance, a person with a mild to moderate conduction aphasia may want to give a toast at her sister's wedding. She can work with her clinician to develop a script that integrates her humor, her love for her sister, and her appreciation for her sister's support. She can practice her toast in front of her clinician, and other familiar and unfamiliar people to make sure she feels comfortable giving the toast on the wedding day. As Garrett and Lasker (2013) suggested, clinicians should work with these specific-need communicators by suggesting and practicing strategies that help them overcome specific communicative challenges. Koul (2011) suggested that AAC interventions for these communicators may include analyzing the requirements of the specific communication tasks and providing techniques that can help them communicate with greater accuracy, efficiency, and confidence.

Summary

This section presented AAC intervention based on PWA's communication needs, competences, and participation levels. To help PWA transit from being partner-dependent communicators to independent communicators, clinicians should collaborate with PWA and their caregivers to complete needs assessments, suggest communicative modalities, organize messages on their AAC systems, create supportive practicing opportunities and make ongoing outcome measurements.

At each stage of the PWA's recovery, it is essential for clinicians to fully understand the PWA's communication needs and competencies. Also, they need to match the PWA's profile with the appropriate AAC intervention.

Conclusion

Several factors contribute to the success of AAC intervention for PWA. It is not only crucial that the PWA's capabilities are carefully matched to specific AAC strategies and techniques, but also that their primary communication partners are trained to implement communication strategies that facilitate communication of PWA. AAC intervention should also be dynamic, so that appropriate strategies are in place as PWA transition from being partner-dependent communicators to independent communicators. For PWA to spontaneously and independently generate novel utterances using AAC methods, clinicians must consider challenges associated with designing interface displays and message enhancement techniques that reduce cognitive effort for PWA. Additionally, partner training and identifying PWA's participatory patterns are key to successful use of AAC strategies for PWA.

■ Case Study

Samuel, a 59-year-old businessman, suffered a left cerebrovascular accident (CVA) in the region of the middle cerebral artery about 3 years ago, resulting in severe Broca's aphasia and apraxia of speech. Associated impairments included right hemiplegia that caused him to use a wheelchair. Prior to his stroke, Samuel was employed as a lawyer and was active in a community chess club and church. After his stroke and subsequent hospitalization, Samuel moved in with his daughter and son-in-law. He received speech-language therapy through a home health agency for 6 months. Treatment techniques included mapping therapy and melodic intonation training (Helm-Estabrooks & Albert, 2004; Thompson, 2001). Currently, Samuel communicates through pointing, gestures, and head movements accompanied by speech output in the form of "yes" and "no." Other verbalization attempts result in perseveration of approximation (i.e. "water, water, water") rather than the target word. Samuel's basic needs and wants are known to his daughter and son-in-law and are communicated using the previously mentioned nonverbal communication strategies. His daughter expressed that they often "have to play 20 questions" before knowing Samuel's actual request or thought. His daughter would like him to be able to clearly and efficiently express his needs, wants, and thoughts to both familiar and unfamiliar communication partners. Samuel would like to participate in chess meets again, but he expressed concern due to his lack of ability to communicate with others (e.g. competitors, friends). To help Samuel communicate more effectively in his home and community settings, technologically based AAC intervention was considered.

Studies comparing the efficacy of technology based AAC intervention approaches to no-technology AAC intervention approaches in persons with chronic severe Broca's aphasia across experimental and non-experimental settings were reviewed to make an informed recommendation. Results indicated that both technology based and no-technology-based AAC intervention options appeared to be effective. The findings were discussed with Samuel and his primary communication partners.

Their viewpoints, preferences, concerns, and expectations were considered when making the decision regarding which AAC interventions to try. Samuel and his daughter and son-in-law indicated that they were interested in trying a technology based AAC intervention approach. Samuel thought this approach may help him increase the number of social interactions with both familiar and unfamiliar communication partners.

After the decision was made to try an SGD, an assessment and intervention protocol was developed which included participation of both Samuel and his daughter and son-in-law. A predictive assessment that involved matching the capabilities of Samuel using several criterion-referenced tasks was implemented to select an SGD that best met his communication needs and goals (Glennen, 1997). Samuel tried several different SGDs from a university laboratory over a period of four weeks, and an SGD was selected that fit his capabilities and preferences. Following the trial period, an assessment report for Medicare funding for the SGD was prepared documenting his communication impairment, motor capabilities, sensory-perceptual capabilities, cognitive linguistic capabilities, as well as his ability to assess the SGD using a touch screen. The report also summarized Samuel's communication needs and communication goals.

After receiving the recommended SGD, Samuel participated in AAC intervention that focused on increasing his ability to share information with others through specific techniques and strategies, which increased his ability to share information with others. With input from Samuel and his family and friends, easily accessible messages were programmed in his device so that he can continue to maintain interactions with his friends and acquaintances. His primary communication partners (i.e., daughter and son-in-law) were also trained using Kagan's (1995) partner-dependent approach. This approach involved training and teaching communication partners skills so that they can in turn reveal the communicative competence of the PWA. The intervention program measured the frequency of the use of his SGD outside the clinical context by checking the log files in the device and the effectiveness of his communication by administering the Communicative Effectiveness Index (CETI) scale (Lomas et al., 1989) to his daughter and son-in-law. This scale measures the effectiveness of functional communication of the persons with aphasia as reported by the caregiver.

An informal interview was conducted to measure intervention outcomes for Samuel. Samuel and his family members reported that he was able to use his devices to make basic requests, express emotions, and make comments. He demonstrated higher level of independence regarding communication in new settings. Family and friends also supported and accepted Samuel's use of the device and suggested that it was easier to communicate with Samuel.

■ References

Ball, L. J., & Lasker, J. (2013). Teaching partners to support communication for adults with acquired communication impairment. *SIG 12 Perspectives on Augmentative and Alternative Communication, 22*(1), 4–15.

Beck, A., & Fritz, H. (1998). Can people who have aphasia learn iconic codes? *Augmentative and Alternative Communication, 14*(3), 184–196.

Beeson, P. M., & Ramage, A. E. (2000). Drawing from experience: The development of alternative communication strategies. *Topics in Stroke Rehabilitation, 7*(2), 10–20.

Beukelman, D. R., Hux, K., Dietz, A., McKelvey, M., & Weissling, K. (2015). Using visual scene displays as communication support options for people with chronic, severe aphasia: A summary of AAC research and future research directions. *Augmentative and Alternative Communication, 31*(3), 234–245.

Beukelman, D., & Mirenda, P. (2013). *Augmentative and alternative communication: Supporting children and adults with complex communication needs.* Brookes.

Brock, K., Koul, R., Corwin, M., & Schlosser, R. (2017). A comparison of visual scene and grid displays for people with chronic aphasia: A pilot study to improve communication using AAC. *Aphasiology, 31*(11), 1282–1306.

Brookshire, R. H., & McNeil, M. R. (2014). *Introduction to neurogenic communication disorders* [E-Book]. Elsevier Health Sciences.

Brown, J. A., Wallace, S. E., Knollman-Porter, K., & Hux, K. (2018). Comprehension of single versus combined modality information by people with aphasia. *American Journal of Speech-Language Pathology, 28*(1S), 278–292.

Corwin, M. (2011). Social validation of augmentative and alternative communication interventions in aphasia. In R. Koul (Ed.), *Augmentative and alternative communication for adults with aphasia: Science and clinical practice* (pp. 129–154). Brill.

Cress, C., & King, J. (1999). AAC strategies for people with primary progressive aphasia without dementia: Two case studies. *Augmentative and Alternative Communication, 15*(4), 248–259.

Dada, S., Stockley, N., Wallace, S. E., & Koul, R. (2019). The effect of augmented input on the auditory comprehension of narratives for people with aphasia: A pilot investigation. *Augmentative and Alternative Communication, 35*(2), 148–155.

Erickson, R. J., Goldinger, S. D., & LaPointe, L. L. (1996). Auditory vigilance in aphasic individuals: Detecting nonlinguistic stimuli with full or divided attention. *Brain and Cognition, 30,* 244–253.

Farias, D., Davis, C., & Harrington, G. (2006). Drawing: Its contribution to naming in aphasia. *Brain and Language, 97*(1), 53–63.

Fonner, K., & Marfilius, S. (2011). *Sorting through AAC apps.* Retrieved from http://www.spectronics.com.au/conference/2012/pdfs/handouts/kelly-fonner/Sorting%20AAC%20aaps%20OCT302011.pdf

Fox, L. E., Sohlberg, M. M., & Fried-Oken, M. (2001). Effects of conversational topic choice on outcomes of augmentative communication intervention for adults with aphasia. *Aphasiology, 15*(2), 171–200.

Frankoff, D. J., & Hatfield, B. (2011). Augmentative and alternative communication in daily clinical practice: Strategies and tools for management of severe communication disorders. *Topics in Stroke Rehabilitation, 18*(2), 112–119.

Garrett, K. L., & Huth, C. (2002). The impact of graphic contextual information and instruction on the conversational behaviours of a person with severe aphasia. *Aphasiology, 16*(4/5/6), 523–536.

Garrett, K. L., & Kimelman, M. D. Z. (2000). AAC and aphasia: Cognitive-linguistic considerations. In D. R. Beukelman, K. M. Yorkston, & J. Reichle (Eds.), *Augmentative and alternative communication for adults with acquired neurologic disorders* (pp. 339–374). Brookes.

Garrett, K., & Lasker, J. (2005). Adults with severe aphasia. In D. R. Beukelman & P. Mirenda (Eds.), *Augmentative and alternative communication: Supporting children and adults with complex communication needs* (3rd ed.). Brookes.

Garrett, K., & Lasker, J. (2013). Adults with severe aphasia and apraxia of speech. In D. R. Beukelman, & P. Mirenda (Eds.), *Augmentative and alternative communication: Supporting children and adults with complex communication needs,* (4th ed., pp. 404–446). Brookes.

Glennen, S. (1997). Augmentative and alternative communication assessment strategies. In S. L. Glennen & D. C. DeCoste (Eds.), *Handbook of augmentative and alternative communication* (pp. 149–192). Singular Publishing.

Goodglass, H., & Kaplan, E. (1983*). Boston Diagnostic Examination for Aphasia*. Lea & Febiger.

Gosnell, J., Costello, J., & Shane, H. (2011). Using a clinical approach to answer "What communication apps should we use?" *Perspectives on Augmentative and Alternative Communication, 20*(3), 87–96.

Griffith, J., Dietz, A., & Weissling, K. (2014). Supporting narrative retells for people with aphasia using augmentative and alternative communication: Photographs or line drawings? Text or no text? *American Journal of Speech-Language Pathology, 23*(2), S213–S224.

Harrington, G. S., Farias, D., Davis, C. H., & Buonocore, M. H. (2007). Comparison of the neural basis for imagined writing and drawing. *Human Brain Mapping, 28*(5), 450–459.

Helm-Estabrooks, N., & Albert, M. L. (2004). *Manual of aphasia and aphasia therapy* (2nd ed.). Pro-Ed.

Ho, K., Weiss, S., Garrett, K., & Lloyd, L. (2005). The effect of remnant and pictographic books on the communicative interaction of individuals with global aphasia. *Augmentative and Alternative Communication, 21*(3), 218–232.

Holland, A. L., Weinberg, P., & Dittelman, J. (2012). How to use apps clinically in the treatment of aphasia. *Seminars in Speech and Language. 33*(3), 223–233.

Hung, P. F., & Ostergren, J. (2019). A comparison of drawing and writing on facilitating word retrieval in individuals with aphasia. *Aphasiology, 33*(12), 1462–1481.

Jacobs, B., Drew, R., Ogletree, B. T., & Pierce, K. (2004). Augmentative and alternative communication (AAC) for adults with severe aphasia: Where we stand and how we can go further. *Disability and Rehabilitation, 26*(21–22), 1231–1240.

Johnson, J. M., Inglebret, E., Jones, C., & Ray, J. (2006). Perspectives of speech-language pathologists regarding success vs. abandonment of AAC. *Augmentative and Alternative Communication, 22*, 85–99.

Kagan, A. (1995). Revealing the competence of aphasic adults through conversation: A challenge to health professionals. *Topics in Stroke Rehabilitation, 2*, 15–28.

Kertesz, A. B. (1982). *Western Aphasia Battery*. Grune & Stratton.

Koul, R. K. (Ed.). (2011). *Augmentative and alternative communication for adults with aphasia: Science and clinical practice*. Brill.

Koul, R. K., & Corwin, M. (2011). Efficacy of no-technology-based AAC Intervention approaches. In R. K. Koul (Ed.), *Augmentative and alternative communication for adults with aphasia: Science and clinical practice*. Brill.

Koul, R., Corwin, M., & Hayes, S. (2005). Production of graphic symbol sentences by individuals with aphasia: Efficacy of a computer-based augmentative and communication intervention. *Brain and Language, 92*, 58–77.

Koul, R., Corwin, M., Nigam, R., & Oetzel, S. (2008). Training individuals with severe Broca's aphasia to produce sentences using graphic symbols: Implications for AAC intervention. *Journal of Assistive Technologies, 2*, 23–34.

Koul, R., & Harding, R. (1998). Identification and production of graphic symbols by individuals with aphasia: Efficacy of a software application. *Augmentative and Alternative Communication, 14*, 11–24.

Koul, R. K., & Lloyd, L. L. (1998). Comparison of graphic symbol learning in individuals with aphasia and right hemisphere brain damage. *Brain and Language, 62*(3), 398–421.

Koul, R., Petroi, D., & Schlosser, R. (2010). Systematic review of speech generating devices for aphasia. In S. Stern & J. W. Mullennix (Eds.), *Computer synthesized speech technologies: Tools for aiding impairment* (pp. 148–160). IGI Global.

Kurland, J., Wilkins, A. R., & Stokes, P. (2014). iPractice: Piloting the effectiveness of a tablet-based home practice program in aphasia treatment. *Seminars in Speech and Language, 35*(1), 51–64.

Lasker, J., Garrett, K. L., & Fox, L. E. (2007). Severe aphasia. In D.R. Beukelman, K.L. Garrett, & K.M. Yorkston. (Ed.), *Augmentative communication strategies for adults with acute or chronic medical conditions* (pp. 163–206). Brookes.

Lasker, J., Hux, K., Garrett, K., Moncrief, E., & Eischeid, T. (1997). Variations on the written choice communication strategy for individuals with severe aphasia. *Augmentative and Alternative Communication, 13*(2), 108–116.

Lee, C.-Y., & Cherner, T. S. (2015). A comprehensive evaluation rubric for assessing instructional apps. *Journal of Information Technology Education: Research, 14*, 21–53.

Lingraphica: The Aphasia Company. (2009). Retrieved from http://www.aphasia.com

Lomas, J., Pickard, L, Bester, S., Elbard, H., Finlayson, A., & Zoghaib, C. (1989). The Communicative Effectiveness Index: Development and psychometric evaluation of a functional communication measure for adult aphasia. *Journal of Speech and Hearing Disorders, 54*, 113–124.

McKelvey, M. L., Dietz, A. R., Hux, K., Weissling, K., & Beukelman, D. R. (2007). Performance of a person with chronic aphasia using personal and contextual pictures in a visual scene display prototype. *Journal of Medical Speech Language Pathology, 15*(3), 305.

McKelvey, M. L., Hux, K., Dietz, A., & Beukelman, D. R. (2010). Impact of personal relevance and contextualization on word-picture matching by people with aphasia. *American Journal of Speech-Language Pathology, 19*, 22–33.

McNeil, M. R., Odell, K., & Tseng, C. H. (1991). Toward the integration of resource allocation into a general theory of aphasia. *Clinical Aphasiology, 20*, 21–39.

Mountcastle, V. B. (1978). An organizing principle for cerebral function: The unit module and the distributed system. In G. M. Edelman & V. B. Mountcastle (Eds.), *The mindful brain: Cortical organization and the group—selective theory of higher brain function* (pp. 7–50). MIT Press.

Muñoz, M. L., Hoffman, L. M., & Brimo, D. (2013). Be smarter than your phone: A framework for using apps in clinical practice. *Contemporary Issues in Communication Science and Disorders, 40*, 138.

Murphy, J., & Oliver, T. (2013). The use of Talking Mats to support people with dementia and their careers to make decisions together. *Health & Social Care in the Community, 21*(2), 171–180.

Nicholas, M., Sinotte, M. P., & Helms-Estabrooks, N. (2005). Using a computer to communicate: Effect of executive function impairments in people with severe aphasia. *Aphasiology, 19*, 1052–1065.

Petroi, D., Koul, R. K., & Corwin, M. (2014). Effect of number of graphic symbols, levels, and listening conditions on symbol identification and latency in persons with aphasia. *Augmentative and Alternative Communication, 30*(1), 40–54.

Pierce, J. E., O'Halloran, R., Togher, L., & Rose, M. L. (2019). What is meant by "Multimodal Therapy" for aphasia? *American Journal of Speech-Language Pathology, 28*(2), 706–716.

Piper, A. M., Weibel, N., & Hollan, J. D. (2014). Designing audio-enhanced paper photos for older adult emotional wellbeing in communication therapy. *International Journal of Human-Computer Studies, 72*(8–9), 629–639.

Porch, B. E. (1981). *Porch index of communicative ability* (3rd ed.). Consulting Psychologists Press.

Purdy, M., & Dietz, A. (2010). Factors influencing AAC usage by individuals with aphasia. *Perspectives on Augmentative and Alternative Communication, 19*, 70–78.

Rispoli, M., Machalicek, W., & Lang, R. (2010). Subject review: Communication interventions for individuals with acquired brain injury. *Developmental Neurorehabilitation, 13*, 141–151.

Rose, M., & Douglas, J. (2008). Treating a semantic word production deficit in aphasia with verbal and gesture methods. *Aphasiology*, *22*(1), 20–41.

Rose, M. L., Raymer, A. M., Lanyon, L. E., & Attard, M. C. (2013). A systematic review of gesture treatments for post-stroke aphasia. *Aphasiology*, *27*(9), 1090–1127.

Sacchett, C., & Black, M. (2011). Drawing as a window to event conceptualisation: Evidence from two people with aphasia. *Aphasiology*, *25*(1), 3–26.

Thompson, C. (2001). Treatment of underlying forms: A linguistic specific approach for sentence production deficits in agrammatic aphasia. In R. Chapey (Ed.), *Language intervention strategies in aphasia and related neurogenic communication disorders* (4th ed., pp. 605–628). Lippincott Williams & Wilkins.

Van de Sandt-Koenderman, M., Wiegers, J., & Hardy, P. (2005). A computerized communication aid for people with aphasia. *Disability and Rehabilitation*, *27*, 529–533.

Wallace, S. E., Dietz, A., Hux, K., & Weissling, K. (2012). Augmented input: The effect of visuographic supports on the auditory comprehension of people with chronic aphasia. *Aphasiology*, *26*(2), 162–176.

Wallace, S. E., & Hux, K. (2014). Effect of two layouts on high technology AAC navigation and content location by people with aphasia. *Disability and Rehabilitation: Assistive Technology*, *9*(2), 173–182.

Weinrich, M., Boser, K. I., McCall, D., & Bishop, V. (2001). Training agrammatic subjects on passive sentences: Implications for syntactic deficit theories. *Brain and Language*, *76*(1), 45–61.

Weinrich, M., Shelton, J. R., Cox, D. M., & McCall, D. (1997). Remediating production of tense morphology improves verb retrieval in chronic aphasia. *Brain and Language*, *58*(1), 23–45.

Zimmerman, G., & Vanderheiden, G. (2008). Accessible design and testing in the application development process: Considerations for an integrated approach. *Universal Access in the Information Society*, *7*(1–2), 117–128.

7

Decision-Making for Access to AAC Technologies in Late Stage ALS

*Deirdre McLaughlin, Betts Peters, Kendra McInturf,
Brandon Eddy, Michelle Kinsella, Aimee Mooney, Trinity Deibert,
Kerry Montgomery, and Melanie Fried-Oken*

■ Introduction

> How important is communication to you?
>
> "There are no words to describe how important it is for me to communicate independently! Personally, I can't imagine life without a communication device. It is as important for me as breathing and nutrition."
>
> —Rich, individual with late stage ALS

Within the past 20 years, augmentative and alternative communication (AAC) intervention has dramatically improved means of expression for people with ALS. Changes have occurred at many levels, from national advocacy and AAC funding policies, to technological advances such as preserving your voice with message and voice banking and the promise of brain-computer interface for computer control. Three significant paradigm shifts have occurred during the past two decades for our global society. First, there is an increased interest in distance or digital communication worldwide. The general population now accesses many services through the Internet, relying on computers for shopping, banking, information retrieval, employment, entertainment, and dyadic communication (Shane et al., 2011). Second, the growth of personal mobile technologies has opened up the acceptability of relying on technology for communication for the general population, reducing the stigma of introducing AAC devices for individuals who cannot use speech for effective message generation (McNaughton & Light, 2013). These advances have benefited people with ALS if they have a means to select content or to interact accurately and efficiently with computers. Finally, access technologies, or the means to physically interact with communication options, have experienced significant attention and development, especially in the past decade (Fager et al., 2012, 2019).

In this chapter, access technologies for people with ALS in the late stages of the disease are highlighted. This population often has very limited or minimal movement and few reliable, consistent options to connect to technology for communication, recreation, environmental control, social connection, and cognitive stimulation. Information is presented on the classification of late stage ALS, including both impairment-based symptoms and function-based perspectives. Then, a clinical example is offered, describing Rich, a man with late stage ALS who has chosen to undergo tracheostomy and extend his life with the support of mechanical ventilation. Current and emerging access technologies, including eye tracking, switch scanning, multimodal access, and the promise of brain-computer interface as means to interact with AAC technologies is also discussed throughout. Guidelines for clinical decision making are proposed and questions are offered to assist individuals with ALS and their clinical teams motor skills worsen. Decision-making guidelines are illustrated with another clinical case, written in collaboration with a person with ALS.

The Presentation of Late Stage ALS

ALS can be discussed according to diagnosis and impairment level, or by function and participation levels. This chapter is grounded in the International Classification of Functioning (ICF) framework (World Health Organization, 2001), using a functional classification. Individuals with the diagnosis of ALS will be referred to as PALS (persons with ALS). The needs and technologies available for PALS in late stages of the disease follow.

There are many staging processes and group classifications that capture ALS disease progression and the resulting functional impairments of activities in daily living. In clinical neurology, late stages of ALS are defined in terms of how many system regions or system functions (respiratory, swallowing, movement, communication) are impacted by the disease. For instance, scales for staging the disease progression using four to five steps range from no functional impairment to death (Chiò et al., 2015; Roche et al., 2012) King's clinical staging system stipulates five stages based on clinical regions of involvement ranging from stage 1, involvement of one clinical area (e.g., movement, breathing, swallowing, communication), to stage 5, death (Roche et al., 2012). The MiToS functional staging system also includes 5 stages, but is based on loss of independence rather than neurophysiology (Chiò et al., 2015). The six discrete steps progress from stage 0, functional involvement (but not loss of independence) in a single domain, to stage 5, death. Figure 7–1 (adapted from Fang et al., 2017) compares the two rating scales. Late ALS, or the stage prior to death in these frameworks, is defined as either a need for gastrostomy and respiratory support (ventilation) (Roche et al., 2012) or as loss of independent function in the following four domains: swallowing, communicating, breathing, and movement (Chiò et al., 2015).

Within the field of communication sciences and disorders, PALS have been grouped by the level of reliance on AAC supports secondary to loss of speech,

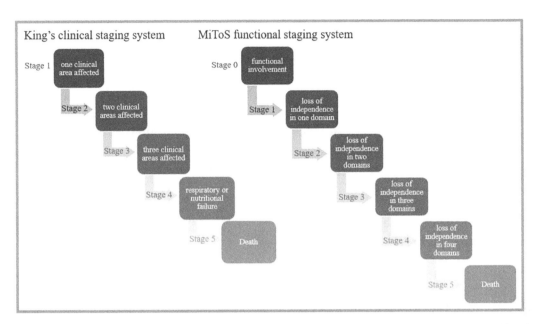

Figure 7–1. This figure depicts two ALS staging scales from neurology literature that captures physiological changes associated with the disease and resulting functional impairment. This figure is adapted from a scientific journal article comparing the scales (Fang et al., 2017). King's clinical staging system stipulates (*right*) five stages based on clinical regions of involvement, ranging from stage 1, involvement of one clinical area (e.g., movement, breathing, swallowing, communication), to stage 5, death (Roche et al., 2012). The MiToS functional staging system (*left*) progress from stage 0, functional involvement (but not loss of independence) in a single domain, to stage 5, death (Chiò et al., 2015).

hand, or mobility functions associated with disease progression. Using a six-group model, Yorkston and colleagues (1993) classify PALS according to speech, hand functioning, and mobility. The six groups are:

Group 1: Adequate Speech and Adequate Hand Function. This group is comprised of individuals with either no detectable motor speech disorder, a motor speech disorder without changes to speech intelligibility, or a motor speech disorder with reduced speech intelligibility that does not require the use of AAC. Hand functioning is considered to be adequate to accomplish self-help tasks with minimal assistance.

Group 2: Adequate Speech and Poor Hand Function. This group is composed of individuals with either no detectable motor speech disorder, a motor speech disorder without changes to speech intelligibility, or a motor speech disorder with reduced speech intelligibility that does not require the use of AAC. Hand functioning to support written communication is severely impaired.

Group 3: Poor Speech, Adequate Hand Functioning, Adequate

Mobility. This group is composed of individuals with a motor speech disorder characterized by poor speech intelligibility and reliance on AAC. Hand functioning and mobility are adequate to accomplish activities of daily living with minimal assistance.

Group 4: Poor Speech, Adequate Hand Functioning, Poor Mobility. This group is composed of individuals with a motor speech disorder characterized by poor speech intelligibility and reliance on AAC. Mobility is impacted for long distances and individuals require the use of an assistive device (e.g., cane, wheelchair, walker). Hand functioning is considered to be adequate to accomplish self-help tasks with minimal assistance.

Group 5: Poor Speech, Poor Hand Functioning, and Good Mobility. This group is composed of individuals with reduced speech intelligibility, requiring the use of AAC. Hand functioning to support written communication is severely impaired. Ambulation is independent without assistive equipment (e.g., cane, wheelchair, and walker).

Group 6: Poor Speech, Poor Hand Functioning, and Poor Mobility. This group is composed of individuals with a motor speech disorder characterized by poor speech intelligibility and reliance on AAC, hand functioning to support written communication that is severely impaired, and mobility difficulties that require the use of assistive equipment (e.g., cane, wheelchair, and walker). This is the population that this chapter is focused around given the significant complex access challenges

that are posed by functional changes at this stage.

What are the clinical challenges presented by PALS in group 6? Below, Rich is described as an example of a PALS presenting in Group 6. Afterward, motor, vision, cognition and language, and psychosocial conditions common to PALS in Group 6 are reviewed in order to determine how best to generate consistent and reliable access methods for these individuals.

One PALS' Challenge

Rich is a 40-year-old retired physician who was diagnosed with spinal-onset ALS five years ago. He lives at home with his wife and three school-age children, and receives caregiving help from in-home nursing staff and other family members who live nearby. Soon after his diagnosis, he had difficulty with computer access and began using a head mouse and speech-recognition software instead of a mouse and keyboard. Approximately two years later, Rich received a tracheostomy to provide full-time invasive respiratory support and was no longer able to speak. A speech-language pathologist helped him obtain a speech-generating device, which he controlled using the head mouse. As his ALS progressed, Rich's head control became increasingly unreliable. He fatigued quickly and made frequent errors when using the head mouse with his SGD. Rich and his family wondered whether there were other alternative access options that would work better for him, and how he could continue to communicate as his motor function deteriorated.

Challenge: What factors need to be considered to help Rich communicate effectively at this stage in his disease process?

Motor Challenges in ALS

Changes in motor function, with upper and lower motor neuron signs and symptoms, are clinical hallmarks of ALS. Presentation and progression vary considerably from person to person. A majority of PALS present with spinal-onset ALS, in which the initial symptoms involve weakness or stiffness in the upper or lower extremities. The alternative presentation is bulbar-onset ALS, in which speech or swallowing difficulties develop first (Kiernan et al., 2011). Weakness and atrophy, stiffness, slowness and incoordination lead to difficulties with hand and/or arm movements that affect performing activities of daily living and manipulation of small objects, typing, or writing. Regardless of the type of onset, ALS is a progressive disease, and therefore, its characteristic upper and lower motor neuron changes will eventually spread to other muscle groups (Borasio & Miller, 2001). Eventually, most or all voluntary motor function is affected, though eye movement is typically preserved (Mitsumoto & Rabkin, 2007). Motor speech skills, as part of motor function changes in ALS, decline during the disease progression (Green et al., 2013). According to Ball, Beukelman, and Pattee (2004) 95% of the people with ALS in the Nebraska ALS Database have

reduced speech intelligibility at some time prior to death.

As a result of these progressive changes, many PALS use multiple access methods for AAC or other technologies over the course of the disease. Individuals with bulbar-onset ALS may lose the ability to speak early on, but still may be able to type effectively on a physical keyboard or touch screen. By contrast, those with spinal-onset ALS may maintain some functional speech for months or years, but require alternative access such as a joystick, head mouse, or eye tracker to type on a computer. By the later stages of the disease, most PALS will experience severe impairments in both speech and limb function. Some eventually progress to a locked-in state, in which only eye movements are preserved, or a completely locked-in state, in which all voluntary motor function is lost (Murguialday et al., 2011). These individuals require AAC to meet their communication needs, but may have limited options for alternative access due to their reduced motor capabilities.

Cognition and Language Challenges in Late Stage ALS

Cognitive and behavioral changes in PALS have been consistently documented (Elamin et al., 2013; Goldstein & Abrahams, 2013) and are accepted as common features of the disease. Recent estimates note that approximately 50% of PALS experience cognitive impairment, of whom 15% present with frontotemporal dementia (FTD) (Crockford et al., 2018) as measured with the King's Clinical Staging System, and cognitive and behavioral change, measured with the Edinburgh Cognitive and Behavioural ALS Screen (ECAS). Changes vary widely and may range from mild impairments detected on neuropsychological testing, to profound FTD. Executive function, behavior, and language are the most likely areas to be involved (Achi & Rudnicki, 2012). Clinicians report that if PALS pursue all treatment measures to live as long as possible, the risk for developing FTD is higher. Crockford et al. (2018) conducted a large multicenter observational cohort of 161 patients with ALS and report that cognitive deficits and behavior impairment are more prevalent in severe disease stages, and by the end stages of the disease, only a small percentage of PALS present with no neuropsychological impairment. The impact of cognitive impairment affects both acceptance of, and ability to learn, initiate, and use AAC (Ball et al., 2007).

It is very difficult to determine if language functions, separated from cognition, are affected in late stage ALS, because motor skills, including oral motor speech skills for responding and upper extremity motor skills for pointing or typing, are significantly impacted. The ALS Functional Communication Scale (Table 7–1) lists seven communication abilities and activities that change over the course of the disease progression (http://www.amyandpals.com/als-communication-scale/). The scale was designed to document, longitudinally, the cognitive communication skills to be targeted as treatment goals for intervention, from initial diagnosis through late stage of the disease.

Vision Challenges in End Stage ALS

It is critical to consider visual skills in PALS, especially in late stages of the disease, since AAC frequently involves visual interfaces (Chen & O'Leary, 2018). PALS who choose mechanical ventilation, thereby prolonging life in the face of continuing deterioration of motor function, may rely on eye gaze or BCI when other muscle groups are no longer capable of serving as control sites. Extraocular motor neurons are often spared until late stage ALS. There are some reports, however, of visual impairments presenting in ALS. Moss and colleagues (2012) compared neuro-ophthalmic evaluations of 37 PALS followed in a multidisciplinary ALS clinic with matched participants in the control group without disabilities. They found that visual acuity was lower in PALS versus participants in the control group. Some PALS also presented with gaze impersistence, moderately to severely restricted voluntary up-gaze, and moderate-to-severe eyelid opening apraxia, or severely saccadic horizontal smooth pursuits. Additionally, oculomotor abnormalities, including smooth pursuit eye movements, optokinetic nystagmus, and visual suppression of vestibular nystagmus were noted in a sample of nine patients with ALS in the early stages (Ohki et al., 1994). AAC clinicians should seek assistance from professionals who can conduct a visual screening and a comprehensive ophthalmologic evaluation when appropriate when considering eye tracking and eye gaze as an access technology in late stage ALS (Fried-Oken et al., submitted for publication).

Psychosocial and Emotional Challenges in Late Stage ALS

Coping with the late stages of ALS, where activities of daily living are significantly restricted by the functional limitations of

Table 7–1. ALS Functional Communication Scale*

Communication Ability	Short-Term Goals	Baseline	Projected	Achieved Today
1. Alerting/ Emergency	Patient (and caregiver) can demonstrate/describe the method by which patient can alert others, not in his/her immediate environment, to a need or emergency	+/−	+/−	+/−
2. Communication Strategies	Patient (and caregiver) demonstrate patient and partner strategies that improve communication success, efficiency, speed, and reduce fatigue	+/−	+/−	+/−
3. Nonvoiced (Low Tech) Communication	Patient demonstrates the ability to communicate novel messages via spelling or combining words using a low tech AAC method	+/−	+/−	+/−
4. Speech Generation	Patient demonstrates the ability to communicate a novel message with a voice (speech or SGD)	+/−	+/−	+/−
5. Communicate with Those at a Distance	Patient demonstrates abilities to use all methods s/he requires to communicate with partners at a distance	+/−	+/−	+/−
6. Independently Set Up and Customize AAC systems	Patient (and caregiver) demonstrate the ability to independently use, set up, and customize low and/or high tech augmentative communication equipment	+/−	+/−	+/−
7. Prepare for Future Changes	Patient (and caregiver) can describe one or more proactive strategies designed to prepare for typical changes associated with ALS in speech/access.	+/−	+/−	+/−
Total Functional Communication Score		/7	/7	/7

*The ALS Functional Communication Scale developed by Amy Roman (2004) lists seven communication abilities and activities that change over the course of the disease progression (http://www.amy andpals.com/als-communication-scale/). The scale was designed to document, longitudinally, the cognitive communication skills that should be targeted as treatment goals for intervention, from initial diagnosis through late stage of the disease.

the disease process is challenging both for PALS and their families. In a large sample of PALS, 37% of patients reported mild-to-moderate depression symptoms, 13% reported moderate-to-severe depression symptoms, 6% reported severe depression symptoms, and 18% reported clinical-level anxiety symptoms (Wicks et al., 2007). Likewise, in a separate sample, depression and anxiety levels were reported in 20% of the family members of PALS (Lillo et al., 2012). Perceived social support and appraisal of one's coping potential and independence is a predictor of depressive symptom severity for PALS (Matuz et al., 2015). The most important stressors identified by PALS and family members are existential concerns (e.g., worries about the future, loss of faith in religion, worries about disease progression), and physical concerns (e.g., muscle weakness, mobility problems, ADL) (Trail et al., 2004). Caregiver burden affects the psychosocial well-being of PALS and their family members. The strongest predictor of caregiver burden appears to be cognitive/behavior changes (reported between 10% to 40% of sample) rather than physical limitations of the disease (Lillo et al., 2012).

AAC clinicians must consider the significant emotional and psychosocial burdens on PALS and their families that present challenges in the later stages of the disease process. Often, the multidisciplinary team includes a social worker, psychologist, or palliative care specialist who can work with the family and patients at this time. Costello (2009) suggests that common roles for speech-language pathologist on palliative care teams and in end of life care include: (1) supporting autonomy whenever possible; (2) providing care information and encouraging questions; (3) encouraging

patients to talk about their experience of illness; (4) supporting self-expression through use of unaided and aided communication strategies; (5) selecting vocabulary for aided communication systems that is personalized and reflects medical, social-connectedness, and psychosocial needs; (6) assisting with message and voice banking; (7) supporting maintenance of social and emotional ties through communication; and (8) supporting patients to express concerns for those left behind.

■ Possible AAC Solutions

Finding appropriate AAC technology solutions for PALS and their care providers, even in late stage ALS, remains an important clinical goal. Ball et al. (2004) reported that about 96% of people with ALS in the Nebraska ALS Database who were recommended AAC in a timely manner accepted and used AAC, with only 6% delaying but eventually accepting technology use. Those who rejected AAC presented with compounding severe health challenges, such as cancer, or concomitant dementia (Ball et al., 2004). The availability of access technologies has been shown to improve quality of life for adults with ALS and has the potential to reduce the burden placed on care providers (Hwang et al., 2014). It is important to note that low-tech solutions with different access options are critical to present, and often are preferred by PALS during the final stage of the disease. Possible access technologies (both high tech and low tech) appropriate for AAC for people who experience late stage ALS are discussed below.

Using Eye Gaze Technologies in Late Stage ALS

Eye tracking technologies have been widely used internationally with PALS (Käthner et al., 2015; Pasqualotto et al., 2015; Spataro et al., 2014) and evaluated via electrooculography (EOG). These technologies range from eye transfer boards (also known as ETRAN) (Fried-Oken, 2000), and the Speakbook, an eye gaze flip book (Joyce, 2011), to digitized speech devices, such as the Megabee™ Eye Pointing Communication Tablet (*MegaBee: Electronic hand-hand communication tablet*, 2010), and finally to computer-based speech generating devices. All eye gaze-based technologies require PALS to look at different parts of the page or screen, and a partner or the computer speaks out what is selected by eye gaze.

The ETRAN board and SpeakBook both involve printed letters or messages, typically presented on a piece of paper or Plexiglas frame. A communication partner looks at the PALS through a hole in the paper or frame, and observes the PALS' gaze as she or he looks at letters or phrases. A coding system is typically used, for example, looking at the top left corner and then the pink dot selects the pink letter in the top left corner. The Megabee™ is an electronic version of the same concept. A communication partner holds up the Megabee and watches as the PALS looks at colored targets in different locations around the central window, then the communication partner presses a colored button for each selection. The Megabee decodes these button-press inputs and prints the resulting message on a small screen.

High-tech eye tracking technologies that provide direct selection to language on communication devices typically collect data on eye gaze position using infrared pupil-corneal reflection. Devices that utilize these methods often include an eye tracking module with a built in infrared light source and camera. As the user looks at various points on the display during a calibration, the camera detects the changing distance between the pupil and a "glint" or reflection of the infrared lightsource from the cornea.

Challenges With Eye Tracking Technologies

> What is challenging about using your eye tracker?
>
> "[Using eye tracking with dwell click is] mentally and physically stressful, frustrating, and exhausting. There is so much strain involved that it increases my heart rate and respiratory rate. I have to take frequent breaks before continuing."
>
> —Rich

Eye tracking technologies are prone to error at various levels including user eye-conditions, shifting position of the user or device, and environmental factors. For example, changes in the ambient light conditions in the environment can significantly impact performance, and PALS regularly report difficulties accessing their eye tracking speech-generating devices outdoors due to competing infrared light sources. Even when indoors, changing lighting conditions can result in problems with reliable eye gaze use.

Positioning changes also have the potential to significantly alter performance of eye gaze technologies. People with late stage ALS experience regular positioning changes as care providers must shift their positioning to prevent bedsores or manage incontinence. Sometimes the device itself must be moved away from the PALS for care activities. Chen and O'Leary (2018) point out that a device positioned too high will result in eyelid fatigue or eyestrain due to looking upward, yet an eye gaze device positioned too low may not read the angle of the user's eyes correctly due the upper lid obscuring part of the pupil from the camera.

Several tools and strategies may support reliable and consistent positioning for use of eye tracking speech-generating devices. Mounting solutions may affix the device directly onto a hospital bed and offer the ability to swing away to a locked position to address the PALS' medical needs, then to swing back and lock in the original position. Some PALS benefit from a rolling-floor mount that allows the device to be positioned more flexibly. A challenge of these tools is to return them to the same position after being removed. Historically, clinicians adjusted multiple levers to approximate the necessary position. Novel float arm mounts have been developed that allow the clinician or caregiver to easily move the device into the necessary position without adjusting multiple levers. Although current mounting solutions are somewhat limited, emerging solutions are in development that may detect a user's head position and adjust the position of the device to match.

Person-centered factors may also result in reduced reliability in eye gaze technology for PALS. Many PALS who utilize eye gaze technologies use a dwell-to-select method of button selection. That is, PALS will look at a button for a predetermined period of time that causes the button to activate. For those using this method, Chen and O'Leary (2018) suggest an ideal dwell time of 0.5 seconds for general eye tracking use, but optimal dwell times have not been explored for PALS. It is likely that PALS with reduced ocular motility will have difficulty directing their gaze from target to target quickly enough to avoid frequent errors with a short dwell time. For example, a PALS who is able to consistently move a body part, such as their finger, toe, jaw, or eyebrow, can activate a switch for a click-to-select method of activation (much like using a computer mouse). As an alternative to activating a switch, a PALS may utilize a blink-to-select activation method. In this case, the user looks at a desired button then blinks their eyes to select it (blinks for selection are longer in duration than normal involuntary blinks). However, PALS often report that this activation method as fatiguing and can become less reliable as the disease progresses.

A critical factor associated with effective use of eye tracking technologies is the quality of the PALS' visual skills as it relates to visual access. Visual skills such as fixation, acuity, ocular motility, binocular vison, convergence, field of vision, and perceptual abilities have all been identified as fundamental for successful use of visually based assistive technology such as AAC (Federici & Scherer, 2012). Specifically, an impairment of one or more of these visual skills may affect the ability of the PALS to effectively analyze and manipulate visual information in the environment, influencing their ability to also understand, problem solve, and execute a plan when utilizing AAC technologies (Warren, 1993).

Using Switch Scanning in Late Stage ALS

Another common access method to a speech-generating device for PALS is scanning. This is the process where items are presented in a pattern and the user makes a selection indirectly by selecting a switch. Scanning on a speech-generating device involves many features that a clinician has to consider during the feature matching process including number of switches, switch placement, switch type, scanning pattern, and page set organization. These features may all be optimized for a person with late stage ALS.

When considering switch scanning as an access method, three questions must be asked: (1) What muscles have consistent, reliable movements for placement of the switch? (2) What switches are available that can be reliably activated with the residual movement? (3) What type of scanning settings should be offered for indirect selection? Often in late stage ALS, PALS may produce only a single consistent, reliable movement, such as protrusion of the jaw or movement of a thumb, for motor control. Either automatic or inverse single switch scanning may be options. However, due to fatigue associated with keeping a switch in an activated position, inverse scanning is often not a feasible option.

To optimize automatic scanning for those with late stage ALS, it is necessary to consider that these individuals often present with long latencies in motor responses. As such, when utilizing automatic scanning with a PALS with late stage ALS, it may be beneficial to significantly reduce the scan speed to improve selection accuracy. However, in trading accuracy for speed, it may take PALS significantly longer to express desired messages. When this is the case, clinicians may consider prioritizing high-frequency vocabulary and messages to be presented early in the scan cycle.

To optimize speed, organizing vocabulary by frequency of use may be beneficial. The placement of vocabulary is based on the frequency of their selection with commonly used words or phrases placed such that they will be offered earlier in the scanning pattern, reducing the time required for selection. For example, consider a PALS who utilizes linear automatic scanning. To select the first symbol, the user has to wait only for the first presentation. To select the second symbol, the PALS has to wait twice until the desired symbol is offered. Letter frequency patterns are commonly used with row/column scanning. In quadrant scanning, the user is presented first with a quadrant, then may be presented with a linear scan pattern of individual symbols. For both of these scan patterns, the lowest number of presented stimuli is two. Thus, the most frequently used message should be presented in the upper left of the display. Some quadrant scanning patterns utilize row-column scanning after a selection of a quadrant. As a result, the user is presented with a minimum of three stimuli including the quadrant, the row, and the individual stimulus.

When scanning using a high-tech communication device, many people with late stage ALS experience difficulty selecting items that are presented first (e.g., if row/column scanning, then the first row; if linear scanning, then the first-item). This is often due to minimal time available to anticipate a selection that needs to be made, or having to visually reorient to the scan location after having cycled through all options and returning to the first presented item. As a potential solution to this issue, many high-tech AAC devices include a feature to increase the scan time of the first presented item or item group.

When it comes to accessing communication devices using scanning, there are a variety of switches that can be used to detect even the most minimal movements. This is particularly critical for late stage ALS as movements can become so limited that they may not close the distance necessary for a proximity switch, or further limited to even a single muscle twitch. Fager, Fried-Oken, Jakobs, and Beukelman (2019) developed a novel access method involving a custom 3-D printed housing containing accelerometers, gyroscopes, and magnetometers. This tool was "trained" such that given several repetitions of intentional and unintentional movements, it could learn when the user meant to activate their switch. These custom-made solutions likely represent the future of switch access technologies, though the availability of these tools is currently limited to participants in research studies.

Switch solutions that clinicians may currently access include mechanical switches, as well as those that detect movements by electromyography (EMG), electrooculography (EOG), proximity sensors, or fiber-optic sensors. The switch solution selected depends on the residual motor control of the individual. For those with the ability to generate a movement, but who lack the strength to use a mechanical switch, proximity switches are often used. These switches require the user to create a movement of a body part within a certain distance of the switch. If the user is unable to generate the movement

necessary to activate a proximity switch, an alternative switch type may include fiberoptic switches. These switches emit a beam of light from the end of the switch. The clinician may select to have the switch activate when the beam of light is interrupted, such as the user moving their finger into the light), or when the beam of light is uninterrupted, such as the user keeping their finger in the light and moving it out to make a selection.

An EMG switch may be a solution for PALS with single muscle control. The EMG switch is placed over the area where the muscle fiber is active. Once the PALS initiates activation of the muscle, the switch is closed. Alternatively, for individuals who have residual eye gaze movements, but with conditions such as ptosis interfering with accurate eye gaze tracking, an EOG switch may be used.

Assessing the appropriateness of a particular switch type can be challenging for clinicians. Even for clinicians who regularly practice with PALS who have complex access needs, objective assessments of switch access are often not completed. Clinicians may develop their own criterion-referenced measures, evaluating reliable switch access to some percentage of acceptability. However, this can be a very time-consuming process, and if not completed, can result in low reliability of switch activation. Koestner and Simpson (2019) recommend the use of Scanning Wizard software, an iOS application and Web-based application used to improve the setup of switch scanning systems.

Scanning Wizard software guides the PALS as well as the clinician through a series of tasks evaluating the user's (1) optimal switch placement/setup, (2) optimal scanning time, (3) the need for an extra delay during scanning tasks, (4) optimal scanning initiation pattern (automatic or manual), (5) scanning loop count, and lastly (6) optimal keyboard setting. A small study of ten people with severe physical and communication needs demonstrated that use of Scanning Wizard software was an effective resource to objectively improve the configuration of their scanning system (Koester & Simpson, 2019).

Challenges to Switch Scanning

Extremely slow rates of selection, leading to reduced speed of communication, offer the greatest challenge to PALS who rely on switch scanning. Even when more than one switch is used, the rate of message generation does not come close to directly selecting letters on a keyboard (Koester & Arthanat, 2017). Many PALS reject scanning because of this challenge. Additionally, poor switch placement, unintentional movement of the switch or the body part used to activate it, and difficulty finding an adequate mounting solution at the switch site also cause frustration. Currently, most switches do not offer any feedback or information to support problem solving when challenges arise. If there is a problem in the setup, it is difficult to know if it is at the SGD level, the switch level, or the PALS level. With this degenerative disease, it is difficult to know when to change switches or locations, and often failure is the only indication, leading to frustration and even abandonment of the SGD. There are many creative and unique switch placement solutions, where the clinician, family, and PALS experimented with materials to increase the reliability of switch placement or mounting reliability. The AAC clinician, working with PALS with late stage ALS will need to consider many different

solutions for switch use if the PALS agrees to stick with this access technology.

Using Multimodal Access Technologies

Although access methods have been presented in isolation, it is critical to recall that many PALS will use multiple input methods across the day. For example, the PALS who has strong eye gaze function in the morning and worsening ptosis across the day might utilize eye gaze access in the morning and scanning in the afternoon and evening. Further, if switch access movements become unreliable, partner assisted auditory scanning may be another method to express desired messages without the operational demands of a high-tech communication system.

Historically, AAC devices have only been designed to expect input from a single access method (e.g., eye gaze only, switch access only). There are significant challenges associated with the use of only a single access modality to access a communication device, including fatigue, over-use injuries, change in positioning, and inefficiency (Fager et al., 2019). In complex access challenges such as in late stage ALS, individuals often require the use of more than one access method to reduce fatigue, conserve energy, and to optimize the speed and accuracy of the communicative exchange.

Fager and colleagues at the Rehabilitation Engineering Research Center on Augmentative and Alternative Communication propose the development of systems that can expect input from more than one access method, such as voice recognition and typing, or single switch scanning and eye gaze (Fager et al., 2019). Fager, Beukelman, Jakobs, and Hosom (2010) have designed a typing system where an individual first uses eye gaze to locate a target on the screen (whether that is a group of symbols or single symbol), activating a switch to begin a scan thereby switching from eye gaze to switch scanning, and then activating the switch a second time to select the target. This type of system accounts for difficulties with dwell activations such as reduced range of motion and precision in ocular movements.

Multimodal access methods are currently available in some commercially available dedicated speech generating device systems. This allows for trialing of possible combinations of access methods with people with late stage ALS. Important considerations for trialing include (1) accuracy and efficiency of a multimodal access method in comparison to a single access method alone; (2) effort and fatigue associated with a single access method in comparison to a multimodal access method; (3) cognitive demands of a multimodal access method in comparison to a single access method; and (4) user preference. Implementation of multiple access methods also has considerations for clinical practice, especially in regard to care team training, such as identifying with a PALS and their care team when specific access methods are challenging (due to time of day, circumstantial considerations, medication, pain, etc.), coming up with communication strategies to request assistance for changing an access method, and training the care team in positioning and implementation of multimodal access methods.

Challenges to Multimodal Access Technologies

As multimodal access options are relatively new within AAC technologies, many speech-generating devices currently have limited access to these features. It can be difficult to determine the advantages of one access method over another given the complex inherent variability in the contributing factors to access challenges (e.g., fatigue, medication, pain, alertness, mood). This can also make it difficult to determine when and if it is appropriate to change access methods. There is not yet software with dynamic recognition of these changes in functioning throughout the day that might be used as a tool by a clinician to change access methods or to prompt the individual with the option to change access methods themselves.

The Potential of Using Brain-Computer Interface (BCI) in Late Stage ALS

"If I could converse as close to normal as possible, I could be myself and express my personality much more than I'm currently able to. I hope that the BCI system can accomplish that. Otherwise, my dreams will stay as dreams."

—Rich

Some individuals with ALS eventually will lose all voluntary motor function, leaving them unable to use eye tracking or switch scanning for AAC access. Brain-computer interface (BCI) technology is being investigated as a new alternative access method that bypasses the motor system, supporting computer control with brain signals alone. As the name suggests, a brain-computer interface system involves three main components: (a) the brain, (b) the computer, and (c) the interface. The user, of course, supplies the brain and the intention to control an assistive technology.

The computer may be a laptop, desktop, tablet, or even a smartphone, and runs software that analyzes brain signals and converts them into signals for controlling the desired application. The interface is the means of recording the brain signals and sending them to the computer. For most noninvasive BCIs, this involves electrodes that detect brain activity, and hardware that amplifies the signals and converts them to a format that can be processed by the computer. Figure 7–2 provides a schematic of the basic design of a BCI for AT control.

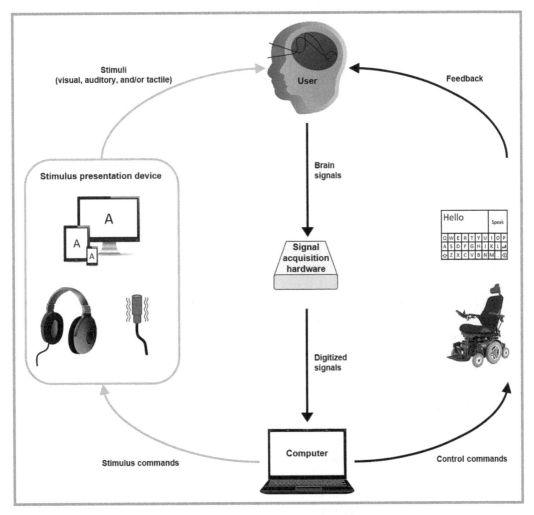

Figure 7–2. This figure provides a schematic of the basic design of a BCI for AT control. A BCI system involves three main components: (a) the brain, (b) the computer, and (c) the interface. The user, of course, supplies the brain and the intention to control an assistive technology. The computer may be a laptop, desktop, tablet, or even a smartphone, and runs software that analyzes brain signals and converts them into signals for controlling the desired application. The interface is the means of recording the brain signals and sending them to the computer. For most noninvasive BCIs, this involves electrodes that detect brain activity, and hardware that amplifies the signals and converts them to a format that can be processed by the computer.

In some BCIs, auditory or tactile stimuli are presented to the user via a presentation device (e.g., display, headphones, or tactors), and the user's reactions produce brain signals related to the intention or lack of intention to select a given stimulus. This is analogous to automatic switch scanning, with brain activity taking the place of muscle activity that would typically be used to activate a switch. Other BCIs require the user to spontaneously produce brain signals (e.g., imagined movements of the left and right hands to move a cursor left and right). Depending on the system, control may work similarly to either multiple-switch scanning or to cursor control with mouse emulation, again with brain signals replacing movement-based signals. In either case, the brain signals are collected and digitized by signal acquisition hardware and sent to the computer for analysis. If the computer has sufficient evidence to infer the user's intent, it sends a control command to the AT software or device. If not, it awaits additional information from the user. In many systems, the user simultaneously receives input from the stimulus presentation device and feedback from the AT.

Brain signals for BCI may be acquired either invasively or noninvasively. Invasive BCI systems require surgery to implant an electrode array directly onto the cerebral cortex. Noninvasive systems capture brain signals from outside the scalp using a variety of methods. Electroencephalography (EEG), which involves electrodes placed against the scalp, often in a cap or headset, is the most common method of noninvasive brain signal acquisition. Research studies have investigated the use of BCI to control both integrated, custom-built BCI communication software and off-the-shelf, commercially-available AAC programs (Gosmanova, Carmack,

Goldberg, & Vaughan, 2017; Thompson, Gruis, & Huggins, 2014). Below, some of the invasive and noninvasive BCI systems that have been explored for use by PALS are reviewed.

A variety of brain responses have been used as control signals in noninvasive BCIs for AAC (Akcakaya et al., 2014; Brumberg, Nguyen, Pitt, & Lorenz, 2019). Many rely on the detection of the P300 event-related potential, a positive change in EEG signals elicited by a rare or unique stimulus in a stream of stimuli. Perhaps the best-known P300-based BCI is the P300 speller that is based on Farwell and Donchin's (1988) original mental prosthesis. The P300 speller interface consists of a matrix of letters and other symbols or words (e.g., space, backspace, or commands for computer control), with rows and columns (or individual characters) flashing in random order. The user focuses on the desired symbol and mentally counts each time it flashes; the flashing of the desired symbol should elicit a P300 response. Each row or column is flashed multiple times in order to elicit repeated P300 responses, providing enough information for the computer to determine the desired letter (Farwell & Donchin, 1988). As of this writing, the BCI communication systems currently available to consumers rely primarily on the P300 paradigm.

A number of studies have demonstrated successful use of a P300 matrix speller by individuals with ALS (Guy et al., 2018; Schettini et al., 2015; Silvoni et al., 2013; Thompson et al., 2014). In a study of long-term independent home use of a P300 BCI system, PALS and their caregivers reported that the benefits outweighed the burdens, and most participants elected to keep the system at the study's end (Wolpaw et al., 2018). Another study demonstrated that some PALS can maintain the ability to operate a P300 BCI over a period of several years (Silvoni et al., 2013). In addition to spelling interfaces, PALS have used BCI systems (using the P300 and/or other brain responses) to answer yes/no questions, activate emergency call bells (Lim et al., 2017), select predetermined phrases (Hwang et al., 2017), and create visual art (Zickler, Halder, Kleih, Herbert, & Kübler, 2013).

PALS also have participated in invasive BCI research studies, though these are less common due to the need for surgical implantation of the electrodes. BrainGate is a long-term, multicenter project exploring invasive BCI for communication and computer control. As part of the BrainGate program, individuals with ALS and other conditions have intracortical micro-electrode arrays implanted directly onto the motor cortex. Study participants, including PALS, have successfully used this invasive BCI system to control a cursor for text-based communication and other applications on a commercial tablet (Nuyujukian et al., 2018). Another research group has reported on a PALS who successfully used her invasive BCI system in her home over a period of 3 years (Pels et al., 2019; Vansteensel et al., 2016).

Challenges to BCI Research and Development

"When BCI reaches a more advanced stage, my main concern would be the placement of the cap, the electrodes and calibration of the equipment to make it effectively functional. The current system, in my opinion, is practically impossible to use by patients without significant assistance."
—Rich

Several studies have found that some PALS are unsuccessful with BCI communication systems (McCane et al., 2014; Wolpaw et al., 2018) though it is unknown whether these same PALS might perform better with a different type of BCI or interface. Studies involving both PALS and healthy control participants often demonstrate significant differences in results between the two groups, with better BCI performance for participants in the control group (Geronimo, Simmons, & Schiff, 2016; Ikegami, Takano, Kondo, Saeki, & Kansaku, 2014; Oken et al., 2014). However, this performance gap is absent in other studies (e.g., McCane et al., 2014; Thompson et al., 2014). Individuals with ALS may take medications that affect attention, vigilance, or brain signals (Meador, 1998; Polich & Criado, 2006). Fatigue, cognitive changes, or visual impairments associated with ALS may also affect BCI performance (Geronimo et al., 2016; McCane et al., 2014). Disease progression or overall level of disability (as measured by the ALS Functional Rating Scale-Revised) does not appear to correlate with BCI performance (McCane et al., 2014; Silvoni et al., 2013), and studies involving PALS in a locked-in or completely locked-in state have produced mixed results (De Massari et al., 2013; Okahara et al., 2018).

In addition to patient factors, system as well as environmental factors may present potential barriers to successful clinical implementation of BCI technology. Many noninvasive systems use wet electrodes, which require a small amount of gel to be added to each electrode to improve signal quality. This gel can be a problem for users who have their hair washed infrequently. Dry electrodes can have inferior signal quality and may cause discomfort for some users. The setup, configuration, and electrode application required for BCI use may be complicated and challenging for caregivers and clinicians (Peters et al., 2015). PALS at end stages of the disease may have electrical equipment that interferes with the data acquisition system of the BCI system. The technical support required by BCIs that are being developed and evaluated is not trivial, as these are sophisticated devices. The coordination required between the signal acquisition hardware and software, the signal processing software, and the assistive technology outcomes can cause challenges at many levels (Chavarriaga et al., 2017). Having a knowledgeable team is of paramount importance if this new access technology is going to be available for PALS. Comfort, ease of use, training for PALS, caregivers, and clinicians must be addressed to facilitate clinical implementation of BCI technology.

The Future for Access Technologies in Late Stage ALS

Access to AAC technologies is challenging in late stage ALS due to the complex interaction of contributing disease factors. Although recent advancements in technology have made AAC systems more accessible, additional research and development of AAC/AT tools for increasing access to technology in this population are needed.

The need is particularly great in increasing the flexibility and adaptability of existing technology to meet the complex access needs of this population. Proposals for new advancements in access technologies are grounded in a multimodality theory of AAC using multiple input signals (e.g., eye gaze, EMG, EEG, switch, direct selection) at one time. Possible advancements include: (1) increas-

ing machine learning techniques in AAC software (active querying) with the goal of improving the system detection of selection versus non-selections; (2) optimizing multimodal signal fusion to dynamically use the most reliable physiological intent evidence by a user, including brain-based signals (EEG, SSVEP, P300, VEP, SMRS, EOG), neural impulses given by muscle activation (EMG), eye gaze (position, velocity of movement), head tracking and other inputs; and (3) providing new vocabulary sources to SGD language models based on partner input to personalize language enhancements and reduce message generation time for functional communication.

The ethics of offering access technologies to PALS in late stage ALS must be considered by the AAC clinician and treating team. Earlier in this chapter, it was questioned whether failure with an access technology is the only way to know that it's time to change that option and explore others. It is paramount to honor PALS preferences in this process with the role of the speech-language pathologist to present information and answer questions. Are there other ways to determine best fit that may not lead to frustration and abandonment even for a clinician with limited experience in AAC?

■ Decision-Making Guidelines

Up to this point, this chapter has presented access technology options and challenges. What follows is a list of clinical questions that should be considered when making decisions about which access technologies to introduce to PALS in late stages of the disease. Many of these guiding questions should be asked during every full AAC evaluation. For late stage ALS access questions, the chapter focuses on unique, specific considerations for PALS. The questions are presented in three categories: (1) PALS-focused, (2) environment-focused, and (3) clinician-focused skills and competencies. The rule here is flexibility and creativity. PALS in late stage ALS present with complex communication needs that are not easily addressed with a standard intervention timeline. A basic knowledge of disease history, motor progression and timing, the PALS' trajectory, past treatment choices, and reported functional variability are the principles that guide decision making. Throughout the decision-making guide, an illustrative case example is highlighted using an individual with late stage ALS.

I. PALS-Focused Considerations

- What are the PALS' **goals** for communication and alternative access?
- What is the PALS' **medical status & plan of care**?

> Marty is a 60-year-old man with late ALS. Approximately 12 years ago, he noticed instability in his balance, followed by mild dysarthria a few months later. He received a formal diagnosis of ALS one year after his initial symptom presentation. The following year, he elected to undergo tracheostomy and has used mechanical ventilation since then. He relies on AAC to meet his communication needs in all situa-

tions, including social interaction, maintaining relationships with family and friends, interacting with health care providers, and directing his everyday care.

- What are the PALS' **motor skills**? Consider history, timing of progression, trajectory, and variability.
- What are the PALS' **hearing acuity** and **auditory skills**? Consider history, timing of progression, trajectory, assistive technologies (e.g., hearing aids) and variability.
- What are the PALS' **visual acuity and oculomotor skills**? Consider history, timing of progression, trajectory, assistive technologies (e.g., single vision or bifocal glasses) and variability.
- What are the PALS' **cognition** & **language skills**? Consider history (including cultural and linguistic considerations), timing of progression, trajectory, and variability.
- What is the PALS' **emotional/ psychosocial** status? Consider relationships with family and friends, stability of care team and staff turnover, and familiarity with technology.

> Marty now has limited remaining voluntary motor function, but can produce small movements of his eyes, chin, and left thumb. These movements are restricted in range and have significant (>1 second) and variable latency. Marty uses horizontal eye movements to give yes/no responses, but has limited

vertical eye movement. He can protrude his chin slightly to activate a proximity switch to control a calling device to alert care providers he needs assistance, though the switch requires frequent repositioning due to trach-care activities or small, unintentional changes in Marty's head position. Finally, Marty can activate a proximity switch by abducting his left thumb, though this switch also requires frequent repositioning. His eye movements and switch activations movements become slower and more unreliable with fatigue.

Marty's cognitive and language skills have remained relatively stable since his diagnosis. However, members of his care team have recently noticed inconsistency with yes/no responses, increased latency in following spoken directions, and occasional lack of response to care provider's questions. Although it is difficult to formally assess cognitive status at this stage given Marty's significant motor impairment, these changes represent a noticeable difference when compared to his skills a few months ago. Marty's team is continually asking whether his inconsistent lack of response is due to FTD progression, changes in motivation,

hearing, or some other communication breakdown.

Marty has reduced visual acuity and wears glasses during all of his waking hours, for both distance and reading. They often slide down the bridge of his nose and must be adjusted by a caregiver. Marty also reports light sensitivity and intermittent double vision, requiring modifications to font sizes, contrast, and brightness of the SGD screen. He has bilateral hearing loss that is corrected with hearing aids, which he wears consistently with support from his care providers.

Marty is known to have an upbeat personality and has had many years to adjust to his diagnosis and the changes in his physical function. In the past, he has welcomed information and advice from his medical team and has taken a proactive approach to symptom management and decisions about his care. However, he is wary of making changes to his current SGD or access method and is not always interested in trying new things. It is critical to continually evaluate the input and value of changes or suggestions made by every team member (including family, clinicians and care team), and to honor Marty's choices.

- What is the PALS' **familiarity with and previous use of technology** and assistive technology?
- What **communication platforms** (face-to-face, social media, texting, email, etc.) does the PALS use now and plan to use in the future?
- What are the PALS' **message needs** now and what might they be in the future?
- What are the PALS' **positioning needs** and what equipment are they using to address these needs now and for the future?
- What **access methods** were used in the past and present, and when/how are they changed?

Marty is a retired information technology professional with a long-standing interest in computers and technological innovations. Before his diagnosis, he used computers daily for work, communication, entertainment, social interaction, shopping, managing finances, and other purposes. Currently, he is primarily interested in using his speech-generating device for face-to-face communication and email. He frequently uses both generic and customized prestored messages for social interaction and directing his care, but also requires access to a keyboard for novel messages. At one point, Marty used his speech-generating device to type an eight-page caregiver manual to direct his care and communicate his preferences. In addition to communication, he would like to use his speech-generating device to access the Internet and control his TV. For many years, Marty has used yes/no responses and partner-assisted scanning as additional communication methods.

Marty spends his time either lying in bed with his head elevated, or in a tilted and reclined position in his power wheelchair. He is unable to drive the chair, which is fitted with attendant controls. His speech-generating device is mounted to his hospital bed on an arm that can swing aside or be removed entirely to provide care providers with easy access to Marty, and to other medical equipment when needed. One proximity switch is positioned near his chin on a flexible arm, while another is near his left thumb, attached to a custom-made foam arm

support. A second speech generating device mount is attached to Marty's wheelchair, though he often prefers to use partner-assisted scanning when seated in the chair to avoid the inconvenience of moving and positioning the speech generating device and switches.

Marty received his first speech-generating device soon after his ALS diagnosis, and accessed it using direct selection on the touch screen. After his tracheostomy and significant decline in motor function, he was no longer able to activate the touch screen, and accessed the speech-generating device with a USB joystick. As his motor function continued to decline, he trialed both eye tracking and single-switch scanning. Marty experienced inconsistent accuracy with eye tracking, apparently related to both his glasses, and reduced ocular motility. He preferred single-switch scanning with hand movements, and used this method reliably for several years, with periodic changes to the switch (e.g., mechanical switch to proximity switch) and its positioning.

After several years of successful switch scanning, Marty's switch activation became increasingly unreliable, and his speech-language pathologist initiated trials of both eye tracking and a BrainFingers™ switch. BrainFingers™ activation was inconsistent, and this was ruled out as an access method. Eye tracking was also inconsistent, but was both faster and more reliable than switch scanning with the thumb switch. Marty's speech-language pathologist customized an eye tracking page set to accommodate his reduced tracking accuracy. He continued to prefer switch scanning, but began using eye tracking as a backup access method at times when he had difficulty activating the switch.

II. Environment-Focused Considerations

■ Who are the members of the PALS' **social circle and care team**? Consider level of familiarity with communication partners for each member of team, level of support for communication provided by team members including communication advocacy, presence. or lack of communication partner training for members of PALS circle, and other social factors contributing to communication from members of social circle.

■ Consider the **impact of the physical environment on access technologies** (e.g., light sources and reflective surfaces for eye gaze, electrical "noise" for brain-based signals, and insufficient space for all DME, difficult environment for attending to competing sensory sources to use speech-generating device).

■ Consider the **technical support** available for AAC technologies through manufacturers and other sources and the competence of members of the PALS' social circle or care team to program, set up, or troubleshoot assistive equipment.

Marty currently lives in an adult foster home specializing in caring for people using mechanical ventilation. His wife, daughter, and extended family members and friends visit him often. His care team includes the foster home nursing staff, a home health speech-language pathologist with expertise in AAC, and other home health care providers. His family, friends, speech-language pathologist, and the foster home staff are well versed in interpreting Marty's unaided communication signals (eye movements for yes/no responses, as well as facial expressions) and in repositioning his speech generating devices and switches as needed. The foster home staff often helps facilitate interaction between Marty and less familiar communication partners.

Marty spends much of the day lying in a hospital bed or seated in his power wheelchair in his private room. The room is small and must accommodate an array of medical equipment such as a medicine cabinet, ventilator, enteral feeding pump, charting station for caregiving team, and suctioning machine, while allowing adequate space for a Hoyer lift for transfers. Marty's speech generating device-mounting system must be low-profile and easy to swing aside or remove entirely to facilitate daily care activities. Reflective surfaces, including switch mounts and IV poles, have at times had to be moved from behind his bed or modified to reduce interference during use of eye gaze access. His room is dimly lit given his light sensitivity.

Speech generating device technical support is available by phone or e-mail from the device manufacturer. Marty also has a device company representative that lives locally and is available for in-person trainings and technical support as needed. Marty's home-health speech-language pathologist visits him regularly. She has extensive experience and expertise in AAC, and often works with individuals with complex access needs. The foster home staff is committed to maintaining Marty's communication access and has received training in positioning and troubleshooting the speech-generating device, mount, and switches. Laminated signs are positioned around his room to communicate his yes/no response ("I look left for 'yes' and right for 'no.'").

III. Clinician-Focused Skills and Competences

- Does the clinician have competence in **disease-specific knowledge** about ALS to provide disease education and counseling regarding both AAC and care structures and systems (e.g., palliative care, hospice, team discussion, and support groups)?
- Does the clinician have proficient knowledge of the **use, programming, and modification of AAC technology**? What training or mentorship is required to gain proficiency?
- Does the clinician have **knowledge of health care systems** (e.g., insurance funding, alternative funding sources, loaner equipment, and timing of funding) in order to obtain equipment and appropriate related support services ideally within an interdisciplinary care team and model)?

Soon after his diagnosis, Marty began receiving care through an ALS Association Certified Treatment Center of Excellence. He received education about AAC options even before his speech had changed, and his speech and communication were monitored at clinic visits every three months. When he began to experience dysarthria, he met with a speech-language pathologist employed by the ALS Association, who completed an AAC evaluation, pursued insurance funding for a speech-generating device, and provided support with training and device programming. After his tracheostomy and changes in his physical function and access needs, Marty worked with a home health speech-language pathologist who specializes in AAC evaluation and treatment.

Both speech-language pathologists were knowledgeable about ALS, AAC (including the latest technology for speech generating devices and alternative access), and the systems involved in obtaining and funding AAC equipment. Both reported gaining expertise in these areas through self-study (including textbooks, journal articles, and speech generating device manufacturer websites), conference workshops/

trainings, guidance from mentor speech-language pathologists, support from peer speech-language pathologists (including via message boards, listservs, and AAC interest groups on social media), and on-the-job experience working with PALS and AAC technologies and techniques.

Discussion of Case Study

Finding optimal access technologies is a challenge that constantly changes within the decision-making framework. The overarching question that remains for Marty and his clinicians is, "How will Marty access technology today?" This question is daunting in the face of a progressive disease. Every AAC clinician who works with individuals with changing health conditions, either progressive diseases such as ALS or improving conditions such as traumatic brain injury has been faced with this question many times. The authors of this chapter recommend using the patient's aspirations and goals in an attempt to improve quality of life as they define it. Access requirements of current assistive technology options are often difficult, if not impossible, for patients to meet. All providers should: (1) strive to try to do their best with available information and technology, (2) promote the use of new options, and (3) center care around patient needs and priorities. Even with optimal effort, answers can be elusive. Sometimes there are only more questions. Other times our best option is to consult the literature or other providers who may know the answer. Sometimes, questions simply remain unanswered.

Be creative. Try your best. Strive to give your patient every option. Try to answer questions that you and they have. Do not be afraid to feel like a novice clinician. Contribute to research efforts and research teams to help develop new options. Advocate with assistive technology companies for the needs of your patients. Together, providers can promote the health and well-being of people with late stage ALS.

■ Conclusions

People with late stage ALS often have difficulty using access technologies that reliably and efficiently meet their complex communication and computer access needs. There are many contributing factors to this difficulty, including disease factors (e.g., symptoms, presentation, progression, trajectory), environmental factors (e.g., positioning limitations, interference of other equipment), equipment factors (e.g., limited technological advancement to deal with unreliable user input), and treating clinician skills and competences. Given the complex interaction of contributing variables to AAC access challenges in people with late stage ALS, it can often be challenging for clinicians working with this population to identify possible solutions.

Although there is no clear answer to access challenges for this population, clinicians may address this difficulty in several ways. They can stay informed on disease-specific contributions to late stage ALS and the current state of access technologies that are available. Second, clinicians can increase their comfort and competence in operating access technologies through training and consultation with related AT professionals (e.g., ALS associations, local AT resources/groups, online AT communities). Finally, they can increase their understanding of health care systems in order to provide appropriate equipment and intervention.

The ultimate hope for the future of access technologies as it applies to this clinical population is to make technology more adaptable, accurate, and efficient for many people with late stage ALS through additional research and development. Future technological advancements will hopefully improve not only the user's experience with the technology, but also the clinician's ability to find the most optimal solution when faced with complex access challenges. These necessary advancements, no doubt, will improve the overall ability for the user to access essential communication tools, thereby improving quality of life in late stages of disease.

■ References

Achi, E. Y., & Rudnicki, S. A. (2012). ALS and frontotemporal dysfunction: A review. *Neurology Research International, 2012*, 806306. https://doi.org/10.1155/2012/806306

Akcakaya, M., Peters, B., Moghadamfalahi, M., Mooney, A., Orhan, U., Oken, B., &

Fried-Oken, M. (2014). Noninvasive brain-computer interfaces for augmentative and alternative communication. *IEEE Reviews in Biomedical Engineering, 7*, 31–49.

Ball, L., Beukelman, D. R., & Bardach, L. (2007). Amyotrophic lateral sclerosis. In *Augmentative communication strategies for adults with acute or chronic medical conditions* (p. 287). Brookes.

Ball, L. J., Beukelman, D. R., & Pattee, G. L. (2004). Acceptance of augmentative and alternative communication technology by persons with amyotrophic lateral sclerosis. *Augmentative and Alternative Communication, 20*(2), 113–122. https://doi.org/10.1080/0743461042000216596

Borasio, G. D., & Miller, R. G. (2001). Clinical characteristics and management of ALS. *Seminars in Neurology, 21*(2), 155–166. https://doi.org/10.1055/s-2001-15268

Brumberg, J. S., Nguyen, A., Pitt, K. M., & Lorenz, S. D. (2019). Examining sensory ability, feature matching and assessment-based adaptation for a brain–computer interface using the steady-state visually evoked potential. *Disability and Rehabilitation: Assistive Technology, 14*(3), 241–249. https://doi.org/10.1080/17483107.2018.1428369

Chavarriaga, R., Fried-Oken, M., Kleih, S., Lotte, F., & Scherer, R. (2017). Heading for new shores! Overcoming pitfalls in BCI design. *Brain Computer Interfaces (Abingdon, England), 4*(1–2), 60–73. https://doi.org/10.1080/2326263X.2016.1263916

Chen Szu-Han Kay, & O'Leary Michael. (2018). Eye gaze 101: What speech-language pathologists should know about selecting eye gaze augmentative and alternative communication systems. *Perspectives of the ASHA Special Interest Groups, 3*(12), 24–32. https://doi.org/10.1044/persp3.SIG12.24

Chiò, A., Hammond, E. R., Mora, G., Bonito, V., & Filippini, G. (2015). Development and evaluation of a clinical staging system for amyotrophic lateral sclerosis. *Journal of Neurology, Neurosurgery, and Psychiatry, 86*(1), 38–44. https://doi.org/10.1136/jnnp-2013-306589

Costello, J. (2009). Last words, last connections: How augmentative communication can support children facing end of life. *ASHA Leader, 14*(16), 8–11. https://doi.org/10.1044/leader.FTR2.14162009.8

Crockford, C., Newton, J., Lonergan, K., Chiwera, T., Booth, T., Chandran, S., . . . Abrahams, S. (2018). ALS-specific cognitive and behavior changes associated with advancing disease stage in ALS. *Neurology, 91*(15), e1370–e1380. https://doi.org/10.1212/WNL.0000000000006317

De Massari, D., Ruf, C. A., Furdea, A., Matuz, T., van der Heiden, L., Halder, S., . . . Birbaumer, N. (2013). Brain communication in the locked-in state. *Brain: A Journal of Neurology, 136*(Pt. 6), 1989–2000. https://doi.org/10.1093/brain/awt102

Elamin, M., Bede, P., Byrne, S., Jordan, N., Gallagher, L., Wynne, B., . . . & Hardiman, O. (2013). Cognitive changes predict functional decline in ALS: A population-based longitudinal study. *Neurology, 80*(17), 1590–1597. https://doi.org/10.1212/WNL.0b013e31828f18ac

Fager, S., Beukelman, D., Fried-Oken, M., Jakobs, T., & Baker, J. (2012). Access interface strategies. *Assistive Technology, 24*(1), 25–33. https://doi.org/10.1080/10400435.2011.648712

Fager, S. K., Beukelman, D. R., Jakobs, T., & Hosom, J. P. (2010). Evaluation of a speech recognition prototype for speakers with moderate and severe dysarthria: A preliminary report. *AAC: Augmentative and Alternative Communication, 26*(4), 267–277.

Fager, S. K., Fried-Oken, M., Jakobs, T., & Beukelman, D. R. (2019). New and emerging access technologies for adults with complex communication needs and severe motor impairments: State of the science. *Augmentative and Alternative Communication, 35*(1), 13–25. https://doi.org/10.1080/07434618.2018.1556730

Fang, T., Al Khleifat, A., Stahl, D. R., Lazo La Torre, C., Murphy, C., Young, C., . . . Al-Chalabi, A. (2017). Comparison of the King's and MiToS staging systems for ALS. *Amyotrophic Lateral Sclerosis & Frontotemporal Degeneration, 18*(3–4), 227–232. https://doi.org/10.1080/21678421.2016.1265565

Farwell, L. A., & Donchin, E. (1988). Talking off the top of your head: Toward a mental prosthesis utilizing event-related brain potentials. *Electroencephalography and Clinical Neurophysiology, 70*(6), 510–523. https://doi.org/10.1016/0013-4694(88)90149-6

Federici, S., & Scherer, M. (2012). *Assistive Technology Assessment Handbook.* CRC Press.

Fried-Oken, M. (2000). *Eye transfer communication.* Retrieved from https://www.ohsu.edu/sites/default/files/2018-11/Eye-Transfer-Communication.pdf

Fried-Oken, M., Kinsella, M., Peters, B., Eddy, B., & Wojciechowski, B. (submitted for publication). Human visual skills for brain computer interface use: A tutorial.

Geronimo, A., Simmons, Z., & Schiff, S. J. (2016). Performance predictors of brain-computer interfaces in patients with amyotrophic lateral sclerosis. *Journal of Neural Engineering, 13*(2), 026002. https://doi.org/10.1088/1741-2560/13/2/026002

Goldstein, L. H., & Abrahams, S. (2013). Changes in cognition and behaviour in amyotrophic lateral sclerosis: Nature of impairment and implications for assessment. *The Lancet. Neurology, 12*(4), 368–380. https://doi.org/10.1016/S1474-4422(13)70026-7

Gosmanova, K., Carmack, C. S., Goldberg, D., & Vaughan, T. M. (2017). EEG-based brain-computer interface access to Tobii Dynavox Communicator 5. RESNA. In *Proceedings of the annual 2017 RESNA conference; 2017 June 26–30.* REGNA New Orleans, LA; Arlington, VA.

Green, J. R., Yunusova, Y., Kuruvilla, M. S., Wang, J., Pattee, G. L., Synhorst, L., . . . Berry, J. D. (2013). Bulbar and speech motor assessment in ALS: Challenges and future directions. *Amyotrophic Lateral Sclerosis & Frontotemporal Degeneration, 14*(7–8), 494–500. https://doi.org/10.3109/21678421.2013.817585

Guy, V., Soriani, M.-H., Bruno, M., Papadopoulo, T., Desnuelle, C., & Clerc, M. (2018). Brain computer interface with the P300 speller: Usability for disabled people with amyotrophic lateral sclerosis. *Annals of Physical and Rehabilitation Medicine, 61*(1), 5–11. https://doi.org/10.1016/j.re hab.2017.09.004

Hwang, H.-J., Han, C.-H., Lim, J.-H., Kim, Y.-W., Choi, S.-I., An, K.-O., . . . Im, C.-H. (2017). Clinical feasibility of brain-computer interface based on steady-state visual evoked potential in patients with locked-in syndrome: Case studies. *Psychophysiology, 54*(3), 444–451. https://doi.org/10.1111/psyp.12793

Hwang, C.-S., Weng, H.-H., Wang, L.-F., Tsai, C.-H., & Chang, H.-T. (2014). An eye-tracking assistive device improves the quality of life for ALS patients and reduces the caregivers' burden. *Journal of Motor Behavior, 46*(4), 233–238. https://doi.org/10.1080/00 222895.2014.891970

Ikegami, S., Takano, K., Kondo, K., Saeki, N., & Kansaku, K. (2014). A region-based two-step P300-based brain-computer interface for patients with amyotrophic lateral sclerosis. *Clinical Neurophysiology, 125*(11), 2305–2312. https://doi.org/10.1016/j.clin ph.2014.03.013

Joyce, P. (2011). *Speak book* (4th ed.). Acecentre. Retrieved from https://acecentre.org .uk/wp-content/uploads/2018/11/speak book-4th-ed.pdf

Käthner, I., Kübler, A., & Halder, S. (2015). Comparison of eye tracking, electrooculography and an auditory brain-computer interface for binary communication: A case study with a participant in the locked-in state. *Journal of Neuroengineering and Rehabilitation, 12*(76). https://doi.org/10 .1186/s12984-015-0071-z

Kiernan, M. C., Vucic, S., Cheah, B. C., Turner, M. R., Eisen, A., Hardiman, O., . . . Zoing, M. C. (2011). Amyotrophic lateral sclerosis. *Lancet, 377*(9769), 942–955. https://doi .org/10.1016/S0140-6736(10)61156-7

Koester, H. H., & Arthanat, S. (2017). Text entry rate of access interfaces used by people with physical disabilities: A systematic review. *Assistive Technology, 30*(3), 151–163.

Koester, H. H., & Simpson, R. C. (2019). Effectiveness and usability of Scanning Wizard software: A tool for enhancing switch scanning. *Disability and Rehabilitation: Assistive Technology, 14*(2), 161–171. https://doi.org /10.1080/17483107.2017.1406998

Lillo, P., Mioshi, E., & Hodges, J. R. (2012). Caregiver burden in amyotrophic lateral sclerosis is more dependent on patients' behavioral changes than physical disability: A comparative study. *BMC Neurology, 12*(1), 156. https://doi.org/10.1186/1471-2377-12-156

Lim, J. H., Kim, Y. W., Lee, J. H., An, K. O., Hwang, H. J., Cha, H. S., . . . Im, C. H. (2017). An emergency call system for patients in locked-in state using an SSVEP-based brain switch. *Psychophysiology, 54*(11), 1632–1643. https://doi.org/10.1111/psyp.12916

Matuz, T., Birbaumer, N., Hautzinger, M., & Kübler, A. (2015). Psychosocial adjustment to ALS: A longitudinal study. *Frontiers in Psychology, 6*, 1197. https://doi.org/10.33 89/fpsyg.2015.01197

McCane, L. M., Sellers, E. W., Mcfarland, D. J., Mak, J. N., Carmack, C. S., Zeitlin, D., . . . Vaughan, T. M. (2014). Brain-computer interface (BCI) evaluation in people with amyotrophic lateral sclerosis. *Amyotrophic Lateral Sclerosis & Frontotemporal Degeneration, 15*(3–4), 207–215. https://doi.org/ 10.3109/21678421.2013.865750

McNaughton, D., & Light, J. (2013). The iPad and mobile technology revolution: Benefits and challenges for individuals who require augmentative and alternative communication. *Augmentative and Alternative Communication, 29*(2), 107–116. https://doi. org/10.3109/07434618.2013.784930

Meador, K. J. (1998). Cognitive side effects of medications. *Neurologic Clinics, 16*(1), 141–155. https://doi.org/10.1016/s0733-86 19(05)70371-6

MegaBee E2L Products (2010). *MegaBee: Electronic hand-hand communication tablet.* Retrieved from http://www.e2l.uk.com/ data/J369.Manual.1.04.pdf

Mitsumoto, H., & Rabkin, J. G. (2007). Palliative care for patients with amyotrophic lateral sclerosis: "Prepare for the worst and hope for the best." *JAMA*, *298*(2), 207–216. https://doi.org/10.1001/jama.298.2.207

Moss, H. E., McCluskey, L., Elman, L., Hoskins, K., Talman, L., Grossman, M., . . . Liu, G. T. (2012). Cross-sectional evaluation of clinical neuro-ophthalmic abnormalities in an amyotrophic lateral sclerosis population. *Journal of the Neurological Sciences, 314*(1), 97–101. https://doi.org/10.1016/j.jns.2011.10.016

Murguialday, A. R., Hill, J., Bensch, M., Martens, S., Halder, S., Nijboer, F., . . . Gharabaghi, A. (2011). Transition from the locked in to the completely locked-in state: A physiological analysis. *Clinical Neurophysiology, 122*(5), 925–933. https://doi.org/10.1016/j.clinph.2010.08.019

Nuyujukian, P., Albites Sanabria, J., Saab, J., Pandarinath, C., Jarosiewicz, B., Blabe, C. H., . . . Henderson, J. M. (2018). Cortical control of a tablet computer by people with paralysis. *PloS One, 13*(11), e0204566. https://doi.org/10.1371/journal.pone.0204566

Ohki, M., Kanayama, R., Nakamura, T., Okuyama, T., Kimura, Y., & Koike, Y. (1994). Ocular abnormalities in amyotrophic lateral sclerosis. *Acta Oto-Laryngologica. Supplementum, 511*, 138–142. https://doi.org/10.3109/00016489409128318

Okahara, Y., Takano, K., Nagao, M., Kondo, K., Iwadate, Y., Birbaumer, N., & Kansaku, K. (2018). Long-term use of a neural prosthesis in progressive paralysis. *Scientific Reports, 8*. https://doi.org/10.1038/s41598-018-35211-y

Oken, B. S., Orhan, U., Roark, B., Erdogmus, D., Fowler, A., Mooney, A., . . . Fried-Oken, M. B. (2014). Brain–computer interface with language model–electroencephalography fusion for locked-in syndrome. *Neurorehabilitation and Neural Repair, 28*(4), 387–394. https://doi.org/10.1177/1545968313516867

Pasqualotto, E., Matuz, T., Federici, S., Ruf, C., Bartl, M., Belardinelli, M. O., . . . Halder, S. (2015). Usability and workload of access technology for people with severe motor impairment: A comparison of brain-computer interfacing and eye tracking. *Neurorehabilitation and Neural Repair, 29*(10), 950–957.

Pels, E. G. M., Aarnoutse, E. J., Leinders, S., Freudenburg, Z. V., Branco, M. P., van der Vijgh, B. H., . . . Ramsey, N. F. (2019). Stability of a chronic implanted brain-computer interface in late-stage amyotrophic lateral sclerosis. *Clinical Neurophysiology, 130*(10), 1798–1803. https://doi.org/10.1016/j.clinph.2019.07.020

Peters, B., Bieker, G., Cach, M., Do, A., Fritz, A., Guger, C., . . . Fried-Oken, M. (2016). *What does BCI stand for? The 2016 Virtual Forum of BCI Users*. Presentation at the Sixth International Brain-Computer Interface Meeting. Pacific Grove, CA.

Peters, B., Bieker, G., Heckman, S. M., Huggins, J. E., Wolf, C., Zeitlin, D., & Fried-Oken, M. (2015). Brain-computer interface users speak up: The Virtual Users' Forum at the 2013 International Brain-Computer Interface meeting. *Archives of Physical Medicine and Rehabilitation, 96*(3), 833–837.

Polich, J., & Criado, J. R. (2006). Neuropsychology and neuropharmacology of P3a and P3b. *International Journal of Psychophysiology, 60*(2), 172–185. https://doi.org/10.1016/j.ijpsycho.2005.12.012

Roche, J. C., Rojas-Garcia, R., Scott, K. M., Scotton, W., Ellis, C. E., Burman, R., . . . Shaw, C. E., & Al-Chalabi, A. (2012). A proposed staging system for amyotrophic lateral sclerosis. *Brain, 135*(3), 847–852. https://doi.org/10.1093/brain/awr351

Roman, A. (2004). *ALS Communication Scale*. Retrieved from https://Amyandpals.com/

Schettini, F., Riccio, A., Simione, L., Liberati, G., Caruso, M., Frasca, V., . . . Cincotti, F. (2015). Assistive device with conventional, alternative, and brain-computer interface inputs to enhance interaction with the environment for people with amyotrophic lateral sclerosis: A feasibility and usability study. *Archives of Physical Medicine and Rehabilitation, 96*(3 Suppl.), S46–S53. https://doi.org/10.1016/j.apmr.2014.05.027

Shane, H. C., Blackstone, S., Vanderheiden, G., Williams, M., & DeRuyter, F. (2011). Using AAC technology to access the world. *Assis-*

tive Technology, 24(1), 3–13. https://doi.org/10.1080/10400435.2011.648716

Silvoni, S., Cavinato, M., Volpato, C., Ruf, C. A., Birbaumer, N., & Piccione, F. (2013). Amyotrophic lateral sclerosis progression and stability of brain-computer interface communication. *Amyotrophic Lateral Sclerosis & Frontotemporal Degeneration, 14*(5–6), 390–396. https://doi.org/10.3109/21678421.2013.770029

Spataro, R., Ciriacono, M., Manno, C., & La Bella, V. (2014). The eye-tracking computer device for communication in amyotrophic lateral sclerosis. *Acta Neurologica Scandinavica, 130*(1), 40–45.

Thompson, D. E., Gruis, K. L., & Huggins, J. E. (2014). A plug-and-play brain-computer interface to operate commercial assistive technology. *Disability and Rehabilitation. Assistive Technology, 9*(2), 144–150. https://doi.org/10.3109/17483107.2013.785036

Trail, M., Nelson, N., Van, J. N., Appel, S. H., & Lai, E. C. (2004). Major stressors facing patients with amyotrophic lateral sclerosis (ALS): A survey to identify their concerns and to compare with those of their caregivers. *Amyotrophic Lateral Sclerosis and Other Motor Neuron Disorders, 5*(1), 40–45. https://doi.org/10.1080/14660820310016075

Vansteensel, M. J., Pels, E. G. M., Bleichner, M. G., Branco, M. P., Denison, T., Freudenburg, Z. V., . . . Ramsey, N. F. (2016). Fully implanted brain–computer interface in a locked-in patient with ALS. *New England Journal of Medicine, 375*(21), 2060–2066. https://doi.org/10.1056/NEJMoa1608085

Warren, M. (1993). A hierarchical model for evaluation and treatment of visual perceptual dysfunction in adult acquired brain injury, part 1. *American Journal of Occupational Therapy, 47*(1), 42–54. https://doi.org/10.5014/ajot.47.1.42

Wicks, P., Abrahams, S., Masi, D., Hejda-Forde, S., Leigh, P. N., & Goldstein, L. H. (2007). Prevalence of depression in a 12-month consecutive sample of patients with ALS. *European Journal of Neurology, 14*(9), 993–1001. https://doi.org/10.1111/j.1468-1331.2007.01843.x

Wolpaw, J. R., Bedlack, R. S., Reda, D. J., Ringer, R. J., Banks, P. G., Vaughan, T. M., . . . Ruff, R. L. (2018). Independent home use of a brain-computer interface by people with amyotrophic lateral sclerosis. *Neurology, 91*(3), e258–e267. https://doi.org/10.1212/WNL.0000000000005812

World Health Organization. (2001). *International classification of functioning, disability and health.* Author.

Yorkston, K. M., Strand, E., Miller, R., Hillel, S., & Smith, K. (1993). Speech deterioration in amyotrophic lateral sclerosis: Implications for the timing of intervention. *Journal of Medical Speech/Language Pathology, 1*(1), 35–46.

Zickler, C., Halder, S., Kleih, S. C., Herbert, C., & Kübler, A. (2013). Brain painting: Usability testing according to the user-centered design in end users with severe motor paralysis. *Artificial Intelligence in Medicine, 59*(2), 99–110. https://doi.org/10.1016/j.artmed.2013.08.003

8

Access to AAC for Individuals with Acquired Conditions: Challenges and Solutions in Early Recovery

Susan Koch Fager, Jessica E. Gormley, and Tabatha L. Sorenson

■ Introduction

Myriad acquired communication disorders may cause individuals to become temporarily or permanently unable to meet their daily communication needs using natural speech or written communication and, instead, rely on meeting these needs using augmentative and alternative communication (AAC). Acquired communication disorders can result from a wide range of acute or chronic medical conditions, illnesses, or injuries such as: traumatic brain injury, spinal cord injury, brainstem stroke, Guillain Barré syndrome, respiratory tract intubation (e.g., tracheostomy), or facial trauma. Some individuals not only experience impairments that limit their ability to produce speech, but also experience severe physical impairments that significantly limit their ability to access AAC systems using direct selection (e.g., pointing or touching a written communication board or speech-generating device). Instead, they require alternative access methods (e.g., eye gaze, switch control) to use AAC systems for effective communication. A multitude of alternative access options exist and continue to grow with the advent of new technology. This chapter presents available access options and strategies that can be used to support adults who experience both complex communication needs and severe physical impairments to use AAC tools effectively with their families, friends, and health care team, through all levels of the recovery process.

■ Inpatient Experiences of Adults With Complex Communication Needs (CCN)

> "I was terrified. I had questions about what was going on, was I going to live? No one could understand me with that tube in my mouth"
>
> —Patient with Guillain Barré
>
> " . . . I just don't know what to do when they ask me an open question like 'what do you need?' I would just stare at them until they realized they had to ask me a question I could respond yes or no to."
>
> —Patient with Brainstem Stroke

The preceding quotes provide insight into the experiences and feelings of adults with acquired communication impairments. Clearly, the inability to communicate effectively can be both frightening and isolating. Limited communication also creates significant challenges to those with complex communication needs (CCN) and their communicative partners.

All patients have the basic human right to receive high quality health care services regardless of their speech and motor skills (United Nations, 2006; The Joint Commission, 2010). Without alternative access strategies, many people with severe speech and motor impairments may not be able to actively participate in their health care, leading to negative experiences, prolonged hospital lengths of stay, and decreased patient satisfaction (Bartlett, Blais, Tamblyn, Clermont, & MacGibbon, 2008; Blackstone, Beukelman, & Yorkston, 2015; Blackstone &

Pressman, 2016; El-Soussi, Elshafey, Othman, & Abd-Elkader, 2014).

During hospitalizations, many patients report feelings of loneliness, powerlessness, fear, and uncertainty. Patients often wonder: *"Will this procedure hurt? "Will I feel this way forever? Is this treatment my best option? Where is my family? Will I be able to go back to work ?"* But what happens when patients are not able to use speech to ask these questions to providers and their loved ones? Some patients may write their questions on a white board or pad of paper, whereas others may type on a text-to-speech app; however, when patients are not able to use their hands due to a severe motor impairment, these methods are not viable options. Without access to a functional communication system, patients are unable to effectively and consistently participate in their care. Unfortunately, individuals with CCN and severe motor impairment frequently report negative communication experiences during their recovery when interacting with health care providers (Blackstone, Beukelman, & Yorkston, 2015; Hemsley et al., 2001; Hemsley & Balandin, 2014; Holm & Dreyer, 2018a, 2018b). With no way to effectively express their questions, opinions, and thoughts, as is often the case for these patients, negative feelings often intensify and contribute to unnecessary patient suffering.

If patients are not able to use a nurse call system to alert their nurse that they are in severe pain from excessive pressure on their elbow, they may experience a pressure ulcer. If patients are not able to describe their symptoms following the administration of a new medication, they may suffer repeated allergic reactions caused by a medication error. In each of these situations, patients would experience a preventable adverse medical event—"an unintended injury or complication caused by the delivery of medical care rather than by the patient's condition" (Bartlett et al., 2008, p. 1555)—due to their lack of access to a communication system to solicit staff attention or communicate discomfort. Adults with communication disabilities are three times more likely to experience a preventable adverse event (e.g., medication error, fall) relative to adults without a communication disability (Bartlett et al., 2008) that can prolong hospital stays, increase patient discomfort, and present increased financial burden on both the patient and health care system. It is estimated that addressing hospital communication barriers with this population through increased access to speech-language pathology services, increased use of AAC systems that include alternative access options, and increased trained communication partners may reduce over 650,000 preventable adverse events and save over $6.8 billion in the United States annually (Hurtig, Alper, & Berkowitz, 2018).

Fortunately, with skilled interventions provided by a knowledgeable healthcare team comprised of speech-language pathologists, occupational therapists, and nurses, patients can use AAC systems with alternative access methods to communicate critical information starting in acute care hospitals and extending throughout the entire continuum of care. The remainder of this chapter will: (a) describe health care settings where AAC should be introduced early in the patient's recovery process, (b) discuss challenges experienced by adults with severe speech and physical limitations, and (c) provide solutions to support patient communication through all stages of patient recovery. Specific AAC access strategies will be presented starting with skills/strategies that may be especially relevant to patients at the early stages of their recovery process then

expanding to strategies that can be used as patients continue to progress through healthcare settings and gain new skills.

Health Care Settings Where Alternative Access to AAC Systems Should First be Introduced and Implemented

Adults with acquired communication disorders need access to an effective communication as early as possible in their recovery process. However, different settings inherently present different combinations of challenges and supports to the therapy process. Similarly, the goals of each setting will also impact how often a patient receives services and what those services look like. The next section will discuss two health care settings where AAC services should be provided—acute care hospitals and rehabilitation facilities.

AAC in Acute Care Hospitals

The course of treatment for individuals with acquired injuries often begins in intensive care units (ICUs) and acute care hospitals. In these settings, the goal is to perform life-sustaining procedures to ensure that the patient is medically stable. Because of the critical and emergent state of patients' conditions, their ability to use natural speech to support communication can be significantly impacted by factors such medications, consciousness, cognitive status, or mechanical ventilation, or a combination of these (Carruthers, Astin, & Munro, 2017; Garrett, Happ, Costello, & Fried-Oken, 2007). Some patients are medically sedated, whereas others may have significant brain swelling impairing consciousness. It is important to understand the underpinnings of the inability to communicate and to remember that each patient's condition and ability to communicate using AAC can rapidly change. This is a challenge in units where the SLP may not have a regular or consistent presence (e.g., ICU). In addition to fluctuating and severe medical status, intervention needs to occur around critical medical care needs and AAC strategies and techniques need to be quickly and easily implemented by all care staff and family members.

AAC in Acute Rehabilitation Facilities

As individuals with severe acquired impairments begin to recover, they often transition to long-term acute care or acute rehabilitation settings to continue their recovery process. In these settings, the goal is to increase participation, develop strategies to compensate for current deficits, and begin to plan for future/ongoing needs. Typically, the intensity and frequency of skilled therapy services also increase as the patient becomes more medically stable and able to sustain alertness and engagement in daily activities. Recovery can be rapid or slow and AAC assessment and intervention is often dynamic in nature and best completed on an ongoing basis as the patient's needs and abilities progress over time. Challenges in this setting are often rooted in the changing abilities of the individual, as well as the establishment of consistent support for communication needs among a wide range of care providers, family, and friends. It is often in acute rehabilitation facilities where clinicians must make decisions involving more long-term communication solutions and prepare patients for discharge to home or long-term care settings.

■ Common Challenges Experienced by Patients Who Require Alternative Access in Health Care Settings

The organization of this chapter centers not on where the AAC intervention occurs but on specific intervention targets that are driven by patient strengths and needs. Before solutions can be effectively implemented, clinicians must first consider what challenges are impacting patients and their communication skills. Many of the challenges discussed in this chapter exist in both the acute care environment and rehabilitation environment; however, some barriers may be more pronounced in one setting relative to the other. For example, due to the critical nature of medical complexities faced by patients in acute care settings, challenges with sedation or delirium may be of major concern. Although the contexts affecting AAC interventions differ across acute care and rehabilitation settings, the intervention targets often remain the same. Clinicians must skillfully match the interventions to patient needs throughout the recovery process.

Challenge: Determining if the Patient Will Demonstrate Temporary or Permanent AAC Communication Needs

Clinicians in acute care setting and rehabilitation facilities commonly ask, "*When should I establish an AAC system in the patient's recovery? What if they only need the system for a few days or weeks before they regain their speech?*" Many patients may experience temporary communication difficulties throughout their recovery process; however, it is challenging to accurately determine which patients will fully recover their natural speech and how long the process might take for the patient to regain their natural speech function. Clinicians should take the necessary steps to ensure that patients can access an effective communication system in their current state regardless if this state persists over time. Even one day without the ability to communicate can traumatize patients and put them at significant risk for adverse events. It is worth the time and effort to ensure that patients have access to this basic human right throughout their entire recovery. The solutions listed in this chapter can help clinicians quickly assess and implement AAC strategies to support these patients.

Challenge: Tracheostomy or Ventilator Dependency

Many patients in the acute care environment experience respiratory challenges and require interventions such as mechanical ventilation, placement of long-term or short-term alternative airways (e.g., tracheostomy, endotracheal intubation), or use of respiratory equipment that disrupts the patient's ability to speak (e.g., CPAP, BiPAP). In the United States alone, over 800,000 individuals are mechanically ventilated each year (Wunsch et al., 2010), which involves the placement of an alternate airway either through the mouth (i.e., endotracheal tube) or neck, following the placement of a tracheostomy. If a patient is intubated orally, patients are not able to speak and often have difficulty communicating with staff and family members. When questioned about their experience with mechanical ventilation, patients com-

monly report difficulty communicating as a factor that negatively impacted their care (Baumgarten & Poulen, 2015; Hurtig & Downey, 2009).

Patients who are mechanically ventilated in the ICU/acute care hospitals are often completely dependent on others to perform life-sustaining tasks (e.g., breathing) and daily activities (e.g., hygiene), have limited access to information about their care, and of necessity, must be subject to frequent, uncomfortable procedures (Baumgarten & Poulsen, 2015; Hurtig, Nilsen, Happ, & Blackstone, 2015; Jansson, San Martin, Johnson, & Nilsson, 2019; Mobasheri et al., 2016). Unsurprisingly, these patients frequently report feelings of anxiety, loneliness, and fear, and that not being able to communicate using either speech or AAC led to anger, frustration, and the feeling of "not being seen as a human being" (Baumgarten & Poulsen, 2015, p. 209). However, the frequent presence of staff and family members can be a calming influence during hospital stays, as these individuals can orient patients to place, time, and activity, provide updates about their care, and speak words of comfort. Increased staff and family presence also provides ample opportunity for others to observe and respond quickly to patient communication signals to gain attention that can be later shaped to access AAC systems (Holm & Dreyer, 2018a, 2018b; Hosseini, Valizad-Hasanloei, & Feizi, 2018; Noguchi, Inoue, & Yokota, 2019).

Challenge: Co-Occurring Cognitive Deficits

Many patients who have CCN and severe physical impairments often experience co-existing conditions that affect their cognitive skills, either temporarily or on a long-standing basis. Cognitive deficits can negatively impact patients' ability to participate in AAC services, understand what is happening around them, and learn new information. Clinicians must understand the implications of cognitive deficits on the patient's ability to participate in sessions and attempt to minimize the cognitive demands of AAC interventions.

Delirium frequently affects individuals who are critically ill and is marked by acute fluctuations in inattention and awareness, with an additional disturbance in at least one cognitive skill (e.g., memory, orientation) that cannot be attributed to another medical condition or medication effects (American Psychiatric Association, 2013). Although this condition is often reversible, long-standing cognitive deficits may persist throughout the patient's recovery process, especially in older adults (Tate et al., 2013). A team approach is required to identify and treat individuals who experience delirium, and evidence suggests that providing patients' access to a communication system may mitigate the effects of delirium (Balas, Happ, Yang, Chelluri, & Richmond, 2009; Blackstone et al., 2015).

Patients with acquired communication disorders and physical impairments may, in addition, take medications that make it difficult to stay alert for extended periods of time. Furthermore, the nature of their acquired injury may also present co-occurring cognitive deficits (e.g., TBI) affecting the patient's alertness, attention, memory, behavioral regulation, and problem solving skills. Determining periods of time when the patient is alert and able to engage in AAC assessment and intervention may prove difficult. Coordination across the interdisciplinary team members

to cluster patient care, offer co-treatments, establish a schedule, and minimize cognitive demands to support patient alertness and engagement is key to supporting these patients.

Challenge: Limited Time

Time constraints are one of the most widely cited barriers to providing AAC services in health care centers and to communicating with adults with acquired disabilities (e.g., Finke, Light, & Kitko, 2008; Gormley & Light, 2019; Hemsley & Balandin, 2014). In many acute care hospitals, speech-language pathologists work with patients on a consultative basis and only have 15 minutes at a time to work with the patient while addressing the patient's swallowing function, cognitive-linguistic skills, and communication skills. In rehabilitation facilities, clinicians often have longer time periods to work with patients relative to acute care hospitals; however, due to patients' complex medical and therapy needs of patients, it may be difficult to schedule the necessary time dedicated to providing AAC intervention, developing systems, and training communication partners (Gormley & Light, 2019). Adults with acquired communication disabilities and severe physical impairments often need significant amounts of time to learn and use AAC systems, especially during early recovery phases. For instance, it may take patients over five minutes to generate a sentence using switch scanning on their AAC system. Nurses have reported that the lack of time needed to communicate with these patients is a significant barrier, as these caregivers may need to care for multiple patients in a short period of time (e.g., medication administration times, answering alarms; Hemsley & Balandin, 2014).

Challenge: Untrained Communication Partners

Another common challenge to supporting the communication of patients with acquired communication disorders and severe physical impairment is that of training the patients' communication partners to use AAC strategies effectively. Many health care providers (e.g., nurses, physicians, allied health professionals) do not receive any preservice training on how to communicate with individuals who rely on AAC (Burns, Baylor, & Yorkston, 2017; Finke, Light, & Kitko, 2008). When these providers have a patient on their caseload that requires AAC, most of the training must occur through in-services and hands-on experiences, which introduces additional time burdens for providers to learn how to set up and maintain the AAC system, as well as the use of appropriate interaction techniques (e.g., Gormley & Light, 2019). Further, family members also must learn how to support their loved one to effectively communicate which requires clinicians to devote additional time to provide adequate support and training.

■ Access and Communication Solutions

Serving adults with acquired communication disorders within the health care environment presents many challenges; however, several solutions exist to support patients and health care providers in this task. So how can we help patients meet

their communication goals, increase their participation in their own recovery process, and improve satisfaction? To start, solutions must be introduced at multiple levels—the patient, the communication partners, and the health care system. Patients experience unique and frequently changing conditions that affect their communication skills Families and other communication partners have different skills and experiences interacting with individuals with CCN, and health care systems policies, procedures, and services all influence the patient's recovery process. Although many factors impact the communication process, with the systematic assessment of each system and systematic selection of interventions to address each area of need, the strengths of patients, partners, and health care organizations can be leveraged to support recovery. The remainder of this chapter provides specific solutions that can be used to help support effective communication with adults who have CCN and motor challenges. Solutions range from interventions that teach patients and their communication partners (e.g., health care providers, families) specific strategies to support effective communication to interventions that address larger systemic barriers through all stages of recovery (Table 8–1).

A range of access solutions exists for individuals with severe physical impairments that support the use of AAC early in recovery. The following describes a general progression of how to establish and meet short-term needs with an eye to developing and implementing solutions that will meet progressing needs over time. Although patients' physical abilities and needs vary, ensuring that the following areas are addressed and considered will support temporary and long-term communication needs as they recover.

Table 8–1. Challenges and Solutions for Adults With Acquired Communication Disorders and Physical Access Difficulties

Challenges	Solutions
Untrained partners	• Teach partner to identify patient's intent to communicate and unique communication signals • Teach partners how to operate/set up the patient's AAC system • Teach interaction skills (e.g., offer communication opportunities, wait, etc.)
Limited involvement of AAC specialists	• Referral protocol changes (automatic communication orders, etc.) • Creating "communication champions"
Limited access to AAC materials in inpatient units	• Creation of communication toolkits that include a wide range of access options (high-tech and low-tech options)

Solution: Identifying a Communication Advocate and Training Communication Partners

As adults with acquired communication disorders and severe physical impairment often rely on others to complete daily activities, they also rely on others to help manage and implement AAC into their lives (Beukelman, Garrett, & Yorkston, 2007). Communication advocates know how to use the AAC system, perform daily maintenance on the system if it requires specialized positioning or charging, assist with adding vocabulary, and can train others how to communicate with the patient (Beukelman et al., 2007). Identifying communication advocates early in recovery can assist in the establishment and implementation of AAC strategies, particularly in settings where the SLP may only be present on a consultative basis (e.g., ICU). This person can be a family member or close friend who is present with the

patient throughout the day or frequently visits the individuals in the medical setting in which they are currently residing.

Regardless of the setting, a multitude of communication partners needs to be trained to achieve effective communication and support the patient's recovery process. Although the communication advocate can lead the efforts on managing the patient's system, other caregivers and family members must also have a basic understanding of these skills to set the patient up for communication success. They must also understand and use basic interaction strategies such as offering frequent communication opportunities, waiting an appropriate amount of time for the patient to respond, and responding appropriately to the patient (Gormley & Light, 2019). Families and health care providers, who are frequent communication partners, must be involved through all steps of AAC assessment and intervention to effectively support the establishment and implementation of AAC strategies.

Example communication partner targets include: (a) teaching health care providers to direct questions to the patient and not just to the family, (b) teaching family members and caregiver "how" to ask yes/no questions to maximize patient involvement and to minimize patient frustration, (c) providing staff with lists of common care-related questions and vocabulary can be helpful along with any other useful information that will increase the likelihood of successful communication, and (d) teaching all partners to provide sufficient wait time for the individual to give a motor response. Use of specialized trainings is also an option to train health care providers. For instance, a free, computer-based training called the Study of Patient-Nurse Effectiveness with Assisted Communication Strategies (SPEACS) intervention is available to teach nurses who work within the intensive care unit to communicate with adults who require mechanical ventilation (Happ, Sereika, Garrett, & Tate, 2008; Happ et al., 2010; Happ et al., 2014).

Health Care Systems Level Solutions

In many ICU and acute medical settings, the SLP receives specific orders for swallowing or speaking valve assessment and intervention (Beukelman & Nordness, 2015, 2017; Hemsley & Balandin, 2014). These specific referrals often do not meet the communication needs of patients with complex communication disorders and severe physical impairment, resulting in the outcome that they may not receive AAC intervention until they transition to rehabilitation settings. The lack of a systems level model that includes the SLP in the needed assessment and intervention

of communication needs beyond the PMV perpetuates the challenges many patients face with temporary and long-term communication access needs. A solution to this problem is the implementation of a medical order for scope of treatment, or for standing orders for patients with specific kinds of diagnoses, and care maps or clinical pathways (Beukleman & Nordness, 2015, 2017). These kinds of referral models broaden the scope of the intervention and allow for the SLPs to freely address the patient communication needs of these individuals beyond the PMV and swallowing interventions. The implementation of these order and referral processes occurs at health care systems models and require facility/organization and administrative support, and are essential in meeting the needs of patients with CCN and severe physical impairment.

Another solution includes the implementation of ongoing screenings to identify individuals who are not able to use speech to communicate. Nursing staff have the most consistent and ongoing contact with patients throughout their recovery and can play an instrumental role in referring the patient for appropriate services. One tool to support the screening and assessment of individuals with CCN in the inpatient setting is the "Inpatient Functional Communication Interview" (O'Halloran, Worrall, Toffolo, & Code, 2020). Nursing can complete the screening tool to identify patients with complex communication early in their hospitalization to establish an AAC system to support patients.

An additional solution includes stocking "communication kits" in hospital units to quickly and easily trial a variety of access methods. These kits should be stocked with a variety of low-tech and high-tech AAC tools to meet each patient's unique clinical profile. Examples of items that could be included in the kit are: paper/laminated communication boards of various sizes and complexity, stylus, white board, tablets with speech-generating apps, switches (e.g., button, light touch, sip-and-puff, eyeblink, etc.), laser pointer, and instructional materials for partners to use partner-assisted scanning, how to ask yes/no questions, low tech eye gaze techniques, and instructions to customize communication boards. Descriptions and examples of these materials are presented throughout the chapter.

Solution: Development of Yes/No Physical Response

Being able to communicate a yes/no response is often foundational to establishing communication early in recovery. When an individual demonstrates substantial physical impairments, access to these communication options and tools can be difficult. Looking for physical signals to symbolize yes/no can be an ongoing process, particularly early in recovery when patients' level of consciousness and fatigue can change. It is important to first look for physical movements that are as intuitive and natural as possible. For example, many people nod and shake their heads to indicate yes/no. If physically able, this is often a movement patients will demonstrate. For those who are severely physically impaired, other options will need to be explored. Some have suggested following a yes/no hierarchy, including head nods/shakes, thumbs up/down, eye blinks, and finally other variations of movement (DeRuyter & Kennedy, 1991; Fager, Doyle, & Karantounis, 2007; Fager & Karantounis, 2011). For individuals with brainstem

impairment, initial movements are often restricted to vertical eye movement (Culp, Beukelman, & Fager, 2007; Culp & Ladtkow, 1991; Papadopoulou et al., 2019). If possible, these individuals may be able to indicate yes/no using an up/down eye movement. Eye blinks are another option for these individuals; however, they can be easily misinterpreted as eye blinks are also ongoing and reflexive, which often requires an adjustment to be made to the blink (e.g., long eye blinks versus short eye blinks). When eye movement is not restricted to a vertical plane, using eye gaze to yes/no targets (e.g., note cards, picture symbols) can be a successful tool. Other potential movements, depending on diagnosis include eyebrow, mouth movements, thumb/finger movement, toe movement, and facial muscle twitches. The key to establishing a physical signal to indicate yes/no is to systematically evaluate the patient's ability to control different physical movements, starting with the most natural/intuitive responses (e.g., head nods/shakes, mouth movement), to other physical movements (e.g., eyebrow, facial twitches, movements in the extremities). In addition to identifying movement options, important considerations include stamina or level of fatigue demonstrated by movement, motor response delay (remembering to give sufficient wait time for the patient to provide the physical response to command), any reflexive movements that interfere with volitional control over this movement, and ability to replicate these movements during different times of day. Establishing a consistent and reliable yes/no response, depending on the specific condition of the individual, may be relatively fast to establish, or may take several trials over time to determine.

In medical settings, individuals recovering from acquired injuries, encounter numerous care providers throughout the day. This can be particularly challenging when attempting to establish a consistent and reliable yes/no communication method. Confusion of care staff as to the yes/no signals the patient is most successful using can cause severe miscommunications with care staff looking for different physical signals, requiring the patient to demonstrate yes/no signals that they are not able to consistently execute, and trialing new yes/no methods that they are most familiar with. This can have devastating consequences for the individual with severe physical impairment in that they are unable to consistently respond to important care questions or communicate critical care needs. Education to all care staff as to the most consistent and reliable yes/no signal system is critical. This can be accomplished through signs, written instructions, demonstration during rounding, and demonstration during shift changes. Documentation, as well as face-to-face education, is important to ensure continuity.

Solution: Access to Nurse Call Systems

The "nurse call button" provides a basic, functional way for an individual to be able to communicate or signal a need early in recovery. Access to signaling help and communication has been shown to substantially reduce anxiety and psychological distress among individuals who are critically ill (Balandin, Hemsley, Sigafoos, & Green, 2007; Bartlett et al., 2008; Costello, 2000; Zubow & Hurtig, 2013). However, traditional nurse call systems have been primarily developed for access by individuals with hand dexterity. Alternative access is often required by individuals with severe physical impairment.

Options exist to accommodate these different access modalities. For example, many standard nurse call systems integrate with flat (pancake) switches and sip-and-puff. Some wireless switch options can be plugged into the nurse call board in a patient room allowing access to a wide array of capability switches. Others have developed integrated nurse call, room control, and communication options. If the patient is already using a high tech AAC device, technology is available to allow for the AAC device to turn on the nurse call system with an IR interface. Assessment for access using alternative methods needs to include not only the identification of the most reliable and consistent movement, but also the reliability of this movement over time, with fatigue and changes in medication, and with changes in positioning (Culp et al., 2007; Zubow & Hurtig, 2013). For individuals with severe physical impairments, this access may not be consistent due to one or more of the aforementioned factors. In these cases, it is often required to implement a regular nurse-rounding schedule to ensure that patient needs are being met. Research has indicated positive effects of a consistent nurse-rounding schedule on patient satisfaction and safety and is now a part of regular clinical care in many medical settings (Meade, Bursell, & Ketelsen, 2006).

Solution: Low-Tech AAC Options—Extending Beyond Yes/No

Access to low-tech AAC systems is frequently the first intervention that many with severe physical impairment receive early in recovery. Table 8–2 reviews low-tech access considerations. Once a consistent/reliable yes/no or signaling method

Table 8–2. Physical Access Options and Considerations for Assessment and Access Option Selection

Access Option	*Considerations for Assessment and Selection*
High-Tech	
Eye tracking	<ul><li>Eye motor control sufficient to move cursor across communication display</li><li>Adequate support for positioning necessary for successful calibration and use of technology</li><li>Eye health issues (e.g., dry eyes)</li><li>Context where eye gaze is used (lighting and positioning can impact accuracy)</li><li>Ptosis (eye droop—certain eye trackers incorporate algorithms to manage ptosis)</li><li>Selection option<ul><li>Dwell: timing and inadvertent activations</li><li>Blink: ability to perform sufficient blink while using device to construct messages</li><li>Switch: other physical movements can be harnessed as selection method, often preferred over dwell as it does not require timing</li></ul></li></ul>
Head tracking	<ul><li>Sufficient range of motion without pain or excessive fatigue</li><li>Absolute versus relative tracking technologies (some head tracking devices can be calibrated and scaled up to accommodate minimal movements)</li><li>Selection methods<ul><li>Dwell: timing and inadvertent activations</li><li>Switch: other physical movements can be harnessed as selection method and often preferred over dwell as does not require timing</li></ul></li></ul>
Switch scanning	<ul><li>Wide range of switch options available to capture available movement capabilities</li><li>One or two switch scanning</li><li>Automatic scanning versus directed scanning</li><li>Motor planning and execution required to make switch selection impacts scanning type and rate</li></ul>
Touchscreen access	<ul><li>Direction selection of touchscreen interface with hand, finger, elbow, or other body part</li><li>Use of adaptive equipment to increase accuracy (e.g., stylus, digit isolation glove, keyguards)</li><li>Modification of communication software layout to increase accuracy (e.g., size, number of targets, location of targets on screen)</li><li>Adaptations to touchscreen access to improve accuracy (e.g., touch exit versus touch enter)</li></ul>

Table 8–2. *continued*

Access Option	Considerations for Assessment and Selection
Low- or No-Tech Access Options	
Facial expressions and gestures (e.g., pointing)	▪ Additional equipment is not always required; however, use of adaptive equipment to increase accuracy (e.g., stylus) can be used ▪ Direct selection of printed, static communication boards with hand, finger, elbow, or other body part
Eye pointing	▪ Screening for eye motor control and potential visual processing issues (consultation of occupational therapy and/or neuro-optometrist may be needed) ▪ Assess for fatigue/stamina using this access method (may need brief interactions at first) ▪ Optimize displays to accommodate for eye motor control/range of eye movement (vertical vs horizontal) ▪ Position visual content to accommodate for field cuts/neglects
Laser pointer	▪ Ensure access method is safe/appropriate for environment ▪ Minimal movements can still be used by placing communication board farther away from patient ▪ Not limited to head movement (can be accessed via hand, foot, etc.)

has been established, expansion of AAC beyond yes/no is often the next focus of intervention. Low-tech options vary and are often impacted by factors such as attention, cognitive status, fatigue, vision, and/or hearing issues. Additionally, a range of options may be developed for use with different communication partners or within different contexts. For example, communication boards might be developed with the patient, care staff, and family to communicate the most salient basic needs, messages related to clinical care needs and care-planning, social/closeness messages, feelings, and environmental control options (Bardach, 2015; Broyles, Tate, & Happ, 2012; Happ, Tuite, Dobbin, DiVirgilio-Thomas, & Kitutu, 2004; Radtke, Baumann, Garrett, & Happ, 2011). These

boards, depending on the visual and cognitive abilities of the patient, might include pictures, line drawings, and/or words to represent this information (Beukelman & Light, 2020). Figures 8–1 and 8–2 provide examples of communication boards.

Because the patients we are discussing lack the ability to point to these boards with their hands, alternative access to low tech communication is required. The following provides a description of common access methods and considerations for using these options.

Solution: Partner Dependent Scanning

Often, low-tech communication options can be navigated auditorily with a partner.

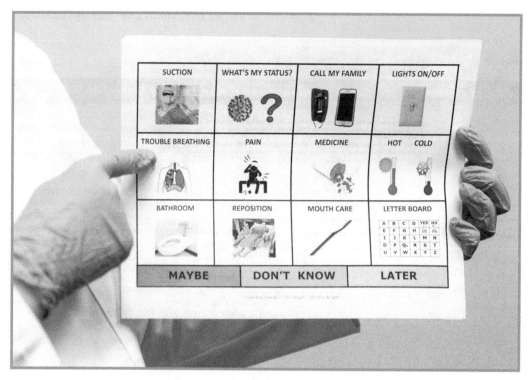

Figure 8–1. Example of low-tech communication board with pictures and words.

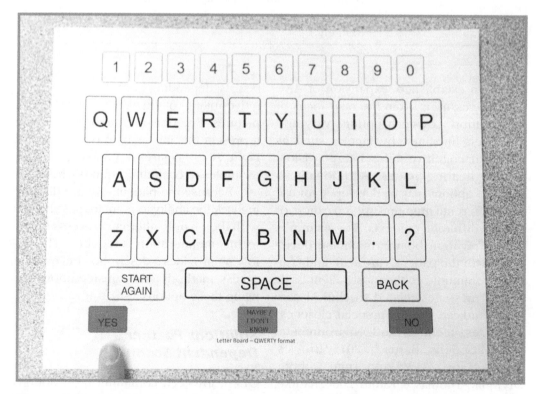

Figure 8–2. Example of low-tech communication board to support spelling of messages.

In this process, options are scanned out loud by the communication partner and the patient uses a specific signal to indicate when the desired target has been reached (e.g., eye blink or physical signal that is being used to indicate "yes"). This technique can be used to narrow down categories and specific messages within the categories or can be used to support spelling of messages (e.g., rows scanned first then individual letters within rows) (Figure 8–3).

Partner-dependent scanning requires attention, stamina, and vigilance on the part of the patient. Some may not be ready for this level of sustained attention due to their medical condition and/or medicine schedule. For those with challenges with attention and fatigue, starting with a small number of critical messages may be appropriate before expanding to larger numbers of messages and spelling to communicate needs. Culp and colleagues (2007) suggested that individuals with severe physical impairment may be ready to construct messages via spelling if they can attend to conversational exchanges of 3 to 5 minutes making up to five to six choices.

Solution: Eye Gaze and Eye Linking

Eye gaze and eye linking can be used as a direct pointing method to binary choices, or to indicate messages on a communication display. Eye motility can be impaired at the early stages of recovery for some individuals, for example, vertical eye gaze early in brainstem stroke recovery (Bauer, Gerstenbrand, & Rumpl, 1979; Culp & Ladtkow, 1992; Culp et al., 2007; Sand et al.,

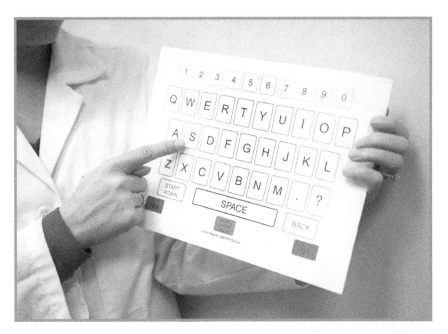

Figure 8–3. Example of partner-dependent scanning using letter board. The communication partner scans (by pointing and speaking aloud each target option) through each row and then column (e.g., letter) after the patient has signaled "yes" to the appropriate row/column.

2013) and should be considered before targeting eye gaze as a low-tech pointing method and boards should be designed to accommodate any eye motor control challenges. Communication boards using for eye gaze access are often constructed of clear/Plexiglass materials (Figure 8–4). Eye gaze access requires the patient to look to the target and the gaze is interpreted by the communication partner. Eye linking is a method where the patient fixes their gaze on a target as the display is being moved until the gaze of the communication partner and the patient "link up" (i.e., both the communication partner and the patient are looking simultaneously at the target). Both methods can be used to communicate single messages, messages nested within categories, and messages constructed via spelling.

Special Considerations for Using Eye Gaze as a Primary Access Method

Visual processing and eye motor control can be impaired early in recovery and remain a long-term challenge (Ciuffreda et al.,2007; Hepworth, Rowe, Walker, Rockliffe, Noonan, Howard, & Currie, 2016; Roman-Lantzy, 2007). Often, consultations with colleagues who have specific training in visual processing, cortical visual impairment, and oculomotor control issues (e.g., occupational therapist, neuro-optometrist) can be of benefit if problems are suspected. Simple scanning tasks (e.g., asking the patient to follow an object with their eyes as it is moved in different planes) can screen for eye motor control issues and help determine if field

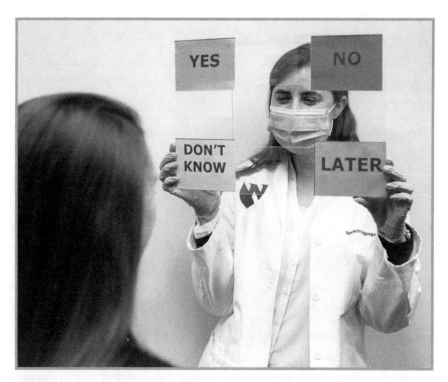

Figure 8–4. Example of low-tech eye gaze board.

cuts or neglects might be present. Visual processing issues might become more apparent as communication boards and displays are being developed and trialed. Changes in size of content, number of targets, color contrast, spacing of targets, and use of words, symbols, or a combination of these might be necessary to overcome challenges (Brown, Thiessen, Beukelman, & Hux, 2015; Light, Wilkinson, Thiessen, Beukelman, & Fager, 2019; Wilkinson & Jagaroo, 2004). Some patients may need auditory cues to interpret some messages and communication content. Light sensitivity may impact their ability to use their eyes as a primary communication method (Greenwald, Kapoor, & Singh, 2012). Additionally, they may fatigue quickly using this method as a primary communication option. For some, the extensive use of eye movement may elicit a pattern of ocular bobbing (particularly for those with brainstem impairment), and may make eye movements difficult for communication partners to accurately interpret (Papadopoulou et al., 2019).

Case Illustration: *Mary was a 53-year-old woman with Guillain Barré syndrome. During her acute care hospital stay, Mary's medical team were uncertain as to whether she was conscious and able to participate in basic communication as she presented as severely flaccid with her eyes continually closed. The team members had been asking Mary to open her eyes for several days in hopes of establishing a yes/no response signal with eye blinks. Once evaluated by the therapy team, it was determined that Mary could use eye movement to communicate when her eyes were manually held open by her communication partner. With physical assistance with eye opening, Mary could*

track moving objects to command and look left, right, up, and down. Mary's first yes/no response method utilized up/down eye movements. However, this method was fatiguing for Mary and the accuracy of her responses tended to degrade after 2 to 3 minutes. Medical staff and Mary's husband were trained on how to use this method to communicate basic care needs and to have brief social interactions with family. Care staff and family were also provided with lists of yes/no questions to increase their ease of communication with Mary and to ensure that they asked her questions in a way she could reasonably respond. As Mary regained the ability to open her eyes, she quickly progressed to using this eye movement to signal yes/no with partner-dependent scanning. A series of full message boards were developed with Mary, her husband, and key care staff and included basic care needs, medical care questions from Mary for her care providers, messages to support expression of emotions, and specific messages related to family and friends for social closeness. As Mary continued to progress, her ability to maintain attention and accurately use this communication access method successfully increased to 5 to 6 minutes with several conversational turns. Partner dependent scanning with an alphabet board was trialed and Mary could successfully spell messages and expand her communication beyond full message communication boards.

Mary's case illustrates some key considerations when implementing eye gaze access with lo-tech AAC options early in recovery. First, Mary did demonstrate the ability to use her eye gaze to communicate; however, she required physical assistance from her communication partners early in recovery to do so. The initial assumption from the medical team was that Mary's consciousness was somehow impaired. Had they waited until Mary regained control of eye opening, she would have been unable to communicate for the first several weeks of her recovery that could have had a devastating effect on her emotional and psychological state. Second, Mary's communication displays were developed and personalized specifically for her. Mary, her family and the care team provided input into the kinds of messages that were critical and of most value during a time where her interactions were required to be brief due to fatigue. As Mary physically recovered control of eye opening, she could continue to use her up/down eye movement to indicate yes/no for expanded communication options. By this time, she was very familiar and accurate with this method as her use of this signal started early in her recovery.

Solution: Light Tech AAC Options

The following describes solutions that begin to bridge the gap from no tech/low tech solutions to high tech solution (see Table 8–2 for light-tech access consideration). These can often be used as intermediate steps to expand communication, provide access to voice output devices, and increase independence of communication without the ongoing dependence on the communication partner.

Laser Pointers

The use of laser pointers has been documented as a direct pointing method to communication boards and communication content within an individual's envi-

ronment (Fager, Beukelman, & Jakobs, 2002; Fager, Beukelman, Karantounis, & Jakobs, 2006; Fager, Bardach, Russell, & Higginbotham, 2012; Fager, Beukelman, Fried-Oken, Jakobs, & Baker, 2012). The laser pointer can be affixed to the head (e.g., via a headband or eyeglasses) or to a body part that the individual has consistent control of (e.g., foot, hand). The range of movement required to move the red dot of the laser across a display is impacted by the distance of the display from the laser. When individuals have severely reduced range of motion, positioning the communication display further away from the laser point can allow for full access to the display. Additionally, the low-tech display can be easily designed to accommodate the available range the patient demonstrates (Fager et al., 2002). The cases and uses of lasers in the literature often describe a prototype technology that was designed to be eye safe. It should be noted that the use of commercially available laser pointers is not eye safe and should be implemented with caution and extensive education of communication partners.

Eye-Blink Switches and Other Switches for Minimal Movement

Other devices might be used as access points to simple digitized speech output device or with high tech AAC devices. Infrared eye-blink switches can be mounted to glasses and connected to simple digitized speech devices (e.g., to communicate yes/no) or connected to AAC devices to support switch-activated scanning if the patient has the stamina and sufficient accuracy to manage this level of access. The infrared eye-blink switch points an eye-safe, infrared beam toward the eye of the patient. When the patient closes his/her eye for a predetermined amount of time, it acts as a switch-closure that activates the device it is connected to. This method may be trialed if a single eye-blink is the most consistent and reliable movement that a patient has. A range of switches are available that can detect subtle muscle movements (e.g., twitch switch, electromyography switches, piezoelectric switches). Many of these kinds of switches can be used to capture subtle facial muscle contractions that are under volitional control of the patient (e.g., eyebrow raise, smirk, shoulder shrug).

Case Illustration: *Joe suffered a severe bout of encephalitis and was in a coma for two weeks. As Joe began to emerge from coma, his gaze would fixate to the left when his eyes were open and he was unable to track any moving objects. However, when asked, Joe could initiate eye blinks to command to indicate yes/no (i.e., long blink for yes and two short blinks for no). This allowed Joe an initial method for answering yes/no questions with medical staff and family. It was determined that the swelling to Joe's brain due to encephalitis had caused significant damage to his occipital lobe and it was unclear what information he could process visually. All low-tech options were presented to him auditorily, and several weeks later, as his stamina and ability to attend and respond to communicative interactions of 5 to 6 turns, he eventually progressed to spelling messages using partner dependent scanning and eye blinks. The team decided to trial access to an AAC device to try to give Joe greater independence with communication. Using an infrared eye-blink switch, Joe used his long eye-blink to communication to initial auditory scanning of communi-*

cation content programmed into an AAC device. The messages included yes/no and a few key basic/urgent needs for medical staff that Joe indicated were important (pain, reposition, wipe face/eyes). Once Joe became proficient with this method, the number of messages was increased. Although this method gave Joe access to voice output and greater independence, he often had misactivations or difficulty activating the switch if he became too fatigued. Joe continued to use a variety of low tech (partner-dependent scanning) and light tech (eye-blink switch activated auditory scanning with AAC device) to meet his communication needs early in recovery.

Joe's case illustrates the challenge of finding a response modality when severe physical impairment (including vision at the motor control and visual processing level) are present. As a result, Joe relied heavily on auditory information to be able to respond and access low and light technology AAC options to communicate. Because alternative access can be challenging when an individual has severe physical impairments, it is important to develop and AAC system that continues to incorporate a variety of options. Trialing an access technology (e.g., infrared eye-blink switch) started Joe down the path of using AAC technology, even if he could not meet all his needs using the device in all contexts. Due to the severity of Joe's condition, he would likely need to rely on AAC long-term and the team started this process early by identifying methods he could use immediately (low-tech partner-dependent scanning) and starting identifying a potential access method (eye-blink switch) that gave him the opportunity to begin independent communication with an AAC device.

Solution: High-Tech AAC in Early Recovery

After ICU and acute care hospitalization when patients become more medically stable, they typically transfer to environments where rehabilitation is the primary focus. The goal of the rehabilitation team is to maximize current ability while planning for and facilitating changes in capability over time. Often for individuals with severe physical impairments, trials of high-tech AAC devices occur at this stage. Some will also have long-term high-tech AAC devices recommended for them at this time. For others, the path to a high-tech AAC device is complicated by rapidly changing abilities and is less clear. For these individuals, high-tech AAC devices may be trialed and a variety of access options may be used as they begin to recover more physical function.

Access to high-tech AAC devices are often described as "direct" and "indirect" alternative access (Beukelman & Light, 2020). Direct options include direct selection from the device interface with a hand, mouth stick, head stick, stylus, or other adaptive equipment. It can also include access methods such as head or eye pointing. Indirect access refers to access methods such as through switch-activated scanning, whereas a switch is selected that causes items on the communication display to be scanned. Early in recovery, some individuals may have more ability to use one access method over the other; however, they may demonstrate the potential to transition to a more efficient method as they recover. Because of this, some access methods may be used to support ongoing daily communication with a wide range of partners because it is the most reliable and consistent method for that individual *at that time*. In addi-

tion, other access methods may be trialed therapeutically in controlled contexts to increase exposure and practice with the method over time in the hopes of developing the capability to rely on this method in the future.

How to Determine What Access Method to Start With

Choosing an access method can be complicated by several issues including attention, medication schedule, fatigue/stamina, physical movement capabilities, communication needs and contexts, and the skills/knowledge of the communication partners. In any medical setting, a patient will encounter a wide array of care-providers with varying levels of skills and knowledge with regard to high-tech AAC. Given these challenges, it is important to look at communication from two perspectives: (1) implementation of tools, devices, and strategies that can meet the patient's daily needs immediately and consistently, and (2) tools, devices and strategies that show potential to meet the patient's needs in the future.

Assessing the patient for reliable and consistent movements as an access method will be key. Note that the access method to the high-tech AAC device may or may not be the same movements the individual has been using to indicate yes/no and signal selections on their low-tech communication system. For example, whereas someone may be using low-tech eye movements to support communication by spelling using partner dependent scanning, they may not have eye motor control capability yet to functionally use eye-tracking technology. Or the patient may demonstrate limited head nods/movement to indicate yes/no, but they do have yet exhibit the range needed to use head tracking access to a high-tech AAC device. It is important to assess movement options at this level and include trials with the access technology to determine the best approach to supporting immediate and daily communication needs (see Table 8–2 for high-tech access selection considerations). Additionally, considering the support personnel available to set-up and trouble-shoot the high-tech AAC device and access method is critical.

Although assessment for the most consistent and reliable access method is occurring, it is important to note and consider input from clinical colleagues as to the potential motor recovery that the patient demonstrates potential for. Although this movement or access method may not yet be functional to meet daily communication needs, practice with the method may be a goal in therapy to transition the patient eventually to this method.

Case Illustration: *Laura was a young woman who had sustained a severe brainstem stroke. Laura came to a rehabilitation hospital with the ability to indicate yes/no through subtle head nods, and spelled messages using partner dependent auditory scanning where she indicated the target row and letter through a subtle head nod. Laura had diplopia (double vision) which required spot patching of her glasses and her eye motor control was beginning to expand from vertical only, to some horizontal movement. The team immediately trialed an eye gaze device but she was unable to accurately use this method and select full messages from a limited communication display of 4 to 6 cells (less than 50% accurate). Laura did exhibit consistent movement in her left thumb. Using automatic row-column scanning, she could successfully navigate a display on a high-tech AAC device to*

not only select full messages, but to also independently spell messages using an onscreen display with word prediction. Although this method was slow, it was highly accurate for Laura. Additionally, the medical support staff could set up the switch and device with relative ease so that she could use it throughout the day. Whereas Laura used this access method to access the high-tech AAC device to meet her daily communication needs during acute rehabilitation, she also demonstrated the potential to transition to two other possible direct access methods, eye gaze, or direct selection with her left hand. These methods might potentially allow Laura more efficient access to a high-tech AAC device than scanning would. Laura was given extensive opportunities to practice using these access methods during therapy. Although her left-hand movement progressed, she found direct access with her hand to be extremely fatiguing and as she recovered, she began to demonstrate increased ataxia with volitional arm extension that decreased her accuracy of selection using this method. As her eye motor control recovered, she could increase her accuracy using eye tracking and could expand from a limited display of six communication messages to using an onscreen keyboard to spell messages. She coupled this direct pointing method with switch access using her left hand to make her selection. This access combination increased her accuracy and efficiency, and overall satisfaction using the high-tech AAC device to support communication. However, eye gaze access required optimal setup and positioning for Laura and was difficult for nursing staff to support throughout the day and in all positions (e.g. wheelchair vs. bed). Therefore, she primarily continued to use switch-activated scanning to control her high-tech AAC device outside of therapy and a communication advocate (her sister) was trained extensively to support optimal positioning and setup of the eye gaze device. Laura's sister agreed to serve as the communication support and trainer for her next level of care so that she could begin utilizing this device in her long-term discharge environment. She could fully transition to this access combination immediately prior to her discharge to a skilled nursing facility near her home and family with the support of her communication advocate. At the time of discharge, she demonstrated the consistent physical ability to successfully use this access method and she had an established support to ensure its carryover and successful implementation in her next level of care.

Laura's case illustrates some key considerations when assessing for and implementing high-tech AAC solutions early in recovery. First, early in her rehabilitation stay, options were trialed with the understanding that Laura would likely change and progress physically over time. This can be challenging when making high-tech AAC recommendations as the "final" recommendation may not come until closer to discharge or after the patient has discharged from inpatient therapy. However, the team found her most consistent and reliable access method that care staff could support successfully (switch-activated scanning) and she used that through much of her rehabilitation stay to meet her daily communication needs. The team then trialed other access methods therapeutically with Laura throughout her rehabilitation stay to help her further develop these physical access alternatives (eye gaze and hand movement control). Although Laura did not regain the ability to successfully use her hand for direct access to her device, she did recover enough eye motor control to use eye gaze access and she could use her hand and a switch as her selection method. Laura preferred this selection method to dwell (e.g., hovering the cursor over a target for a predetermined amount of time in order to make a selection) as she felt she had more control of her selections and made less inadvertent activations while she was constructing messages. Although our focus is often on a single access method, being able to take advantage of other access options is important to implement the most effective solutions for individuals with severe motor impairments. Additionally, Laura's communication advocate (her sister) was identified early in this process and incorporated in the use of Laura's AAC throughout her stay. Eye tracking technology requires time, training, and familiarity with the technology to be able to successfully support its use (Ball et al., 2010; Fager, 2018; Fager et al., 2012; Higginbotham, Shane, Russell, & Caves, 2007). In settings where care providers might frequently change (e.g., hospital or skilled nursing facility) this can be very challenging. Having a communication advocate that can help to ease transitions to different care environments and maintain the use of technology as these changes occur.

Solutions for Transitions— Setting the Stage for Ongoing AAC Support

AAC intervention for individuals early in recovery is a changing and dynamic process. Some will have needs that are temporary, others will need AAC long-term but their access capabilities will change as they recover. Not only do they require support for successful medical environment transitions (e.g., ICU, acute care hospital, rehabilitation hospital) but also as they transition to home and community settings. Research has indicated that often the abandonment of AAC occurs when the support for these strategies and technologies fall away (Fager, Hux, Beukelman, & Karantounis, 2006). Several steps can be taken early in recovery to ensure the successful support of AAC throughout the recovery process and across multiple care environments.

As mentioned earlier in this chapter, identification of a communication advocate or advocates is key to ensuring continuity of AAC implementation and support. Supplying this advocate with the knowledge and tools to share with others as the patient enters new care settings is essential. In addition to the knowledge and skills the communication advocate has regarding the specific access needs and abilities of the patient, providing them with information that they and the patient can easily share with care-providers is helpful. This can come in the form of written instructions and pictures (e.g., communication passports). One resource that provides free, printable downloads of communication materials and strategies to train providers is the Patient-Provider Communication website (http://www.patientprovidercommunication.org). Some access strategies can be difficult to explain in written text for communication partners that are unfamiliar with these strategies (e.g., partner dependent scanning, or when the physical signals that the patient demonstrates are subtle or require context and cues to elicit). In these instances, video illustration of these techniques and strategies may be helpful. Research is beginning to emerge about the positive impact of video supports to help care-providers use AAC techniques and strategies to increase patient-provider communication in medical environments (e.g., Gormley & Light, 2019).

Conclusion

Access to AAC early in recovery is critical for the health and well-being of patients as they recover. Access to AAC tools and strategies allow patients to be able to communicate critical information and be a part of their care planning. Access to AAC also provides a sense of connection with care-givers and family during this stressful and challenging time. Recovery of natural speech for some may be imminent but for others their reliance on AAC will be long-term. In either instance, access to AAC to support communication is an essential component to care and recovery for these individuals. Access can be challenging early in recovery but a wide range of tools and strategies exist that can be implemented to meet individual's communication needs.

Acknowledgement. The authors would like to thank Jessica Thompson CF-SLP for contributing the photos for this chapter.

References

American Psychiatric Association. (2013). *Diagnostic and statistical manual of mental disorders* (5th ed.). Washington, DC: Author.

Balandin, S., Hemsley, B., Sigafoos, J., & Green, V. (2007). Communicating with nurses: The experiences of 10 adults with cerebral palsy and complex communication needs. *Applied Nursing Research, 20*(2), 56–62. https://doi.org/10.1016/j.apnr.2006.03.001

Balas, M. C., Happ, M. B., Yang, W., Chelluri, & Richmond, T. (2009). Outcomes associated with delirium in older patients in surgical ICUs. *Chest, 135,* 18–25. https://doi.org/10.1378/chest.08–1456

Ball, L., Nordness, A., Fager, S., Kersch, K., Mohr, B., & Pattee, G. (2010). Eye gaze access to AAC technology for people with amyotrophic lateral sclerosis. *Journal of Medical Speech-Language Pathology, 18*(3), 11–23.

Bardach, L. (2015). Enhancing communication in hospice settings. In *Patient-provider communication: Roles for speech-language pathologists and other health care professionals* (pp. 271–301). Plural Publishing.

Bartlett, G., Blais, R., Tamblyn, R., Clermont, R. J., & MacGibbon, B. (2008). Impact of patient communication problems on the risk of preventable adverse events in acute care settings. *Canadian Medical Association Journal, 178*(12), 1555–1562. https://doi.org/10.1503/cmaj.070690

Bauer, G., Gerstenbrand, F., & Rumpl, E. (1979). Varieties of locked-in syndrome. *Journal of Neurology, 221,* 77–91. https://doi.org/10.1007/BF00313105

Baumgarten, M., & Poulsen, I. (2015). Patients' experiences of being mechanically ventilated in an ICU: A qualitative metasynthesis. *Scandinavian Journal of Caring Sciences, 29*(2), 205–214. https://doi.org/10.1111/scs.12177

Beukelman, D. R., Garrett, K. L., & Yorkston, K. M. (2007). *Augmentative communication Strategies for adults with acute or chronic medical conditions.* Brookes.

Beukelman, D., & Light, J. (2020). *Augmentative & alternative communication for children and adults.* (5th ed.). Brookes.

Beukelman, D. R., & Nordness, A. S. (2015). Patient-provider communication in rehabilitation settings. In *Patient-provider communication: Roles for speech-language pathologists and other health care professionals.* Plural Publishing.

Beukelman, D.R., & Nordness, A.S. (2017). Patient-provider communication for people with severe dysarthria: Referral policies that lead to systems change. *Seminars in Speech and Language, 38*(3), 239–250. https://doi.org/10.1055/s-0037-1602843

Blackstone, S., Beukelman, D. R., & Yorkston, K. (2015). *Patient-provider communication: Roles for speech-language pathologists and other health care professionals.* Plural Publishing.

Blackstone, S. W., & Pressman, H. (2016). Patient communication in health care settings: New opportunities for augmentative and alternative communication. *Augmentative and Alternative Communication, 32*(1), 69–79. https://doi.org/10.3109/07434618.2015.1125947

Brown, J., Thiessen, A., Beukelman, D. R., & Hux, K. (2015). Noun representation in AAC grid displays: Visual attention patterns of people with traumatic brain injury, *Augmentative and Alternative Communication, 31,* 15–26. https://doi.org/10.3109/07434618.2014.995224

Broyles, L. M., Tate, J. A., & Happ, M. B. (2012). Use of augmentative and alternative communication strategies by family members in the intensive care unit. *American Journal of Critical Care, 21*(2), e21–e32. https://doi.org/10.4037/ajcc2012752

Burns M., Baylor C., & Yorkston K. (2017). Patient–provider communication training for dysarthria: Lessons learned from student trainees. *Seminars in Speech and Language, 38*(3), 229–238. https://doi.org/10.1055/s-0037-1602842

Carruthers, H., Astin, F., & Munro, W. (2017). Which alternative communication methods are effective for voiceless patients in Intensive Care Units? A systematic review. *In-tensive and Critical Care Nursing, 42,* 88–96. https://doi.org/10.1016/j.iccn.2017.03.003

Ciuffreda, K. J., Kapoor, N., Rutner, D., Suchoff, I. B., Han, M. E., & Craig, S. (2007). Occurrence of oculomotor dysfunctions in acquired brain injury: A retrospective analysis. *Optometry, 78,* 155–161. https://doi.org/10.1016/j.optm.2006.11.011

Costello, J. (2000). AAC intervention in the intensive care unit: The children's hospital Boston model. *Augmentative and Alterna-*

tive Communication, 16, 137–153. https://doi.org/10.1080/07434610012331279004

Culp, D., Beukelman, D. R., & Fager, S. K. (2007). Brainstem impairment. In D. R. Beukelman, K. L. Garrett, K. M. Yorkston. (Eds). *Augmentative communication strategies for adults with acute or chronic medical conditions* (pp. 59–90). Brookes.

Culp, D., & Ladtkow, M. (1992). Locked-in syndrome and augmentative communication. In K. Yorkston (Ed.), *Augmentative communication in the medical setting* (pp. 59–138). Psychological Corporation.

DeRuyter F., & Kennedy M. R. T. (1991). Augmentative communication following traumatic brain injury. In D. R. Beukelman & K. M. Yorkston (Eds.), *Communication disorders following traumatic brain injury.* Pro-Ed.

El-Soussi, A. H., Elshafey, M. M., Othman, S. Y., & Abd-Elkader, F. A. (2014). Augmented alternative communication methods in intubated COPD patients: Does it make a difference. *Egyptian Journal of Chest Diseases and Tuberculosis, 64,* 21–28. https://doi.org/10.1016/j.ejcdt.2014.07.006

Fager, S. (2018). Alternative access for adults who rely on augmentative and alternative communication. *Perspectives—SIG 12*(3), https://doi.org/10.1044/persp3.SIG12.6

Fager, S., Bardach, L., Russell, S., & Higginbotham, J. (2012). Access to augmentative and alternative communication: New technologies and clinical decision-making. *Journal of Pediatric Rehabilitation and Medicine, 5,* 53–61. https://doi.org/10.3233/PRM-2012-0196

Fager, S., Beukelman, D. R., Fried-Oken, M., Jakobs, T., & Baker, J. (2012). Access interface strategies. *Assistive Technology, 24*(1), 25–33. https://doi.org/10.1080/10400435.2011.648712

Fager, S., Beukelman, D., Karantounis, R., & Jakobs, T. (2006). Use of safe-laser access technology to train head movement in persons with severe motor impairment: A series of case reports. *Augmentative and Alternative Communication, 22,* 222–229. https://doi.org/10.1080/07434610600650318

Fager, S., Beukelman, D. R., & Jakobs, T. (2002). AAC intervention for locked-in syndrome using the safe-laser access system. *Perspectives in Augmentative and Alternative Communication, 11,* 4–7. https://doi.org/10.1044/aac11.1.4

Fager, S., Hux, K., Beukelman, D.R., & Karantounis, R. (2006). Augmentative and alternative communication use and acceptance by adults with traumatic brain injury. *Augmentative and Alternative Communication, 22,* 37–47. https://doi.org/10.1080/07434610500243990

Fager, S. K., Doyle, M., & Karantounis, R. (2007). Traumatic brain injury. In D. R. Beukelman, K. L. Garrett, & K. M. Yorkston (Eds.), *Augmentative communication strategies for adults with acute or chronic medical conditions* (pp. 131–162). Brookes.

Finke, E., Light, J., & Kitko, L. (2008). A systematic review of the effectiveness of nurse communication with patients with complex communication needs with a focus on the use of augmentative and alternative communication. *Journal of Clinical Nursing, 17,* 2102–2115. https://doi.org/10.1111/j.1365-2702.2008.02373.x

Garrett, K. L., Happ, M. B., Costello, J. M., & Fried-Oken, M. B. (2007). AAC in the intensive care unit. In D.R. Beukelman, K. L. Garrett, K. L. & K. M. Yorkston, (Eds). *Augmentative communication strategies for adults with acute or chronic medical conditions* (pp. 15–77). Brookes.

Gormley, J., & Light, J. (2019). Providing services to individuals with complex communication needs in the inpatient rehabilitation setting: The experiences and perspectives of speech-language pathologists. *American Journal of Speech-Language Pathology, 28,* 456–468. https://doi.org/10.1044/2018_AJSLP-18-0076

Greenwald, B. D., Kapoor, N., & Singh, A. D. (2012). Visual impairments in the first year after traumatic brain injury, *Brain Injury, 26,* 1338–1359. https://doi.org/10.3109/02699052.2012.706356

Happ, M. B., Baumann, B. M., Sawicki, J., Tate, J., George, E. L., & Barnato, A. E. (2010).

SPEACS-2: Intensive care unit "communication rounds" with speech-language pathology. *Geriatric Nursing, 31*, 170–177. https://doi.org/10.1016/j.gerinurse.2010.03.004

Happ, M. B., Garrett, K. L., Tate, J. A., DiVirgilio, D., Houze, M. P., Demirci, J. R., . . . Sereika, S. M. (2014). Effect of a multi-level intervention on nurse-patient communication in the intensive care unit: Results of the SPEACS trial. *Heart & Lung, 43*, 89–98. https://doi.org/10.1016/j.hrtlng.2013.11.010

Happ, M. B., Sereika, S., Garrett, K., & Tate, J. A. (2008). Use of quasi-experimental sequential cohort design in the study of patient-nurse effectiveness with assisted communication strategies (SPEACS). *Contemporary Clinical Trials, 29*, 801–808. https://doi.org/10.1016/j.cct.2008.05.010

Happ, M. B., Tuite, P., Dobbin, K., DiVirgilio-Thomas, D., & Kitutu, J. (2004). Communication ability, method, and content among nonspeaking nonsurviving patients treated with mechanical ventilation in the intensive care unit. *American Journal of Critical Care, 13*(1), 210–218.

Hemsley, B., & Balandin, S. (2014). A metasynthesis of patient-provider communication in hospital for patients with severe communication disabilities: Informing new translational research. *Augmentative and Alternative Communication, 30*(4), 329–343. https://doi.org/10.3109/07434618.2014.955614

Hemsley, B., Sigafoos, J., Balandin, S., Forbes, R., Taylor, C., Green, V. A., & Parmenter, T. (2001). Nursing the patient with severe communication impairment. *Journal of Advanced Nursing, 35*(6), 827–835. https://doi.org/10.1046/j.1365-2648.2001.01920.x

Hepworth, L. R., Rowe, F. J., Walker, M. F., Rockliffe, J., Noonan, C., Howard, C., & Currie, J. (2016). Post-stroke visual impairment: A systematic literature review of types and recovery of visual conditions. *Ophthalmology Research: An International Journal, 5*(1), 1–43. https://doi.org/https://doi.org/10.9734/or/2016/21767

Higginbotham, J., Shane, H., Russell, S., & Caves, K. (2007). Access to AAC: Present, past, and future. *Augmentative and Alternative Communication, 23*(3), 243–257.

Holm, A., & Dreyer, P. (2018a). Nurse-patient communication within the context of non-sedated mechanical ventilation: A hermeneutic-phenomenological study. *Nursing in Critical Care, 23*(2), 88–94. https://doi.org/10.1111/nicc.12297

Holm, A., & Dreyer, P. (2018b). Use of communication tools for mechanically ventilated patients in the intensive care unit. *Computers Informatics Nursing, 36*(8), 398–405. https://doi.org/10.1097/CIN.0000000000000449

Hosseini S. R., Valizad-Hasanloei M. A., & Feizi A. (2018). The effect of using communication boards on ease of communication and anxiety in mechanically ventilated conscious patients admitted to intensive care units. *Iranian Journal of Nursing and Midwifery Research, 23*(5), 358. https://doi.org/10.4103/ijnmr.IJNMR_68_17

Hurtig, R. R., Alper, R. M., & Berkowitz, B. (2018). The cost of not addressing the communication barriers faced by hospitalized patients. *Perspectives of the ASHA Special Interest Groups, 3*, 99–112.

Hurtig, R., & Downey, D. (2009). *Augmentative and alternative communication in acute care and critical care settings*. Plural Publishing.

Hurtig, R., Nilsen, M. L., Happ, M. B., & Blackstone, S. W. (2015). Adult acute and intensive care in hospitals. In *Patient-provider communication: Roles for speech-language pathologists and other health care professionals*. San Diego, CA: Plural Publishing.

Jansson, S., San Martin, T. R., Johnson, E., & Nilsson, S. (2019). Healthcare professionals' use of augmentative and alternative communication in an intensive care unit: A survey study. *Intensive & Critical Care Nursing, 54*, 65–70. https://doi.org/10.1016/j.iccn.2019.04.002

The Joint Commission. (2010). *Advancing effective communication, cultural competence, and patient and family centered care: A roadmap for hospitals*. Oakbrook Terrace, IL.

Light, J., Wilkinson, K. M., Thiessen, A., Beukelman, D. R., & Fager, S. K. (2019). Designing effective AAC displays for individuals with developmental or acquired disabilities: State of the science and future research directions. *Augmentative and Alternative Communication, 35*, 42–55. https://doi.org/10.1080/07434618.2018.1558283

Meade, C. M., Bursell, A. L., & Ketelsen, L. (2006). Effects of nursing rounds: On patients' call light use, satisfaction, and safety. *The American Journal of Nursing, 106*, 58–70. https://doi.org/10.1097/00000446-200609000-00029

Mobasheri, M. H., King, D., Judge, S., Arshad, F., Larsen, M., Safarfashandi, Z., . . . Darzi, A. (2016). Communication aid requirements of intensive care unit patients with transient speech loss. *Augmentative and Alternative Communication, 32*, 261–271. https://doi.org/10.1080/07434618.2016.1235610

Noguchi, A., Inoue, T., & Yokota, I. (2019). Promoting a nursing team's ability to notice intent to communicate in lightly sedated mechanically ventilated patients in an intensive care unit: An action research study. *Intensive and Critical Care Nursing, 51*, 64–72. https://doi.org/10.1016/j.iccn.2018.10.006

Nordness, A. S., & Beukelman D .R. (2017). Patient provider communication across medical settings. *Topic in Language Disorders, 37*, 334–347. https://doi.org/10.1097/TLD.0000000000000133

O'Halloran, R., Worrall, L., Toffolo, D., & Code, C. (2020). *Inpatient functional communication interview: Screening, assessment, and intervention*. Plural Publishing.

Papadopoulou, S., Dionyssiotis, Y., Krikonis, K., Logopati, N., Kamenov, I., & Markoula, S. (2019). Therapeutic approaches in locked-in syndrome. *Folia Medica, 61*(3), 343–351. https://doi.org/10.3897/folmed.61.e39425

Radtke, J. V., Baumann, B. M. Garrett, K. L, & Happ, M. B. (2011). Listening to the voiceless patient: Case reports in assisted communication in the intensive care unit. *Journal of Palliative Medicine, 14*, 791–795. https://doi.org/10.1089/jpm.2010.0313

Roman-Lantzy, C. (2007). *Cortical visual impairment: An approach to assessment and intervention*. American Foundation for the Blind.

Sand, K. M., Midelfart, A., Thomassen, L., Melms, A., Wilhelm, H., & Hoff, J. M. (2013). Visual impairment in stroke patients—a review. *Acta Neurologica Scandinavica, 127*(Suppl. 196), 52–56. https://doi.org/10.1111/ane.12050

Tate, J. A., Sereika, S., Divirgilio, D., Nilsen, M., Demirci, J., Campbell, G., & Happ, M. B. (2013). Symptom communication during critical illness: The impact of age, delirium, and delirium presentation. *Journal of Gerontological Nursing, 39*, 28–38. https://doi.org/10.3928/00989134-20130530-03

United Nations. (2006). *Final Report of the Ad Hoc Committee on a Comprehensive and Integral International Convention on the Protection and Promotion of the Rights and Dignity of Persons with Disabilities.* Author.

Wilkinson, K. M., & Jagaroo, V. (2004). Contributions of principles of visual cognitive science to AAC System Display Design, *Augmentative and Alternative Communication, 20*, 123–136, https://doi.org/10.1080/07434610410001699717

Wunsch, H., Linde-Zwirble, W. T., Angus, D. C., Hartman, M. E., Milbrandt, E. B., & Kahn, J. M. (2010). The epidemiology of mechanical ventilation use in the United States. *Critical Care Medicine, 38*, 1947–1953. https://doi.org/10.1097/CCM.0b013e3181ef4460

Zubow, L., & Hurtig, R. (2013). A demographic study of AAC/AT needs in hospitalized patients. *Perspectives in Augmentative and Alternative Communication, 22*, 79–90.

PART IV

AAC Challenges and Solutions: Special Populations and Issues

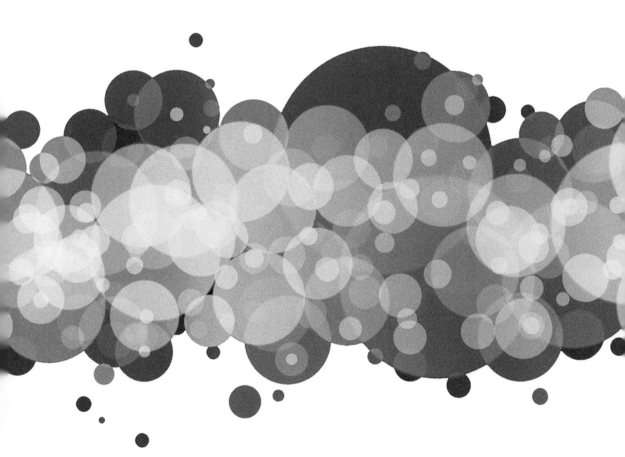

PART IX

AAC Challenges and Solutions: Special Populations and Issues

9

Challenges in Providing AAC Intervention to People With Profound Intellectual and Multiple Disabilities

Jeff Sigafoos, Laura Roche, and Kathleen Tait

■ Introduction

At issue is the challenge of providing augmentative and alternative communication (AAC) intervention to individuals with profound intellectual and multiple disabilities (PIMD). To illustrate the nature of PIMD, we begin by introducing a woman who was recently involved in some AAC intervention research conducted by the first author and several masters students. Sarah,[1] now 28 years old, was born with cerebral palsy affecting all four of her limbs (i.e., spastic quadriplegia). She received subsequent diagnoses of microcephaly, epilepsy, and vision impairment. Sarah is unable to walk and has limited use of her hands. Medically she is very fragile and highly susceptible to colds and infections. Fluids and medicines must be

delivered via a PEG (percutaneous endoscopic gastronomy) tube. Cognitively, she functions in the profound range of intellectual disability. She experiences major limitations in all areas of adaptive behavior functioning. In consequence, she is totally dependent on direct-care staff for feeding, dressing, toileting, and washing. Conventional play and leisure skills are nonexistent and her social skills are limited to the occasional smile and laugh. She is unable to speak and shows little comprehension of speech. Staff report that she communicates pleasure by laughing and will "grizzle" when upset.

Sarah certainly has the diagnostic characteristics associated with the label PIMD. This term is used as a descriptor for individuals who have severe to profound intellectual disability and significant physical impairment (Lyle, 2019; Nakken &

---

[1]Pseudonyms have been assigned to all of the individuals described in this chapter to protect confidentiality.

Vlaskamp, 2007). Many such individuals also have hearing and/or vision impairment (Erickson & Quick, 2017; van Splunder, Stilma, Bernsen, & Evenhuis, 2006). As was the case for Sarah, persons with PIMD also often present with complex health and medical conditions, such as seizures, scoliosis, and respiratory problems (Gulati & Sondhi, 2018). Understandably, such individuals require extremely high levels of life-long care and support (Wehmeyer et al., 2009).

Communication intervention is one obvious area of needed support. Petry and Maes (2007) described the support needs of people with PIMD as including " . . . support and stimulation to acquire . . . communication skills such as demanding something, indicating yes or no, making eye contact, and listening to stories" (p. 133). Expanding on the range of communication supports for people with PIMD, Rensfeldt Flink, Johnels, Broberg, and Thunberg (2020) noted that people with PIMD also need support to (a) promote independent use of language and/ or communication symbols, (b) increase their level of awareness regarding their own communicative intentions, and (c) increase their ability to initiate and maintain social-communication interactions with a range of communicative partners across a range of environments and activities. It is well documented that nearly all people with PIMD have severe communication impairment or complex communication needs, meaning they have limited or no expressive speech and significant receptive language deficits (Belva, Matson, Sipes, & Bamburg, 2012). This alone would seem to make them obvious candidates for AAC intervention. Sadly, obvious needs often go unmet. Several surveys have found considerable unmet needs with respect to providing AAC intervention to persons with intellectual disability and complex communication needs (Siu et al., 2010; Sutherland, Gillon, & Yoder, 2005; Sutherland et al., 2014).

The results of these surveys match our respective clinical experiences. One of the most heartbreaking aspects of our educational, clinical, and research work is encountering people with PIMD who have never received intervention to enhance or advance their communication abilities. Time and again over the past 30 years we meet people like Sarah who are largely dependent on others to anticipate their wants and needs and accurately interpret their laughs, groans, eye movements, and other prelinguistic behaviors. Unfortunately, the meaning or communicative intent of prelinguistic behavior is notoriously difficult to interpret even by familiar listeners, leading to frequent communication breakdowns (Keen, 2014). Figure 9–1 illustrates a scenario we have witnessed many times. The child appears to be attempting to communicate via her arm movements, but the meaning of the act is lost on her listener. Such communication breakdowns are common in people with PIMD who rely on prelinguistic or highly idiosyncratic forms of behavior to communicate. In light of their severe communication impairments, we have struggled to understand why so many people with PIMD—people who clearly need AAC intervention—have either failed to receive AAC intervention or have failed to progress with it.

There are a number of possible reasons for the relative absence of AAC provision in services for people with PIMD. Sadly, limited AAC provision may simply reflect the generally poor quality of support provided to this population overall (Beadle-Brown et al., 2016). Another possibility could simply be a lack of awareness

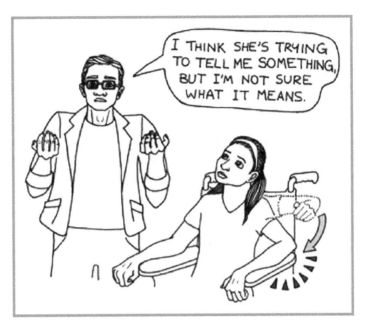

Figure 9–1. The meaning of a person's idiosyncratic/prelinguistic behaviors are often difficult to interpret.

of AAC or lack of training with respect to providing AAC intervention. Data suggest that individuals involved in the education, care, and/or support of people with various developmental disabilities, including people with PIMD, generally lack experience and training in providing AAC intervention. Many such care staff also do not have access to professionals with such expertise (Siu et al., 2010; Sutherland et al., 2005, 2014). Another reason could be the presumption that severe cognitive impairments and apparent lack of communicative intent negate any possibility that persons with PIMD could ever learn to use AAC. We have frequently come across this type of attitudinal barrier. However, intentional/functional communication skills might develop when an appropriately configured AAC mode is combined with a well-designed systematic instructional program (Reichle, York, & Sigafoos, 1991). That is, the intervention process itself

might promote communicative intentionality. However, we are under no illusion that teaching functional/intentional use of AAC to people with PIMD is easy. We have certainly had our fair share of intervention failures. The challenge has been widely recognized in the education and rehabilitation literature more generally. Munde and Vlaskamp (2015), for example, agreed that "Designing activities that fit the abilities and needs of individuals with profound intellectual and multiple disabilities (PIMD) is a challenge . . ." (p. 284).

Fortunately, there is a growing evidence base demonstrating successful procedures for teaching functional/intentional use of AAC to people with PIMD (for reviews see Gilroy, McCleery, & Leader, 2017; Lancioni, O'Reilly, & Basil, 2001; Roche, Sigafoos, Lancioni, O'Reilly, & Green, 2015; Simacek, Pennington, Reichle, & Parker-McGowan, 2018). Lancioni, Sigafoos, O'Reilly, and Singh (2013), for example, identified 54 studies on teaching persons with severe/profound and multiple disabilities to communicate using various types of aided/high-tech AAC devices (e.g., microswitches and computer-based speech-generating devices). Across these 54 studies, a range of communicative functions, intents, or skills were successfully taught, such as recruiting attention/social interaction, requesting preferred stimuli, and rejecting nonpreferred items. AAC modes taught included various aided devices (e.g., microswitches, tape recorders, and computer-based devices) and a range of communication symbols (e.g., line drawing, photographs, and tangible symbols). The overall results from these reviews indicate that relatively well-established instructional procedures—based primarily on behavior analytic principles—can be effective in teaching AAC use to people with PIMD. However, Simacek et al. (2018) noted methodological limitations in some studies (e.g., failure to assess treatment integrity or specify the precise amount and intensity of intervention). In addition, most studies have only targeted requesting skills. Successful demonstrations of teaching more socially oriented communication skills (e.g., initiating and maintaining social interactions) to people with PIMD are less prevalent in the literature, although a few such studies do exist to guide practice (see Lancioni et al., 2013 for several relevant studies).

Despite these limitations, there is a research base to support the viability of AAC intervention for people with PIMD (e.g., Gilroy et al., 2017; Lancioni et al., 2001, 2013; Roche et al., 2015; Simacek, et al., 2018). In line with the evidence-based practice movement (Schlosser & Raghavendra, 2004), clinicians should draw upon this literature to guide their own intervention efforts. However, even highly competent clinicians making use of the best available evidence are likely to encounter a range of challenges when designing and implementing AAC intervention with people with PIMD.

The next sections of this chapter describe three challenges that may arise when designing and implementing AAC intervention with people with PIMD. We selected these three specific challenges because they have been frequently encountered in our respective programs of clinical work and applied intervention research. In what follows, we describe the nature of each challenge, illustrate the main features of each challenge with specific case examples and stakeholder quotes, and offer potential solutions. Some of the solutions offered are derived from the research literature whereas others are more anecdotal and based on our own clinical experiences.

◼ Identifying Reinforcers and Viable Response Topographies

The issue of prerequisites has been roundly debated in the AAC literature (Kangas & Lloyd, 1988; Reichle & Karlan, 1985; Romski & Sevcik, 2005). One position in this debate questions the value of AAC intervention for participants who have yet to achieve certain cognitive milestones, such as object permanence, contingency awareness, and communicative intent. Because people with PIMD often fail to demonstrate such abilities (Woodyatt & Ozanne, 1992), this argument would essentially exclude them from receiving AAC services, despite their obvious need. The alternative and more contemporary view is that there are no prerequisites to AAC intervention. In fact, researchers have suggested that these supposedly prerequisite cognitive abilities might develop and emerge as a result of providing a well-designed AAC intervention (Kangas & Lloyd, 1988; Reichle & Karlan, 1985; Romski & Sevcik, 2005; von Tetzchner, 1997). von Tetzchner (1997), for example, argued for overinterpreting nonintentional behaviors as if these had specific communicative meanings. By doing so, pre-intentional behaviors might acquire communicative intent over time.

Although the absence of certain cognitive abilities should not preclude people with PIMD from receiving AAC intervention, there might, nonetheless, be certain types of pre-intervention assessment information that could facilitate AAC intervention. Reichle et al. (1991), for example, argued for the relevance of gathering two types of assessment data at the beginning stages of AAC intervention. Specifically (a) conducting an assessment to identify at least one reinforcer, and (b) identifying at least one viable response topography. Meeting these two requirements can be challenging. Indeed, we would hazard a guess that most of our thwarted intervention efforts over the past 30 years stem from a failure to identify reinforcers, or failure to find a viable response form that the person could reliably use for communication purposes.

Stakeholder Quote

"Jeremy really likes watching *The Lion King* on DVD. He'll watch it over and over again. He also likes to hold soft things in his hand, such as a stress ball. If he doesn't like something, he'll let us know by moving away."

It has long been known that effective use of reinforcement promotes engagement and skill acquisition (Gutowski, 1996; Martens, Bradley, & Eckert, 1997). With respect to AAC intervention, reinforcers can also be used to create the need and motivation for communication (Sigafoos, 1999). Unfortunately, identifying stimuli (e.g., objects, activities, and/or experiences) that will function as effective types of reinforcement for people with PIMD is rarely straightforward. There are several reasons for this. First, people with PIMD usually cannot tell others what they like or don't like, and reliance on caregiver reports for such information is often invalid (Green et al., 1988). Instead, identification of reinforcing stimuli for people with PIMD often requires use of more direct, structured, and systematic preference assessment techniques, which can present their own implementation challenges.

The basic paradigm for assessing preferences in people with PIMD involves offering different stimuli and observing the person's reaction to each offer (e.g., Did the person reach for or grasp the object? Did the person look intently at the object? Did the person show any signs of happiness when presented with the stimulus, such as smiling or positive vocalizations?). Within this basic paradigm, various configurations or ways of offering stimuli have been evaluated. For example, stimuli might be offered one at a time or in pairs from which the person could then make a choice. Canella, O'Reilly, and Lancioni (2005) reviewed the literature on these approaches and concluded that the basic paradigm represents a valid approach for identifying reinforcers for people with PIMD. Two assumptions underpin the basic preference assessment paradigm, these are: (a) frequently selected stimuli or stimuli that frequently evoke a positive reaction can be classified as preferred, and (b) preferred stimuli will often function as reinforcers. A large amount of intervention research supports the validity of these assumptions (for reviews see Canella et al., 2005; Logan & Gast, 2001; Tullis et al., 2011).

Preference assessment is a critical initial step in the overall AAC intervention process. Fortunately, there are a range of evidence-based preference assessments that are validated for use with people with PIMD (Canella et al., 2005; Logan & Gast, 2001; Tullis et al., 2011). Most preference assessments depend on the person being able to indicate a preference in some obvious way, for example by reaching for and choosing an object (e.g., a toy or snack) and then using that object functionally (e.g., playing with the toy or eating the snack). However, some individuals with PIMD lack sufficient motor skills to directly select and functionally use preferred items. In such situations, assessors will have to consider alternative means by which a person might be able to express his or her preferences and engage with preferred activities. Some possible alternative indications of preference include (a) being engaged (e.g., orienting toward the activity, increased levels of alertness), (b) indications of happiness (e.g., smiling and positive vocalizations), and (c) a general increase in movement. Looking intently at an item might also be an indicator of preference for some people.

In line with this latter possibility, Cannella-Malone, Koss Schmidt, and Bumpus (2018) described the use of eye-tracking technology to assess preferences in three young adults (18 to 19 years old) with PIMD. The technique involved tracking which of two offered items a participant most often directed his or her gaze

towards. Cannella-Malone et al. (2018) found that items associated with more gaze fixation functioned as effective reinforcers. Sigafoos and Dempsey (1992) had previously shown that eye gaze was a valid choice-making response among three children with PIMD. Data of this type further suggest that when individuals with PIMD visually fixate on an object, they might in fact be indicating that they want that item. That is, eye gaze might function as a requesting response. Following this logic, Sigafoos and Couzens (1995) successfully taught a 6-year-old boy with severe intellectual disability and cerebral palsy to use an eye gaze communication board. The boy was taught to gaze at pictures of headphones, a cassette player, and cassette tapes, to request these items so that he could then listen to music. Collectively, these results suggest that eye gaze might not only be a viable means of assessing preferences, but could also be a viable response form that some individuals with PIMD could be taught to use for communication purposes.

Indeed, some behaviors that a person uses to indicate preference might also be used as a means of communication. A child who will consistently and reliably reach for preferred snacks, drinks, or toys, for example, might be taught to use this same reaching response to select communication symbols on an AAC device. An adolescent who leans away from certain sights or activities might learn to use this same response to escape from and avoid nonpreferred objects and activities. For example, the associated body movement could break a circuit beam that triggers output from a speech-generating device. Along these lines, the communication breakdown depicted in Figure 9–1 might be repaired by linking the child's motor response to an AAC device, as depicted in

Figure 9–2. Lancioni et al. (2013) described a number of such assistive technology solutions for enabling people with PIMD to engage in a range of adaptive behaviors, including functional communication.

The responses a person uses to indicate choice and preference might not always represent viable or practical modes of AAC. Without highly specialized and expensive technology, it may be difficult to teach a person to intentionally communicate via some existing general body movement or specific facial expression. In addition, the responses a person uses to make choices and indicate preferences might not necessarily reflect the full range of response forms that the person would be capable of using for communication purposes. In light of this, some additional assessments may be helpful for identifying viable response topographies that could be established as functional communication responses as part of an AAC intervention.

One approach for attempting to identify the range of potential communication acts used by a person with PIMD involves interviews or rating scales completed with or by parents, teachers, and other caregivers acting as informants. Various structured protocols have been developed for this purpose (Brady et al., 2018; Sigafoos et al., 2000; Urbanowicz, Leonard, Girdler, Ciccone, & Downs, 2016). However, such information should be interpreted with caution until its validity can be confirmed via direct observation. To this end, more direct, observation-based assessment protocols have been developed and successfully used to identify communication forms and functions expressed by people with severe/profound and multiple disabilities

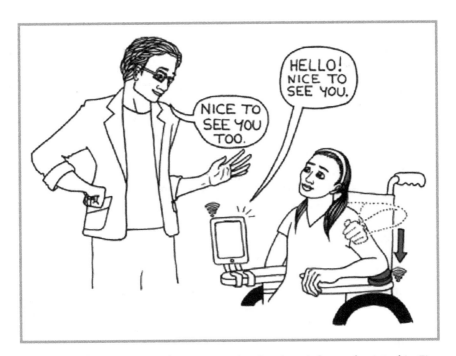

Figure 9–2. Repairing the communication breakdown depicted in Figure 9–1 by linking the child's arm movement to a microswitch-based speech-generating device.

(Atkin & Perlma Lorch, 2016; McLean, Brady, McLean, & Behrens, 1999).

One such direct observational approach was conducted with Sarah, who was described at the start of this chapter. An initial preference assessment suggested that Sarah really liked being pushed in a swinging chair. When she was being pushed, Sarah would often smile and laugh and she also seemed to become more active and animated in her movements. Given that this activity appeared to be highly reinforcing for Sarah, we thought we might be able to teach her to use an AAC device to request continuation of the activity. Once this goal had been selected, we undertook structured observations to identify a response form that Sarah could be taught to use to signal this type of request. For this assessment, we got Sarah swinging in the chair and would then pause the activity for 30 sec. During these 30 sec. interruptions, we noted the behaviors that she emitted. After running 40 such interruptions, we then calculated the percentage of interruptions in which each of several different response topographies were observed.

Stakeholder Quote

Sarah's support staff interpreted many of her vocalizations and facial expressions as forms of communication. For example: "When she makes that droning sound it means she is upset. When she is happy she will laugh and smile."

The results, reported by Gerondis (2019), are shown in Figure 9–3. Sarah was reliably observed to engage in nine different topographies at varying percent-

ages. These results gave us a number of response options to work with. In the end, we decided to use the second most frequently occurring response form (i.e., slapping the left outside panel of the chair with the open palm of her left hand). This response was selected because it occurred frequently and was less likely to be misinterpreted than the head swivel response, which looked as if she was shaking her head NO. To make this slapping response more obviously communicative and easier for listeners to interpret, we affixed a microswitch-based speech-generating device to the same location on the chair that she frequently slapped with her left palm. Her intervention focused on strengthening this response by interrupting the activity, waiting for her to respond by hitting the switch, and then reinforcing this response by resuming her preferred activity.

Although it may often appear that people with PIMD are relatively passive and exhibit very few responses that could provide the raw material from which to build AAC skills, careful observation, such as conducted with Sarah, may reveal a range of potentially viable response forms. Once identified, AAC intervention could aim to develop these responses into intentional/functional communication responses. The existing response forms could be strengthened by reinforcing them and the existing form might also be co-opted into a technology assisted AAC intervention, such as illustrated in Figure 9–2.

■ Fostering Biobehavioral States Conducive to AAC Intervention

People with PIMD will often show widely fluctuating biobehavioral states or levels

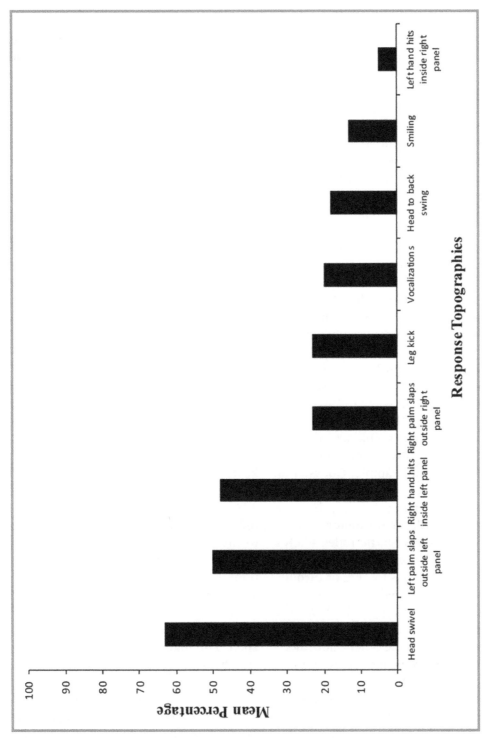

Figure 9–3. Results of Sarah's response topography assessment showing the mean percentage of interruptions in which each response form was observed.

of alertness (Arthur-Kelly, Foreman, Maes, Colyvas, & Lyons, 2018; Guess et al., 1988, 1990; Guess, Roberts, & Rues, 2002; Munde & Vlaskamp, 2015). The concept of biobehavioral state was first articulated by Wolff (1959) to account for the continuum of behavioral and physiological conditions of infants. This continuum ranged from being asleep and inactive to being awake and crying. Later, Helm and Simeonsson (1989) defined the concept as an "expression of the maturity, status, and organization of the central nervous systems . . . which mediates the child's ability to respond to the environment and stimulation (p. 203). Guess and colleagues (Guess et al., 1988, 1990, 2002) were pioneers in the investigation of biobehavioral states in people with PIMD. From this work, researchers have been able to describe a continuum of biobehavioral states that can be reliably observed in people with PIMD (Arthur-Kelly et al., 2018; Foreman, Arthur-Kelly, Bennett, Neilands, & Colyvas, 2014; Guess et al., 1988, 1990, 2002). At the lower (less alert) end of this continuum are states characterized by sleepiness and relatively little functional motor activity. For example, Guess et al. (1988) distinguished between the following less alert states: (a) Asleep-Inactive (eyes closed, little or no motor activity, regular respirations, startle reflex likely), (b) Asleep, yet Active (e.g., showing some motor activity such as tossing or turning, limb movements, rapid eye movements, and irregular breathing), and (c) Drowsy (e.g., heavy eyelids, yet some vocalizations may occur). At the other (more alert) end of the continuum, lay relatively more active and alert biobehavioral states, such as: (a) Awake-Inactive-Alert (e.g., able to localize and track stimuli, will turn heard toward objects, regular respiration, some vocalizations), and (b) Awake-Active-Alert

(e.g., engagement in functional movements, such as reaching, grasping, eating, and play behavior). People with PIMD have been noted to transition along this continuum (e.g., from being active and alert to being drowsy or asleep) rapidly and multiple times per day (Foreman et al., 2014).

Stakeholder Quote

"Imogen spends most of her time asleep. It is very difficult to wake her up and I'm not even sure if I should try to wake her up. Maybe she is just really tired and I should let her keep sleeping."

—Paraphrase of a comment by Imogen's Year 7 classroom teacher

---

Biobehavioral states reflective of the more alert end of the continuum are viewed as optimal conditions for learning and hence optimal conditions for providing intervention. (Arthur-Kelly et al., 2018; Munde & Vlaskamp, 2015). Thus, an important consideration when providing AAC intervention to people with PIMD is the timing of implementation in relation to the person's biobehavioral state. Ideally, it would seem logical that intervention should be implemented when the student is alert and thus more responsive to instruction. Unfortunately, research by Arthur-Kelly and colleagues (Arthur, 2003; Foreman, Arthur-Kelly, Pascoe, & Smyth King, 2004) documented that students with PIMD can spend up to 70% of their classroom time in less optimal (i.e., less alert) states for participating in communication interactions. Consequently, unless more optimal learning states can be induced, there may be relatively few windows of opportunity in which the person is alert enough to likely profit from AAC intervention.

A major challenge in providing effective AAC intervention to people with PIMD is how to promote biobehavioral states that are conducive to learning and conducive to meaningful social-communicative interactions (Munde & Vlaskamp, 2015). Knowledge of the variables that influence a person's level of alertness and transitions along the continuum of biobehavioral states, therefore, could be seen as critically important. Knowledge of this type may enable clinicians to promote and maintain optimal states for learning and communication engagement.

There can be many reasons for the fluctuating levels of alertness associated with PIMD. In some cases, this fluctuation may stem from physiological variables. Seizure activity, for example, can make a person drowsy or sleepy and thus unresponsive to instruction. Such states may last for up to several hours following a seizure incident. Other individuals might be easily fatigued even from seemingly passive activity, such as being fed a meal or given assistance with completing self-care tasks. Sleep disturbances, which are not uncommon in people with PIMD, may also lead to daytime drowsiness. Alertness can also be affected by medication.

Clearly internal physiological factors can have a major influence on the biobehavioral states and state transitions in people with PIMD. However, Guess et al. (1988) noted that external environmental factors may also have a pronounced influence on activity and alertness levels. In fact, some research suggests that external stimulation may have a more significant impact on alertness than internal factors (Munde & Vlaskamp, 2015). Green, Gard-ner, Canipe, and Reid (1994), for example, provided evidence suggesting that biobehavioral state changes in persons with PIMD can stem from environmental, and not just physiological, factors. For example, the level of environmental stimulation and the extent to which the person is assisted to engage with stimulating activities might also determine the amount of time that the person spends in various biobehavioral states. Guess et al. (1990) further suggested that a person's level of alertness might vary in relation to the reinforcing value of the various activities and types of stimulation that are made available to them.

Tait and Sigafoos (2018) explored the influence of different types of environmental stimulation on levels of alertness. The study involved structured observations in classrooms that included children with PIMD. The observation protocol was designed to determine whether the children's biobehavioral states varied across different environmental conditions. Five children with PIMD, aged 9 to 13 years, were observed under three conditions: (a) when they were engaged in game/toy play with the teacher (High Stimulation), (b) when being read a story by the teacher (Moderate Stimulation), and (c) when they were alone with no direct stimulation being provided (Low Stimulation). At regular intervals during each condition, the child was rated as either being alert (i.e., head up, eyes open, and oriented towards the teacher or materials) or not alert (i.e., head down and eyes closed). The results showed that children were more frequently rated as alert in the High and Moderate Stimulation conditions than in the Low Stimulation condition. Specifically, children were rated as being alert about 50% of the time when they were engaged with the storybook or game/toy play activity, but had near zero levels of alertness when they were left alone with no specific stimulation being provided.

The discovery that the type and level of environmental stimulation can influence a person's biobehavioral state has several implications for designing AAC intervention. First, the results suggest that interventionists may find it useful to monitor a person's level of alertness across different activities and when the person is engaged with different types of stimulation. However, it is important to emphasize that the distinction between being more alert versus less alert can often be subtle and hence difficult to detect and measure (Munde & Vlaskamp, 2015). Consequently, judging whether or not a person is sufficiently alert to profit from intervention can be challenging. Tait and Sigafoos (2018) for example, found that having one's eyes open versus closed seemed to be the main indicator of being more versus less alert in the sample of children with PIMD that they studied. Other subtle signs of alertness that might be exhibited by people with PIMD could be orienting towards a visual or auditory stimulus, making eye contact with another person, producing sounds/vocalizations, facial expression, or even subtle changes in the person's muscle tone (Munde & Vlaskamp, 2015; Vlaskamp, de Geeter, Hujismans, & Smit 2003).

Second, people with PIMD may very quickly enter a drowsy/sleepy state when preferred sources of environmental stimulation are withdrawn or reduced. We have even had people with PIMD fall asleep during the inevitable short pauses that occur between communication opportunities while running AAC interventions. Once in this less-alert state, the person might then be left alone. This, in turn,

could exacerbate the person's tendency to remain in a drowsy/sleepy state and thus further reduce his or her opportunities for learning. On this note, Schoen, Miller, Brett-Green, and Neilson (2009) reported that teachers frequently withhold instruction when students with PIMD appear to be sleepy or drowsy. They do so, it seems, because of a presumption that such students will only respond to intervention when they are active and alert. This logic probably does have some merit. However, being in a less alert state could stem from insufficient environmental stimulation. This scenario would seem to indicate the need to increase the level of [preferred] stimulation being provided so as to induce a state of greater alertness.

Providing stimulation—such as socially interacting with the person, reading a story to the person, or presenting food, drink, games, and toys—might be sufficient in some cases to increase a person's level of alertness to a point where he or she would then be more responsive to intervention. For the five children in the Tait and Sigafoos (2018) study, the fact that they were more often rated as being alert under the storybook and game/toy conditions suggests that these activities were stimulating and enjoyable. Such activities might therefore also function as effective types of reinforcement in line with the reasoning of Guess et al. (1990). Based on this rationale, a logical starting point for AAC intervention might be to implement procedures aimed at teaching the person to request access to, or continuation of, such seemingly preferred activities.

More generally, in our clinical work and when conducting applied intervention research, we have used a variety of techniques in an effort to induce and maintain a state of optimal alertness in people with

PIMD. Some of the techniques that we have used, and which anecdotally appear to be of benefit, include (a) acknowledging and responding to even the person's slightest subtle movements or vocalizations, (b) presenting a variety of [hopefully] stimulating objects and activities for a good length of time (e.g., 30 sec. or more) and waiting to see if the person will attend to the offer in some way, such as by looking at or moving toward the offered object, and (c) trying some warm-up/wake-up routines prior to implementing AAC intervention sessions. Other suggested strategies for increasing and maintaining alertness in people with PIMD include choosing activities according to the person's interests and embedding intervention into preferred routines in which the person is most likely to be alert and responsive to instruction (Johnson, Rahn, & Bricker, 2015). Munde and Vlaskamp (2015) also recommended allowing sufficient time for the person with PIMD to respond to stimulation. They suggested that care staff "often act too quickly, whereas they would be better off waiting for a reaction" (p. 284). Warmup activities could include any number of different scenarios, such as simply talking with the person, implementing some passive range of motion exercises, providing a snack or a drink, or presenting potentially enjoyable auditory and/or visual stimulation, such as music or colored lights. Overall, when physiological factors—such as seizure activity, medication side effects, or lack of sleep—can be ruled out, clinicians, teachers, and parents, may be well advised to implement one or more of the above mentioned strategies. Doing so might help to promote and maintain levels of activity and alertness that will make the person more responsive to AAC

intervention. However, although such suggestions seem sensible, there is relatively little research on strategies for promoting greater alertness in people with PIMD. Thus, promoting biobehavioral states that are more conducive to AAC intervention remains a major challenge.

■ Accommodating Developmental Reflexes

Infants enter the world with an extraordinary array of reflexive behavior (Chandradasa & Rathnayake, 2019; Rousseau, Matton, Lecuyer, & Lahaye, 2017). Press your finger into the palm of a newborn and the child automatically grasps it; often with considerable force. Stroke the underside of an infant's foot and the big toe moves upward while the other toes fan out. Gently turn an infant's head to the right or left and the arms will assume what looks like a classic fencing pose. A large number of such developmental (Gulati & Sondhi, 2018) or primitive (Gieysztor, Choinska, & Paprocka-Borowicz, 2018) reflexes have been documented in the repertoire of newborns (Acharya, Jamil, & Dewey, 2019; Chandradasa & Rathnayake, 2019; Grzywniak, 2016; Marques-de-Moraes, Dionisio, Tan, & Tudella, 2017; Rousseau et al., 2017). Several major types of developmental reflexes are described in Table 9–1 and there are many others, such as the stepping reflex, rooting reflex, sucking reflex, and tongue thrust reflex. Developmental reflexes are presumed to have considerable significance in human motor and cerebral development (Rousseau et al., 2017).

Chandradasa and Rathnayake (2019) defined primitive reflexes as "automatic

Table 9–1. Description of Several Developmental Reflexes

Reflex	Description
Asymmetric tonic neck reflex (ATNR)	This reflex, also known as the fencing reflex, is elicited by a head turn to the right or left. When the head is turned to the right, the left arm bends at the elbow and moves upward behind the head while the right arm extends outward in the same direction in which the head is turned When the head is turned to the left, the right arm bends and rises, while the left arm extends outward. This reflex appears around the 18th week of fetal development and usually disappears by four months of age. Presence of the reflex past six months of age is associated with cerebral/developmental disorders.
Babinski/ Plantar	This reflex is elicited by a firm stroking of the sole of the foot which results in the big toe moving upward and fanning of the other toes. This reflex usually appears about one week postdelivery and usually disappears by 2 years of age. Retention past 2 years of age generally indicates neurological problems, such as an upper motor neuron lesion.
Galant/truncal incurvation reflex	This reflex is elicited by stroking the side of the spine when the infant is held face down. A normal reaction is for the child to flex toward the stimulated side. The reflex generally appears during the 18th week of fetal development and is usually integrated (disappears) by 12 months of age. Retention occurs in cases of cerebral injury and can cause posture control problems.
Moro	This reflex is elicited when infants experience a sudden loss of support. The response involves the arms slowly spreading out and then returning toward midline. Crying also usually follows shortly after the response begins. The Moro reflex does not attenuate with repeated elicitation. This reflex is often confused with the startle reflex, which can be elicited by loud noises, for example. Unlike the Moro reflex, the startle reflex involves more rapid abduction (spreading out) of the arms and it does not fully disappear, although it does attenuate with repeated elicitation. The Moro reflex develops at around 25 weeks of gestation and usually disappears by 3 months of age. Retention past 3 months of age may indicate problems with the central nervous system.
Palmar grasp reflex	This reflex is elicited by stimulation of the palm of the hand, such as when the palm is stroked or by placing an object in the infant's hand. The fingers close inward as in grasping an object. The reflex can appear in utero at about 16 weeks and generally disappears by 4 months of age. Retention past 4 months of age can indicate frontal lobe damage.
Symmetrical tonic neck reflex (STNR)	This reflex elicits upper extremity extension and lower extremity flexing when the head is raised (extended) and vice versa when the head is lowered. (flexed). The STNR reflex emerges around 6 to 9 months of age and should diminish by 9 to 11 months of age. The reflex aides in the transition to crawling and walking. The reflex is often retained in children with cerebral palsy. When retained, even in a diminished capacity, this reflex may disrupt fluent movement requiring hand-eye coordination.

Table 9–1. *continued*

Reflex	Description
Tonic labyrinthine reflex/ extensor tone	When held up by the waist or chest, this reflex causes an infant to assume the superman pose. Also, when lying on their backs, a backward head movement will cause the infant's back to stiffen and arch. The legs will also stiffen with the feet and toes pointing forward. This reflex is present from birth and usually disappears by 4 months of age. In people with cerebral palsy and other neurological conditions, this reflex may persist and even become more prominent over time.

Note. Table 9–1 is original with content based on Acharya, Jamil, & Dewey (2019); Chandradasa & Rathnayake (2019); Gieysztor, Choinska, & Paprocka–Borowicz (2018); Marques-de-Morase, Dionisio, Tan, & Tudella (2017); and Rousseau, Matton, Lecuyer, & Lahaye (2017).

involuntary movements that occur in response to a stimulus" (p. 1). Gieysztor et al. (2018) noted that most primitive reflexes develop in utero and are generally fully functional at birth, although some reflexes—such as the Babinski reflex—appear some weeks after birth. One of the more astonishing features of infant development is that most of these developmental or primitive reflexes are temporary. That is, they disappear or become integrated as part of early typical neuromotor development. Indeed, successful integration (or inhibition) of developmental reflexes appears to be essential for the acquisition of purposeful motor actions (Rousseau et al., 2017). Typically, integration of such reflexes generally occurs by 6 months of age (Chandradasa & Rathnayake, 2019).

Retention of developmental reflexes past this age may indicate damage to the central nervous system. The disappearance of developmental reflexes is often significantly delayed or might never fully occur among children with neurodevelopmental disorders, such as cerebral palsy and PIMD (Gieysztor et al., 2018; Gulati & Sondhi, 2018; Kawakami et al., 2013).

Gulati and Sondhi (2018), for example, noted that delayed disappearance and persistence of developmental reflexes are signs of cerebral palsy. Gulati and Sondhi (2018) also noted that developmental reflexes may be more pronounced in children with cerebral palsy and that retained reflexes may even become more exaggerated over time. Developmental reflexes have also been known to re-emerge following traumatic brain injury or stroke (Gieysztor et al., 2018). Interestingly, a fair percentage of typically developing children (Gieysztor et al., 2018) and adults (Jacobs & Gossman, 1980) will exhibit certain developmental reflexes given the right stimulus. This suggests that retention or re-emergence of some such reflexes is not necessarily always associated with cerebral pathology.

Developmental reflexes are postulated to have an important role in advancing typical motor development (Chandradasa & Rathnayake, 2019; Rousseau et al., 2017). Conversely, the exaggerated expression and/or delayed integration of such reflexes may contribute to atypical motor patterns. For example, Gulati and Sondhi (2018) noted that an exaggerated tonic labyrinthine reflex—often seen in children with cerebral palsy—can cause extreme back arching due to muscle spasms. This, in turn, could make it more difficult for the person to achieve a comfortable seated position or rest in the supine position.

Persistence of developmental reflexes might also disrupt intervention efforts. Retention of the asymmetrical tonic neck reflex (ATNR), for example, might make it more difficult to execute the motor actions required to use an aided AAC system, such as activating a microswitch-based speech generating device. A pronounced ATNR response might also make it more difficult to deliver response prompts. For example, it may be quite difficult to physically assist a person to activate a speech-generating device when their preferred or dominant arm and hand is either extended or flexed due to the ATNR.

Sarah—who was introduced at the beginning of this chapter—had a pronounced ATNR reflex that often interfered with her use of a microswitch-based speech-generating device. The microswitch was affixed to the left side of her chair at about hip level. In this position, Sarah could readily access and easily activate the device, which she did to request continuation of her preferred (swinging) activity. However, if Sarah turned her head to the left or right during requesting opportunities, this head movement would often trigger the ATNR, which was incompatible with the arm and hand movements that were required for her to use the microswitch.

To address this challenge, we followed the recommendation of Rousseau et al. (2017), who suggested that interventionists try to avoid eliciting any retained reflexes. In Sarah's case this meant facing her directly during social interactions so that there was no need for her to turn her head. We tried to eliminate, as far as possible, the introduction of any abrupt visual and auditory stimulation at her periphery. We also discovered that gently placing a hand on her arm appeared to reduce the magnitude of the ATNR. When an ATNR had been triggered, it appeared helpful to wait for it to subside and then redirect her arms to a neutral midline position before implementing the next teaching opportunity. Overall, the general approach used with Sarah was to avoid triggering her ATNR and waiting for any such responses to subside before proceeding with intervention.

With other individuals, we have attempted to incorporate developmental reflexes into their AAC intervention program. That is, the aim is to harness the reflex and thus enable the person to use it functionally for communication purposes. A recent intervention conducted with Richard will serve to illustrate this approach.

Richard's intervention began in April 2019 at which time he was 24 years old. His diagnoses included mitochondrial disease, severe epilepsy, scoliosis, and vision impairment. He was unable to walk, had no speech, and had very limited functional use of his arms and hands. Profound intellectual disability was also suspected, although he had not been formally assessed. Because of his lack of motor skills, he was totally dependent on care staff for all of his daily self-care needs. In fact, Richard had such a limited behavioral repertoire that we had been unable to identify a response form that might be easily enlisted for use as a communicative response. He did however have a pronounced palmar grasp reflex.

Stakeholder Quote

In many cases, significant others in the person's life may not realize that the individual exhibits retained reflexes. This seemed to be the case for some of the direct-care workers who supported Richard. In fact, when researchers alerted staff to Richard's persistent palmar grasp reflex, the reply from one staff person was telling: "I didn't know he did that."

Given that Richard showed a pronounced palmar grasp reflex, we decided to see if we could harness this reflex for communicative purposes. To this end, we obtained a grasp switch (Ablenet Inc., https://www.ablenetinc.com). This switch (Figure 9–4) is intended to be held in the palm of the hand and is activated by a

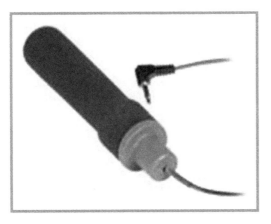

Figure 9–4. Grasp switch used with Richard. The switch is intended to be held in the palm of the hand and is activated by a gentle squeeze. Richard's switch was connected to a speech–generating device that produced a request for assistance (i.e., *"Can somebody help me?"*) when the squeeze switch was activated.

gentle squeeze. For Richard, we plugged this switch into a speech-generating device (i.e., a BIGmack switch, Ablenet Inc., https://www.ablenetinc.com). Each squeeze of the grasp switch produced digitized speech output, *"Can somebody help me?"* Richard's intervention focused on teaching him to use the grasp switch to request help with a familiar self-care routine. The self-care routine involved cleaning his lips and mouth with a cloth treated with mouthwash. This routine occurred prior to and after each meal. Richard seemed to like this self-care routine and the social interaction that accompanied it. He also seemed to show some anticipation of the routine (e.g., looking intently at the staff person and the paraphernalia associated with the self-care routine).

His intervention started with an initial baseline phase. For this, opportunities lasting 60 sec. were arranged immediately prior to undertaking the self-care routine. For each opportunity, the grasp switch was placed in Richard's left hand, as recommended by his care staff, and he was asked to hold it. Staff then wrote down how many times Richard activated the switch during each 60-sec. opportunity. At this baseline stage, activation of the switch had no programmed consequences. The purpose of the baseline phase was to determine how often Richard activated the switch reflexively. Over 13 baseline opportunities, conducted over a period of 11 days, Richard activated the switch an average of 13.8 times per each 60-sec. opportunity. This high rate of switch activation during baseline most likely resulted from the fact that placement of the switch in his hand elicited the palmer grasp reflex.

After the baseline phase, we conducted the intervention phase. This phase was intended to teach Richard to inhibit his palmar grasp reflex so that he would activate the switch once or only a few times during each opportunity. If such a pattern emerged, it would perhaps suggest that switch activation had transitioned from mere reflexive behavior to an intentional act of communication. The intervention procedures were similar to baseline, except that reinforcement was contingent upon the first switch activation that occurred during each 60-sec. opportunity. That is, as soon as the switch was activated, staff initiated the self-care routine and interacted socially with Richard. In addition to contingent reinforcement, antecedent practice trials were implemented. Practice trials consisted of placing the switch in Richard's hand and using gentle hand-over-hand guidance to help him squeeze the switch

once and then relax his grip to prevent further activations. While providing this hand-over-hand guidance, we also talked him through the procedure (e.g., *Yes, that's right. Squeeze it once, then relax.*). With this procedure in place, the number of switch activations per opportunity was reduced. Specifically, across 18 opportunities conducted over a month, the mean frequency of switch activations per opportunity averaged 1.8 responses. This dramatic change from baseline to intervention (Figure 9–5), suggested that Richard was perhaps learning to activate the grasp switch to request the self-care routine and social interaction rather than merely activating the switch due to his palmer grasp reflex.

In addition to Sarah and Richard, we have come across many individuals with PIMD with retained and often exagger-

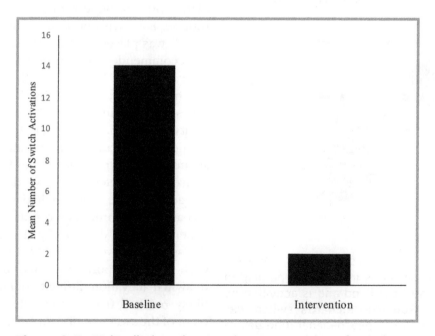

Figure 9–5. Richard's data showing the mean number of switch activations per opportunity during baseline and intervention. The change from baseline to intervention suggests that Richard may have been learning to inhibit his palmar grasp reflex and instead learning to use the switch as a means of communication.

ated developmental reflexes, such as the ATNR and palmar grasp reflex. The presence of such reflexes complicates intervention efforts and certainly presents unique challenges with respect to designing and implementing AAC. The evidence-base regarding successful approaches for addressing such challenges is meager. Approaches involving passive physical movement in an attempt to integrate primitive reflexes have proven to be ineffective (Cummins, 1998). A recent tangentially related study by Soloveichick et al. (2019) points to a potentially promising intervention approach. In this study, four preterm infants who were at risk for developmental disability participated in an early intervention program known as Movement Imitation Therapy. The therapy involves interrupting atypical movement patterns and then using physical guidance to shape more typical general movement patterns. After 10 weeks of therapy at a dosage of approximately 50 min per day, three of the four infants showed improved movement patterns. Even though the focus of this study was on infant's general movement patterns, variations of this therapy may have some relevance to accommodating developmental reflexes exhibited by people with PIMD. This would seem to be an interesting direction for future research.

On the other hand, the approaches we adopted with Sarah and Richard appeared to have been helpful, but they were not rigorously evaluated and therefore must be recommended with caution. For example, we did not collect data on the frequency or intensity of Sarah's ATNR during our interactions with her. With Richard, neither reliability data nor procedural integrity checks were collected during his baseline and intervention opportunities. Overall, although retained primitive reflexes do appear to create unique challenges for AAC intervention, there is a considerable need for future research on how to appropriately and effectively address this particular challenge.

◼ Summary and Conclusion

Providing effective AAC intervention to people with PIMD can be challenging due to the combination of intellectual, physical, sensory, and health impairments that such individuals can experience. Among the many challenges that can complicate intervention efforts, the present chapter considered three: (a) identifying reinforcers and response forms, (b) fostering biobehavioral states conducive to intervention, and (c) accommodating developmental reflexes. Respective solutions to these challenges include (a) undertaking evidence-based assessments to identify reinforcers and potential communication behaviors, (b) providing stimulation to promote greater levels of alertness, and (c) taking steps to avoid elicitation of developmental reflexes or co-opting these responses for communication purposes. The evidence-base related to assessing preferences is strong, but considerably more research is needed to determine how best to overcome the other challenges highlighted in this chapter. Successfully overcoming these challenges is critical for effective provision of AAC intervention for people with PIMD.

◼ References

Acharya, A. B., Jamil, R. T., & Dewey, J. J. (2019). *Babinski reflex*. National Library of Medicine, National Institutes of Health. Retrieved from https://www.ncbi.nlm.nih.gov/books/NBK519009/

Arthur, M. (2003). Socio-communicative variables and behavior states in students with profound and multiple disabilities: Descriptive data from school settings. *Education and Training in Developmental Disabilities, 38*, 200–219.

Arthur-Kelly, M., Foreman, P., Maes, B., Colyvas, K., & Lyons, G. (2018). Observational data on socio-communicative phenomena in classrooms supporting students with profound intellectual and multiple disability (PIMD): Advancing theory development on learning and engagement through data analysis. *Advances in Neurodevelopmental Disorders, 2*, 25–37. https://doi.org/10.1007/s41252-017-0045-1

Atkin, K., & Perlman Lorch, M. (2016). An ecological method for the sampling of nonverbal signaling behaviors of young children with profound and multiple learning disabilities (PMLD). *Developmental Neurorehabilitation, 19*, 211–225.https://doi.org/10.3109/17518423.2014.935822

Beadle-Brown, J., Leigh, J., Whelton, B., Richardson, L., Beecham, J., Baumker, T., & Bradshaw, J. (2016). Quality of life and quality of support for people with severe intellectual disability and complex needs. *Journal of Applied Research in Intellectual Disabilities, 29*, 409–421. https://doi.org/10.1111/jar.12200

Belva, B. C., Matson, J. L., Sipes, M., & Bamburg, J. W. (2012). An examination of specific communication deficits in adults with profound intellectual disabilities. *Research in Developmental Disabilities, 33*, 525–529. https://doi.org/10.1016/j.ridd.2011.10.019

Brady, N. C., Fleming, K., Swinburne Romine, R., Holbrook, A., Muller, K., & Kasari, C. (2018). Concurrent validity and reliability for the Communication Complexity Scale. *American Journal of Speech-Language Pathology, 27*, 237–246. https://doi.org/10.1044/2017_AJSLP-17-0106

Cannella, H. I., O'Reilly, M. F., & Lancioni, G. E. (2005). Choice and preference assessment research with people with severe to profound developmental disabilities: A review of the literature. *Research in Developmental Disabilities, 26*, 1–15. https://doi.org/10.1016/j.ridd.2004.01.006

Cannella-Malone, H. I., Koss Schmidt, E., & Bumpus, E. C. (2018). Assessing preference using eye gaze technology for individuals with significant intellectual and physical disabilities. *Advances in Neurodevelopmental Disorders, 2*, 300–309. https://doi.org/10.1007/s41252-018-0072-6

Chandradasa, M., & Rathnayake, L. (2019). Retained primitive reflexes in children, clinical implications and targeted home-based interventions. *Nursing Children and Young People. 32*(1), 37-42. https://doi.org/10.7748/ncyp.2019.e1132

Cummins, R. A. (1988). *The neurologically-impaired child: Doman-Delacato techniques reappraised.* Routledge.

Erickson, K., & Quick, N. (2017). The profiles of students with significant cognitive disabilities and known hearing loss. *Journal of Deaf Studies and Deaf Education, 22*, 35–48. https://doi.org/10.1093/deafed/enw052

Foreman, P., Arthur-Kelly, M., Bennett, D., Neilands, J., & Colyvas, K. (2014). Observed changes in the alertness and communicative involvement of students with multiple and severe disability following in-class mentor-modelling for staff in segregated and general education classrooms. *Journal of Intellectual Disability Research. 58*, 704–720. https://doi.org/10.1111/jr.12066

Foreman, P., Arthur-Kelly, M., Pascoe, S., & Smyth King, B. (2004). Evaluating the educational experiences of students with profound and multiple disabilities in inclusive and segregated classroom settings: An Australian perspective. *Research and Practice for Persons with Severe Disabilities, 29*, 183–193.

Gerondis, M. (2019). *Identifying and enhancing a potential communicative act in an adult woman with profound intellectual and multiple disabilities.* Unpublished Applied Research Project, Masters of Educational Psychology Programme, School of

Education, Victoria University of Wellington, Wellington, New Zealand.

Gieysztor, E. Z., Choinska, A. M., & Paprocka-Borowicz, M. (2018). Persistence of primitive reflexes and associated motor problems in healthy preschool children. *Archives of Medical Science, 14*, 167–173. https://doi.org/10.5114/aoms.2016.60503

Gilroy, S. P., McCleery, J. P., & Leader, G. (2017). Systematic review of methods for teaching social and communicative behavior with high tech augmentative and alternative modalities. *Review Journal of Autism and Developmental Disorders, 4*, 307–320. https://doi.org/10.1007/s40489-017-0115-3

Green, C. W., Gardner, S., Canipe, V., and Reid, D. H. (1994). Analyzing alertness among people with profound multiple disabilities: Implications for provision of training. *Journal of Applied Behavior Analysis, 27*, 519–531. https://doi.org/10.1901/jaba.1994.27-519

Green, C. W., Reid, D. H., White, L. K., Halford, R. C., Brittain, D. P., & Gardner, S. M. (1988). Identifying reinforcers for persons with profound handicaps: Staff opinion versus systematic assessment of preferences. *Journal of Applied Behavior Analysis, 21*, 32–43. https://doi.org/10.1901/jaba.1988.21–31

Guess, D., Mulligan-Ault, M., Roberts, S., Struth, J., Siegal–Causey, E., Thompson, B, . . . Guy, G. (1988). Implications of biobehavioral states for the education and treatment of students with the most handicapping conditions. *Journal of the Association for Persons with Severe Handicaps, 13*, 163–174. https://doi.org/10.1177/154079698801300306

Guess, D., Roberts, S., & Rues, J. (2002). Longitudinal analysis of state patterns and related variables among infants and children with significant disabilities. *Research and Practice for Persons with Severe Disabilities, 27*, 112–124. https://doi.org/10.2511/rpsd.27.2.112

Guess, D., Siegel-Causey, E., Roberts, D., Rues, J., Thompson, B., & Siegel-Causey, D. (1990). Assessment and analysis of behavior state and related variables among students with severely handicapping conditions. *Journal of the Association for Persons with Severe Handicaps, 15*, 211–230. https://doi.org/10.1177/154079699001500401

Gulati, S., & Sondhi, V. (2018). Cerebral palsy: An overview. *Indian Journal of Pediatrics, 85*, 1006–1016. https://doi.org/10.1007/s12098-017-2475-1

Gutowski, S. J. (1996). Response acquisition for music or beverages in adults with profound multiple handicaps. *Journal of Developmental and Physical Disabilities, 8*, 221–231. https://doi.org/10.1007/BF02578391

Helm, J. M., & Simeonsson, R. J. (1989). Assessment of behavior state organization. In D. B. Bailey & M. Wolery (Eds.), *Assessing infants and preschoolers with handicaps* (pp. 202–224). Merrill.

Jacobs, L., & Gossman, M. D. (1980). Three primitive reflexes in normal adults. *Neurology, 30*, 184–188. https://doi.org/10.1212/WNL.30.2.184

Johnson, J. J., Rahn, N. L., & Bricker, D. (2015). *An activity-based approach to early intervention* (4th ed.). Brookes.

Kangas, K., & Lloyd, L. (1988). Early cognitive skills as prerequisites to augmentative and alternative communication use: What are we waiting for? *Augmentative and Alternative Communication, 4*, 211–221. https://doi.org/10.1080/07434618812331274817

Kawakami, M., Liu, M., Otsuka, T., Wada, A., Uchikawa, K., Aoki, A., & Otaka, Y. (2013). Asymmetrical skull deformity in children with cerebral palsy: Frequency and correlation with postural abnormalities and deformities. *Journal of Rehabilitation Medicine, 45*, 149–153. https://doi.org/10.2340/16501977-1081

Keen, D. (2014). Prelinguistic communication. In J. Arciuli & J. Brock (Eds.), *An introduction to communication in autism: Current findings and future directions* (pp. 11–28). Benjamins.

Lancioni, G. E., O'Reilly, M. F., & Basil, G. (2001). Use of microswitches and speech output systems with people with severe/profound intellectual or multiple disabilities:

A literature review. *Research in Developmental Disabilities, 22,* 21–40. https://doi.org/10.1016/s0891-4222(00)000064-0

Lancioni, G. E., Sigafoos, J., O'Reilly, M. F., Singh, N. N. (2013). *Assistive technology: Interventions for individuals with severe/profound and multiple disabilities.* Springer.

Logan, K. R., & Gast, D. L. (2001). Conducting preference assessments and reinforcer testing for individuals with profound multiple disabilities: Issues and procedures. *Exceptionality, 9,* 123–134. https://doi.org/10.1207/S15327035EX0903_3

Lyle, D. (2019). *Understanding profound intellectual and multiple disabilities in adults.* Routledge. https://doi.org/10.4324/9780429019791

Marques-de-Moraes, M. V., Dionisio, J., Tan, U., & Tudella, E. (2017). Palmer grasp reflex in human newborns. *Pediatrics and Therapeutics, 7*(1). https://doi.org/10.4172/2161-0665.1000309

Martens, B. K., Bradley, T. A., & Eckert, T. L. (1997). Effects of reinforcement history and instructions on the persistence of student engagement. *Journal of Applied Behavior Analysis, 30,* 569–572. https://doi.org/10.1901/jaba.1997.30.569

McLean, L. K., Brady, N. C., McLean, J. E., & Behrens, G. A. (1999). Communication forms and functions of children and adults with severe mental retardation in community and institutional settings. *Journal of Speech, Language, and Hearing Research, 42,* 231–240. https://doi.org/10.1044/jslhr.4201.231

Munde, V., & Vlaskamp, C. (2015). Initiation of activities and alertness in individuals with profound intellectual and multiple disabilities. *Journal of Intellectual Disability Research, 59,* 284–292. https://doi.org/10.1111/jir.12138

Nakken, H., & Vlaskamp, C. (2007). A need for a taxonomy for profound intellectual and multiple disabilities. *Journal of Policy and Practice in Intellectual Disabilities, 4,* 83–87. https://doi.org/10.111/j.1741-1130.2007.00104.x

Petry, K., & Maes, B. (2007). Description of the support needs of people with profound multiple disabilities using the 2002 AAMR system: An overview of literature. *Education and Training in Developmental Disabilities, 42,* 130–143. Retrieved from https://search-proquest-com.helicon.vuw.ac.nz/docview/62041282?accountid=14782

Reichle, J., & Karlan, G. (1985). The selection of an augmentative system in communication intervention: A critique of decision rules. *Journal of the Association for Persons with Severe Handicaps, 10,* 146–156. https://doi.org/10.1177/154079698501000304

Reichle, J., York, J., & Sigafoos, J. (1991). *Implementing augmentative and alternative communication: Strategies for learners with severe disabilities.* Brookes.

Rensfeldt Flink, A., Johnels, J. A., Broberg, M., & Thunberg, G. (2020). Examining perceptions of a communication course for parents of children with profound intellectual and multiple disabilities. *International Journal of Developmental Disabilities.* https://doi.org/10.1080/20473869.2020.1721160

Roche, L., Sigafoos, J., Lancioni, G. E., O'Reilly, M. F., & Green, V. A. (2015). Microswitch technology for enabling self-determined responding in children with profound and multiple disabilities: A systematic review. *Augmentative and Alternative Communication, 31,* 246–258. https://doi.org/10.3109/07434618.2015.1024888

Romski, M., & Sevcik, R. (2005). Augmentative communication and early intervention: Myths and realities. *Infants and Young Children, 18,* 174–185. https://doi.org/10.1097/IYC.0000000000000172

Rousseau, P. V., Matton, F., Lecuyer, R., & Lahaye, W. (2017). The Moro reaction: More than a reflex, a ritualized behavior of nonverbal communication. *Infant Behavior and Development, 46,* 169–177. https://doi.org/10.1016/j.infbeh.2017.01.004

Schlosser, R. W., & Raghavendra, P. (2004). Evidence-based practice in augmentative and alternative communication. *Augmentative and Alternative Communication, 20,*

1–21. https://doi.org/10.1080/07434610310 001621083

Schoen, S. A., Miller, L. J., Brett-Green, B. A., & Nielsen, D. M. (2009). Physiological and behavioral differences in sensory processing: A comparison of children with autism spectrum disorder and sensory modulation disorder. *Frontiers in Integrative Neuroscience, 3*(29). https://doi.org/10.3389/neuro .07.029.2009

Sigafoos, J. (1999). Creating opportunities for augmentative and alternative communication: Strategies for involving people with developmental disabilities. *Augmentative and Alternative Communication, 15,* 183–190. https://doi.org/10.1080/074346199123 31278715

Sigafoos, J., & Couzens, D. (1995). Teaching functional use of an eye gaze communication board to a child with multiple disabilities. *British Journal of Developmental Disabilities, 41,* 114–125. https://doi.org/10.11 79/bjdd.1995.015

Sigafoos, J., & Dempsey, R. (1992). Assessing choice making among children with multiple disabilities. *Journal of Applied Behavior Analysis, 25,* 747–755. https://doi.org/ 10.1901/jaba.1992.25-747

Sigafoos, J., Woodyatt, G., Keen, D., Tait, K., Tucker, M., Roberts-Pennell, D., & Pittendreigh, N. (2000). Identifying potential communicative acts in children with developmental and physical disabilities. *Communication Disorders Quarterly, 21,* 77–86. https://doi.org/10.1177/152574010 002100202

Simacek, J., Pennington, B., Reichle, J., & Parker-McGowan, Q. (2018). Aided AAC for people with severe to profound and multiple disabilities: A systematic review of interventions and treatment intensity. *Advances in Neurodevelopmental Disorders, 2,* 100–115. https://doi.org/10.1007/ s41252-017-0050-4

Siu, E., Tam, E., Sin, D., Ng, C., Lam, E., Chui, M., . . . Lam, C. (2010). A survey of augmentative and alternative communication service provision in Hong Kong. *Augmentative and Alternative Communication, 26*(4), 289–298. https://doi.org/10.3109/0 7434618.2010.521894

Soloveichick, M., Marschik, P. B., Gover, A., Molad, M., Kessel, I., & Einspieler, C. (2019). Movement imitation therapy for preterm babies (MIT-PB): A novel approach to improve the neurodevelopmental outcomes for infants at high-risk for cerebral palsy. *Journal of Developmental and Physical Disabilities, 32,* 587–598. https://doi.org/10 .1007/s10882-019-09707-y

Sutherland, D., van der Meer, L., Sigafoos, J., Mirfin-Veitch, B., Milner, P., O'Reilly, M. F., . . . Marschik, P. B. (2014). Survey of AAC needs for adults with intellectual disability in New Zealand. *Journal of Developmental and Physical Disabilities, 26,* 115–122. https://doi.org/10.1007/s10882-013-9347-z

Sutherland, D. E., Gillon, G. G., & Yoder, D. E. (2005). AAC use and service provision: A survey of New Zealand speech-language therapists. *Augmentative and Alternative Communication, 21,* 295–307. https://doi .org/10.1080/07434610500103483

Tait, K., & Sigafoos, J. (2018). Assessing engagement and responsiveness of children with profound/multiple disabilities. *Journal of Applied Research in Intellectual Disability, 31,* 567. https://doi.org/10.1111/jar.12475 [Abstracts of the IASSIDD European Congress, 17–20 July, 2018, Athens]

Tullis, C. A., Cannella-Malone, H. I., Basbigill, A. R., Yeager, A., Fleming, C. V., Payne, D., & Wu, P-F. (2011). Review of the choice and preference assessment literature for individuals with severe to profound disabilities. *Education and Training in Autism and Developmental Disabilities, 46,* 576–595. https://doi.org/10.1207/S15327035EX 0903_3

Urbanowicz, A., Leonard, H., Girdler, S., Ciccone, N., & Downs, J. (2016). Parental perspective on the communication abilities of their daughters with Rett syndrome. *Developmental Neurorehabilitation, 19,* 17–25. https://doi.org/10.3109/17518423.2013.87 9940 van Splunder, J., Stilma, J. S., Bernsen, R. M. D., & Evenhuis, H. M. (2006). Prevalence of visual impairment in adults with intellectual disabilities in the Netherlands: Cross-sectional study. *Eye, 20,* 1004–1010. https://doi.org/10.1038/sj.eye.6702059

Vlaskamp, C., de Geeter, K. I., Huijsmans, L. M., & Smit, I. H. (2003). Passive activities: The effectiveness of multisensory environments on the level of activity of individuals with profound multiple disabilities. *Journal of Applied Research in Intellectual Disabilities, 16,* 135–143. https://doi.org/10.1046/j.1468-3148.2003.00156.x

von Tetzchner, S. (1997). Communication skills among females with Rett syndrome. *European Child & Adolescent Psychiatry, 6,* 33–37.

Wehmeyer, M., Chapman, T. E., Little, T. D., Thompson, J. R., Schalock, R., & Tassé, M. J. (2009). Efficacy of the Supports Intensity Scale (SIS) to predict extraordinary support needs. *American Journal on Intellectual and Developmental Disabilities, 114,* 3–14. https://doi.org/10.1352/2009-114:3-14

Wolff, P. H. (1959). Observations on newborn infants. In L. J. Stone, H. T. Smith, & L. B. Murphy (Eds.), *The competent infant* (pp. 257–272). Basic Books.

Woodyatt, G., & Ozanne, A. (1992). Communication abilities and Rett syndrome. *Journal of Autism and Developmental Disorders, 22,* 155–173. https://doi.org/10.1007/BF01058148

10

The Challenge of Symbolic Communication for School-Aged Students with the Most Significant Cognitive Disabilities

Karen Erickson, Lori Geist, Penny Hatch, and Nancy Quick

Across U.S. public schools, approximately 566,000 students (National Center for Education Statistics, 2019) have significant cognitive disabilities (SCD) that prevent them from achieving grade level academic standards even with appropriate instruction and accommodations (Office of Special Education Programs [OSEP], 2005). The term SCD, coined by the U.S. Department of Education, is used to describe a group of students who receive special education services under a variety of disability categories (e.g., autism, multiple disabilities, traumatic brain injury, etc.) and have an intellectual disability that is characterized by "significant limitations both in intellectual functioning and adaptive behavior, which covers many every day social and practical skills" (American Association of Intellectual and Developmental Disabilities, 2017, paragraph 1).

Students with SCD compose approximately 1% of the K–12 population and almost 10% of students with disabilities in US public schools (Thurlow & Wu, 2016).

Many students with SCD are described in the research literature as having severe intellectual and developmental disabilities (Snell et al., 2010) or significant support needs (Copeland, Keefe, Calhoon, Tanner, & Park, 2011). All students with SCD have impairments in metacognition, as well as short- and long-term memory that make them learn at rates that are slower than other students with and without disabilities and make it challenging for them to generalize skills (Kleinert, Browder, & Towles-Reeves, 2009; Nash, Clark, & Karvonen, 2015). These characteristics lead students with SCD to require extensive, repeated, individualized instruction and support including, substantially adapted materials and individualized methods of accessing information, to acquire, maintain, demonstrate, and transfer skills across settings (Dynamic Learning Maps Consortium, 2016).

This chapter focuses on the 35% of students with SCD who also have complex communication needs (Erickson & Geist,

2016) and learning profiles that often impede their ability to develop symbolic communication. This group of students is not literate (Erickson & Geist, 2016) and acquires relatively small vocabularies regardless of communication modality (Beukelman, Yorkston, Poblete, & Naranjo, 1984; Cameto et al., 2010). Students with SCD and complex communication needs are a subgroup of the larger population of students with complex communication needs.

As a group, students with SCD in the United States also face systemic barriers that prevent them from learning to use speech, signs, or symbols for personal expression and the exchange of information. These barriers include limited: (a) access to aided augmentative and alternative communication (AAC); (b) access to services from speech-language pathologists with expertise in AAC; and (c) expectations regarding their learning potential. This chapter describes an approach to addressing these challenges through a universal communication intervention that targets classroom teachers and staff.

■ Limited Access to Aided AAC and SLPs with AAC Expertise

Like all people with complex communication needs, students with SCD and complex communication needs have the potential to benefit from aided AAC. Unfortunately, access to aided AAC is extremely limited for most students with SCD. Fewer than a quarter have access to sophisticated speech generating devices (SGDs), and nearly half of students with SCD who use aided AAC have access to only one or two symbols at a time (Erick-

son & Geist, 2016). Access to aided AAC for students with SCD is limited by a number of factors including: (a) policies that require students to demonstrate the ability to use a SGD before one is recommended and approved (Center for Medicare and Medicaid Services, 2017); (b) physical and sensory challenges that may restrict physical access when a device is available (Erickson & Geist, 2016); and (c) intellectual disabilities that carry increased learning challenges (Kleinert et al., 2009; Nash et al., 2015).

In addition to limited access to aided AAC, most students with SCD do not have access to speech and language services at an intensity or duration they require to learn. The vast majority of students with SCD are educated in separate schools or self-contained classrooms (Erickson & Geist, 2016). According to a national survey (American Speech-Language-Hearing Association [ASHA], 2018), speech-language pathologists (SLPs) serving students in these separate schools have average caseloads of 34 students, with significantly higher averages of 50 for elementary and 48 for secondary general education settings where self-contained classrooms are located. Across settings, the majority of students on SLPs' caseloads receive intervention for only an hour or less per week (ASHA, 2018), typically during one or two, short (20 to 30 minutes), small group sessions (Brandel & Loeb, 2011). Given the range of diagnostic, supervisory and support responsibilities SLPs must also assume, their average time to engage in direct intervention ranges from 26 (separate school) to 28.8 (all settings) hours per week (ASHA, 2018). This equates to very limited time devoted to individual students, with few differences in intensity of service based on level of student need (Brandel & Loeb,

2011), which can make it impossible to ameliorate the restricted communication skills of many students with SCD.

A Model for Communication Intervention in the Classroom

Special education teachers serving students with SCD have considerably more time to provide students with direct communication interventions than do SLPs. Although class sizes vary based on students' needs and state guidelines, they are consistently smaller and offer a higher adult to student ratio than general education classroom settings (U.S. Department of Education, 2012). For example, class sizes for students with SCD in North Carolina range from 6 to 12 students, with one teacher and at least one teaching assistant per classroom (North Carolina State Board of Education, 2014). This means that special educators have class sizes that are likely more than 75% smaller than the caseloads of the SLPs who serve their students.

Special education teachers and other classroom staff could dramatically increase the intensity of communication interventions available to students with SCD. Unfortunately, 76% of special education programs fail to offer a single course in AAC (Costigan & Light, 2010). Additionally, many effective approaches to teaching communication are slow to move from controlled research studies to typical settings, commonly referred to as research-to-practice gaps (Olswang & Prelock, 2015). These gaps are largely due to intervention recommendations that are not attuned to the context, poten-

tial barriers, and necessary resources for effective implementation (Fixsen, Blase, Metz, & Van Dyke, 2013). The purpose of the implementation model described in this chapter, Project Core, is to provide classroom teachers and related staff with the materials, professional development, assessment, self-reflection and coaching supports they need to successfully teach symbolic communication to their students with SCD and complex communication needs. The goal is not to eliminate the need for SLPs. Rather, the goal is to help classroom teachers take ownership of their role in teaching communication so that SLPs can build upon and refine their efforts to promote improved communication outcomes and educational access for students with SCD and complex communication needs. To accomplish this, evidence-based solutions were packaged in a way that made them easy to learn and implemented to promote more symbolic communication, as well as autonomy and self-determination.

Project Core: A Universal Solution

Project Core was developed by the authors and a team at the Center for Literacy and Disability Studies in the Department of Allied Health Sciences at the University of North Carolina at Chapel Hill. It is a classroom-based, comprehensive model of communication intervention that supports classroom teachers and teams through a system of professional development, a set of evidence-based practices, supports for lesson planning and self-reflection, and an emphasis on personal access to aided AAC featuring core vocabulary for all students.

The evidence-based practices in Project Core include: (a) leveraging core vocabulary (e.g., Cross, Erickson, Geist, & Hatch, in press); (b) ensuring all students have access to personal AAC systems (e.g., Ganz et al., 2012); (c) identifying and attributing meaning to all acts of communication, including early, nonsymbolic behaviors (e.g., Rowland, 2011; Yoder, McCathren, Warren, & Watson, 2001); (d) showing students what is possible and how to use symbolic communication through the use of aided language input strategies (e.g., Trembath, Balandin, & Togher, 2007); and (e) applying the principles of naturalistic teaching to maximize learning opportunities and promote generalization across contexts and purposes (e.g., Pindiprolu, 2012). Each is described in more detail below.

Core Vocabulary

Project Core takes a *core vocabulary* approach to vocabulary. Core vocabulary is a term used to describe the relatively small set of words that are used most frequently in oral and written language (Banajee, Dicarlo, & Stricklin, 2003; Deckers, Van Zaalen, Van Balkom, & Verhoeven., 2017; Trembath et al., 2007). Core vocabulary words are among the first words typically developing children hear from their parents (Quick, Erickson, & Mccright, 2019), and use most often in their own speech (e.g., Banajee et al., 2003). Core words also overlap with the first words children are explicitly taught to read (e.g., Dolch, 1955) and are predominant in children's early writing (Clendon & Erickson, 2008). Rather than specific nouns, core words are primarily pronouns, verbs, auxiliary verbs, prepositions, adjectives, and determiners. The

fact that core vocabulary words comprise much of spoken language and are essential to the expression of novel messages has been confirmed through a number of studies investigating: typically developing young children (e.g., Banajee et al., 2003), mono and bilingual school-aged children with and without language impairments (e.g., Boenisch & Soto, 2015), children with intellectual disabilities (e.g., Deckers et al., 2017), as well as adults (e.g., Balandin & Iacono, 1998). The core vocabulary approach in Project Core leverages the utility of context-independent words to support receptive and expressive communication across environments, activities, partners, purposes, and functions.

There is growing interest in the use of core vocabulary as an alternative to the exclusive use of concrete, context-dependent vocabulary as an initial lexicon for students with SCD and complex communication needs (Deckers et al., 2017; Cross et al., in press; van Tilborg & Deckers, 2016). Most proponents of core vocabulary acknowledge that it is conceptual and may, therefore, be more difficult to learn because the words themselves have multiple meanings and graphic representations of core words are opaque (Erickson & Koppenhaver, 2020; Snodgrass, Stoner, & Angell, 2013). However, in comparison to concrete vocabulary, core vocabulary allows for a dramatic increase in opportunities for teaching and learning because core words can be used across contexts, purposes, and partners both in isolation and in combination (Adamson, Romski, Deffebach, & Sevcik 1992; Deckers et al., 2017). This increase in opportunities to teach and learn is the basis upon which core vocabulary was selected as the focus of an initial lexicon for students with SCD and complex communication in Project Core.

Historically, initial lexicon considerations for students with SCD and complex communication needs have focused on symbols that represent preferred items or activities (Beukelman, McGinnis, & Morrow, 1991; Schlosser & Sigafoos, 2002; Snell, Chen, & Hoover, 2006) in order to promote requesting (Frost & Bondy, 2002) and functional communication (Adamson, et al., 1992). These items are generally selected through preference assessments (Sigafoos & Reichle, 1992; Snell et al., 2006) and interventions that reinforce successful communication efforts through contingent reinforcement. Vocabulary highlighting student preferences harnesses the power of student attention, increasing the likelihood of joint attention, which is the process assumed to assist learners in mapping words to their referents (Tomasello, 2003). However, the context-specific nature of vocabulary reflecting personal preferences limits opportunities for teaching and learning and restricts purposes for communication primarily to the communicative function of requesting (Dodd & Gorey, 2013).

This emphasis on preferred items and activities is often accompanied by the prioritization of concrete vocabulary over conceptual vocabulary (Van Tatenhove, 2009). Concrete vocabulary generally includes object nouns, as well as some action verbs and descriptors, which are all relatively easy to learn because students can physically interact with the objects and perform or observe the actions associated with the words. Learning concrete vocabulary in aided AAC is further supported by the fact that it is possible to represent many items, especially nouns, with highly transparent graphic symbols that visually resemble their referents and are, therefore, highly guessable (Beukelman & Mirenda, 2013; Schlosser & Sigafoos, 2002).

Although this use of concrete vocabulary has some cognitive and developmental advantages, the context-specific nature of concrete vocabulary limits opportunities for teaching, learning, and use, while restricting opportunities for combining words (Dodd & Gorey, 2013). For example, consider the graphic symbols for a preferred food (e.g., "cracker") and a preferred activity (e.g., "music"). There are few opportunities to use or see others use these symbols throughout the day, as these symbols can only be used to label or request in specific contexts. Further, these words can only be used in meaningful combinations when used with conceptual core words (e.g., "more music" or "want cracker").

For many students with SCD and complex communication needs, the vocabulary that they are provided routinely changes in order to accommodate particular activities or routines (Deckers et al., 2017; Van Tatenhove, 2009). This common approach to presenting individual symbols or creating displays with words and symbols related to a specific activity or environment may promote successful use in specific contexts. However, this practice is likely to create barriers to generalized use and communication access, as words available during one activity are often not available in subsequent activities or routines. When vocabulary does reappear, it is often displayed with different words and in different locations relative to other available symbols (e.g., the graphic symbol representing "ball" appears on the left of an array of four symbols used during free time, and the same symbol appears on the right in an array of four symbols used during a shared reading interaction). As students with SCD require more intense repetition, stability, and predictability for learning (Kleinert et al., 2009;

Nash et al., 2015), continually changing the vocabulary and/or its location to support activity-specific interaction is likely to limit word learning and communication development.

One of the teachers involved in a site where Project Core was developed and evaluated reflected on this contrast between core vocabulary and more concrete vocabulary during an interview. She said:

> "It [core vocabulary] is an effective way for the kids to communicate and to express to us. It has opened up the curriculum like no other way because now we can engage in conversation. It just changes up the whole way we teach because now it flows with the kids, instead of just throwing everything at the kid and asking some narrow question like, *'Is the book about a worm or a dog?'"*

Concerns regarding core vocabulary for use with students with SCD focus on the belief that core words and the symbols representing them are too abstract. A primary argument opposing an emphasis on core vocabulary is based on the fact that the cognitive load for learning the symbols that represent core vocabulary is greater than that of concrete vocabulary because core vocabulary references more abstract concepts (e.g., "want") than concrete objects (e.g., "cookie"). Considering that graphic representations of core vocabulary tend to be more opaque than graphic representations of concrete vocabulary (Beukelman & Mirenda, 2013), children may not immediately recognize the meaning of symbols that represent core words (Light, 2016). However, young children can learn abstract graphic representations with instruction (Worah, McNaughton, Light, & Benedek-Wood, 2015) and students with SCD both use and generalize conceptually abstract words (Snodgrass et al., 2013) across contexts, partners, and purposes (Adamson et al., 1992), even when the symbols are arbitrary (Sevcik, Barton-Hulsey, Romski, & Fonseca, 2018). Project Core builds on this research by emphasizing evidence-based practices in communication intervention and using core vocabulary, which exponentially increases the learning opportunities that are present throughout a typical day. This, in turn, empowers students, teachers, and teams with a repertoire of words that can be used with any topic, across all contexts, partners, and purposes.

Identifying a Universal Core Vocabulary

A primary goal of Project Core is to contribute to the evidence-base regarding the use of core vocabulary with students with SCD and complex communication needs. To address this, we sought to identify a set of core vocabulary words that could be used universally as a starting place. We were specifically interested in identifying a set of core words spanning grades K–12 that reflected the research in core vocabulary in AAC and the vocabulary that is needed to successfully communicate while in academic settings where college and career readiness standards are being taught. Our first step was to compile the vocabulary lists from four seminal studies involving young children (Banajee et al., 2003; Beukelman, Jones, & Rowan, 1989; Marvin, Beukelman, & Bilyeu, 1994; Trembath et al., 2007). Next, widely used commercial and public domain core vocabulary lists were collected and combined with the list compiled from the research. These included core vocabulary lists developed for commercially available AAC systems (i.e., Gateway, GoTalk, TouchChat, and Word Power), by school systems (e.g., Oakland School District in Michigan), and AAC specialists (e.g., Gail VanTatenhove).

The next step involved a careful analysis of the expressive language demands of college and career readiness standards for students in kindergarten through high school. This process identified specific words (e.g., different, equal) and classes of words (e.g. conjunctions, reflexive pronouns) that students are required to use. The two steps resulted in a list of 596 words. These words were then weighted using a scoring system that took into account the number of AAC core vocabulary lists that included the word, the frequency, and dispersion of the word in written English, and the number of expressive language demands that could be addressed by the word. Details of the weighting system can be found in a technical report (found at http://www .project-core.com/technical-reports/). The weighting process resulted in a prioritized list from which 36 words were selected to compose the Universal Core vocabulary (Table 10–1). In selecting the 36 words, our goal was to select a small

set of highly ranked words that fit the following criteria: (a) meaningful as single words; (b) meaningful when combined with one another; and (c) useful across environments, activities, and interactions.

To determine the total number of words to include, we worked to identify the smallest set of words meeting these criteria that also allowed adults to demonstrate aided AAC in every conceivable interaction across a typical school day.

Common Approaches to Aided AAC Organization

Organizing and representing the words in the Universal Core vocabulary involved a variety of choices to make it maximally accessible to the full range of beginning communicators with SCD. For example, the organization had to work for students who could use direct selection as well as those who would need scanning, eye-pointing, and arrays with few symbols in each visual array to accommodate sensory or motor challenges. Similarly, the Universal Core had to be represented with symbols that the full range of students with significant cognitive disabilities could learn and use.

The need to create several formats to address the needs of students with SCD

Table 10–1. The Universal Core Vocabulary in Alphabetic Order

all	can	different	do	finished	get
go	good	he	help	here	I
in	like	it	look	make	more
not	on	open	put	same	she
some	stop	that	turn	up	want
what	when	where	who	why	you

precluded use of the Fitzgerald key, a common organizational approach that would not support the intended consistency across formats and is not supported by research (Beukelman & Mirenda, 2013). A Fitzgerald key organization theoretically supports communicators in their efforts to generate grammatical, multiword utterances, but the students who are the focus of Project Core are learning to communicate using single symbols. By the time they are combining two or more words in grammatical order, they should be using more robust communication systems that support more complex forms of communication than are possible with the Universal Core vocabulary alone.

Another feature that is common to AAC organization, especially with organizations based on part of speech like the Fitzgerald key, is the use of background color-coding. With this approach, words in the same word class all have the same background color or cell outline. The approach is intended to support communicators in locating the desired word. Research in the past decade suggests that background color-coding in grids with fewer than 64 symbols provides limited cues to support locating symbols and can actually interfere with the visual search for symbols in smaller grids (Light et al., 2019; Thistle & Wilkinson, 2009; Wilkinson & Coombs, 2010; Wilkinson & Snell, 2011). In an effort to eliminate potential interference with searching for a desired symbol, the Universal Core vocabulary does not use background color-coding.

The Universal Core Organizations

Design priorities for the Universal Core formats included good usability (i.e., easy to learn and use) for teachers with little to no background in AAC and wide accessibility for students with SCD through direct selection, partner-assisted scanning or eye-pointing. Each of these formats is available for download from the Project Core website. The simple layouts in the various formats are aimed at increasing the teaching and learning opportunities for students who would not otherwise have access to personal AAC systems with the words in the Universal Core vocabulary. The most commonly used formats are displayed and described in Table 10–2.

To reduce the learning demands for teachers and students as they use different formats of the Universal Core, the organization of all of the various formats is related. We created the layouts with fewer symbols on each page by dividing the 36-location format into four 3×3 blocks and nine 2×2 blocks. For the 4-page book layout with 9 medium-size symbols on each page, the layout of each of the four pages matches a 3×3 quadrant from the 36-location format. The first page matches the layout of the symbols in the quadrant in the upper left corner of the 36-location format. The second page matches the layout of the symbols in the quadrant in the upper right corner of the 36-location format, and so on. For the 9-page book for partner-assisted scanning with 4 symbols on each page, the layout of each page of the nine pages matches a 2×2 set of symbols from the 36-location format. The first page is the first 2×2 set of symbols in the upper left corner. The second page is the middle 2×2 set of symbols across the top. The third page is the 2×2 set of symbols in the upper right corner. The fourth page is the 2×2 set of symbols in the middle on the left and so on, moving left to right, top to bottom on the 36-location format.

Table 10–2. Open-Source Universal Core Vocabulary Formats

Format	Description
	This 36-location layout is best suited to students whose language, vision, and access abilities support visually scanning an array of 36 words/symbols and pointing in some way to make selections.
	The 4-page book layout with 9 medium-size symbols on each page is for students who can point in some way to make selections but need a slightly larger target.
	The 9-page layout with 4 large symbols on each page is for students who can point in some way to make selections but need a large target. (Note: This example shows the high saturation/low complexity symbols that are available for all formats to address the needs of some students with visual impairments.)
	The 9-page book for partner-assisted scanning is for students who cannot point to make selections. Four symbols on each page are arranged in an in-line format to promote consistent auditory and/or visual presentation of symbol choices by communication partners.
	This 9-page book is designed for selection via eye-pointing with a symbol in each corner of the see-through pages.
	Each of the words in the Universal Core vocabulary has been created in a 3D representation. Each 3D symbol has a base with a distinct shape, texture, and color for each word class (e.g., adjective, pronoun, verb) as well as the word indicated in braille and print. On each base, there is a tactual symbol representing the specific word.

This design approach is also intended to reduce the learning demands for students who may start with a 4- or 9-location book format and move to a 36-location format as they grow in their communication abilities. This is a deliberately simple approach to offering consistency across the different open-source formats. These formats are not intended to indicate research-based guidance on where to position graphic symbols on similar displays or overlays, but rather serve as one approach to explore and, as appropriate, modify.

Symbol Selection

The research regarding graphic symbols focuses predominantly on the transparency, or the ease with which the meaning of symbols can be determined without instruction. However, in the context of core vocabulary, transparency has little meaning because the words are conceptual rather than concrete. Simply put, the symbols do not represent things, they represent ideas; as such, they are not intended to be transparent. Furthermore, the research suggests that transparency is not especially helpful to individuals who are learning to use graphic symbols but have minimal to no comprehension of spoken language (Stephenson, 2009). Instead of relying on transparency, they learn the symbols they are taught (Romski & Sevcik, 2005), especially when they understand the use of symbols as referents in natural communicative interactions (Stephenson, 2009).

Without much research to guide our decisions, we decided to focus our efforts on representing the Universal Core vocabulary with the most common symbols sets used in AAC, in order to make sure that students have access to communication displays that use symbols like those that are most often used in the environments where they live and learn. As a result, each of the Universal Core displays is available in Picture Communication Symbols™ (standard and high contrast), SymbolStix®, and Widgit Symbols©, three common symbols sets.

Providing Personal Access to AAC

The various formats used to represent the Universal Core vocabulary are intended to maximize personal access to AAC for as many students with SCD and complex communication needs as possible. Meta-analyses (Ganz et al., 2012; Schlosser & Lee, 2000) and systematic reviews (Holyfield, Drager, Kremkow, & Light, 2017; Romski, Sevcik, Barton-Hulsey, & Whitmore, 2015) support aided AAC with personal access to systems as an evidence-based practice. For example, a meta-analysis of 50 single-subject experimental studies supports the effectiveness of aided AAC intervention, generalization, and maintenance (Schlosser & Lee, 2000). Fifty-eight percent of the subjects in the studies were school-aged students with SCD. The meta-analysis determined that 87.5% of the aided AAC interventions were highly effective (44.8%) or fairly effective (42.7%), which means they had at least 70% nonoverlapping data. A second meta-analysis of 24 single case studies of students with autism spectrum disorders who used aided AAC revealed large effect sizes for communication, as well as social skills, academics, and the reduction of challenging behaviors (Ganz et al., 2012). Finally, a recent systematic review of 18 studies related to aided AAC interventions for adolescents and adults with autism spectrum disorder reported that aided AAC intervention appears to be highly effective for this target population (Holyfield et al., 2017).

In summary, numerous sources point to aided AAC as an evidence-based practice. Furthermore, they support the use of aided AAC across ages and disabilities. In fact, the body of evidence continues to support the understanding that all persons who cannot use speech to meet their communication needs are candidates for and can benefit from AAC intervention regardless of the severity of their intellectual or cognitive disability (Snell et al., 2010). The evidence taken as a whole provides strong support for the use of aided AAC, and adds to the concern regarding the limited access to aided AAC reported for many students with SCD and complex communication needs (Erickson & Geist, 2016). Project Core was designed to address this widespread concern.

Identifying and Attributing Meaning to Early Behaviors

Beginning communicators are often dependent on early, nonsymbolic forms of communication that must be interpreted by communication partners (Rowland, 2011). Supporting beginning communicators' understanding that their behaviors can influence and direct the behaviors of other people is an important step along the path to learning to communicate symbolically (Beukelman & Mirenda, 2013). This is especially the case for students who are dependent on nonsymbolic forms of communication like many students with SCD and complex communication needs. Building this understanding relies in part on communication partners consistently: (1) identifying early communication acts, such as body movements, facial expressions and vocalizations, (2) attributing meaning to these early acts, and (3) honoring the communicative intent of all behaviors (Cress, Arens, & Zajicek, 2007; Yoder et al., 2001). Additionally, instruction should build on early forms and develop multimodal approaches to communication that blend the use of forms like vocalizations, gestures, and graphic symbols (Beukelman & Mirenda, 2013). Communication partners can work toward this by using sign language or graphic symbols to demonstrate alternative forms of expression that reflect the intent of nonsymbolic communication acts (O'Neill, Light, & Pope, 2018; Sennott, Light, & McNaughton, 2016). For example, when an adult identifies a student reaching for a desired object, the adult can attribute meaning (e.g., saying, "I see you reaching. You *want* that") and honor the student's intent by providing access to the desired object. As discussed in more detail in the next section, adults can also demonstrate the use of a more conventional form by pointing to the graphic symbol for the word *WANT* on the student's AAC system and telling the student "you could say, *WANT*." The aim is for students to learn to intentionally communicate and connect their early behaviors with more conventional, symbolic forms of communication (Reichle, 1997; Smith, Barker, Barton-Hulsey, Romski, & Sevcik, 2016).

In Project Core, teachers and teams are taught to identify and attribute meaning to all early communication behaviors. They are also taught to demonstrate symbolic equivalents of the perceived meaning of student communication efforts. In addition, teachers and teams are taught to track the development of student communication behaviors from pre-intentional to intentional and conventional use. This is accomplished using the Communication

Matrix (Rowland, 2004, 2011) at least two times each year and more often when the team does not have other evidence of development on a day-to-day basis.

Aided Language Input

All students benefit from models of effective language use (McLean & McLean, 1999). In fact, according to studies of statistical learning, language input is more valuable than expressive practice for both supporting a student's development of internal representations needed for generalization, as well as improving expressive language use (Plante & Gómez, 2018). For students with SCD learning to communicate using aided AAC, models should be provided using forms of communication that are consistent with those the student is learning to use to express novel messages (von Tetzchner, 2015) because spoken models alone do not serve as examples of how and what a student can say using graphic symbols. Communication partners need to both understand the multiple ways a student is currently communicating and be able to demonstrate effective communication using appropriate AAC systems (Shire & Jones, 2014).

There is a strong evidence-base supporting the benefits of demonstrating symbol use during natural communication interactions through aided language input, which builds receptive understanding and expressive use of symbolic language (e.g., O'Neil, Light, & Pope, 2018; Sennott et al., 2016). Whether relevant techniques are described by other names, such as the system for augmenting language (Romski & Sevcik, 1993), aided language stimulation (Brady, Thiemann-Bourque, Fleming, & Mathews, 2013), natural aided language

(Cafiero, 2001), or aided language modeling (Drager et al., 2006), aided language input practices have been found to increase student understanding and use of graphic symbols. Numerous studies have supported gains for beginning communicators in expressive vocabulary (e.g., Drager et al., 2006), receptive vocabulary (e.g., Romski et al., 2010), and turn-taking (e.g., Binger, Kent-Walsh, Ewing, & Taylor, 2010; Romski et al., 2010). Without aided language input, students who use aided AAC systems hear spoken language or see sign language, but have no opportunity to experience others communicating in ways they can use to interact in the turn-taking process of communication.

Providing aided language input is an interconnected process that involves a communication partner: (a) attributing meaning and honoring all efforts to communicate; (b) pointing to graphic symbols on an AAC system while speaking; (c) inviting students to initiate or respond while providing sufficient time for them to do so; and (d) expanding on student attempts using more conventional forms (e.g., "I see you smiling. Do you *like* it?" Or, "You pointed to *DIFFERENT*. Does that *LOOK DIFFERENT?*"). AAC systems used for providing aided language input should be the same or similar to the student's personal AAC system. There is general agreement that simplifying language while preserving grammatical structure improves accessibility (Clendon & Anderson, 2016); and the use of comments versus questions is highly recommended to maximize input without requiring output or expression on the part of the child (Smith et al., 2016).

The potential of aided language input practices is clear. They can improve the communication abilities of students with

SCD and complex communication needs and research supports that with training and support, teachers, and other classroom staff can implement these practices effectively (Clendon & Anderson, 2016; Kent-Walsh, Murza, Malani, & Binger, 2015).

Teaching in Natural Environments

An important element of supporting communication development is ensuring that there are meaningful reasons to communicate. The Project Core implementation model builds on the fact that schools are designed to engage students meaningfully throughout the school day. Further, it builds on a definition of naturalistic teaching that focuses on interventions that occur during daily routine activities and capitalize on students' preferred interests, needs, and abilities as expressed in the moment (Pindiprolu, 2012). Rather than creating specific times for communication intervention, teachers incorporate the strategies throughout the school day and target communication during naturally occurring routines and interactions, such as morning arrival, mealtime, play and leisure activities, and personal care, as well as academic instructional routines. This approach is especially effective for students with the most restricted vocabulary knowledge and expressive communication skills (Yoder, Kaiser, & Alpert, 1991) including those with SCD and complex communication needs (Romski & Sevcik, 1996). Naturalistic teaching is featured in Project Core as it encourages generalization of communication across contexts and communication partners (Cowan & Allen, 2007; Woods, Kashinath, & Goldstein, 2004).

A System of Professional Development and Coaching

Ensuring that the instructional practices discussed above occur in classrooms with regularity and fidelity requires professional development. The field of AAC has long recognized the importance of communication partner training, with many studies reporting successful implementation of targeted intervention practices by communication partners with little to no aided AAC expertise prior to training (Kent-Walsh et al., 2015; Senner & Baud, 2017). Studies support parents, SLPs, teachers, teaching assistants, and peers as successful facilitators who can provide effective communication instruction (Clendon & Anderson, 2016).

Widely held principles of effective professional development include the importance of: (a) alignment of professional development with teachers' goals and needs, as well as school and national standards, often referred to as "coherence"; (b) content focus, considering both content area knowledge and general teaching principles; and (c) active learning situated in classroom contexts (Desimone, 2009; Leko & Brownell, 2009). The importance of active learning strategies to fully engage professionals in the process and provide opportunities to practice new skills in supported contexts is well established (e.g., Binger & Kent-Walsh, 2012; Showers & Joyce, 1996). Engaging teachers and classroom staff in active learning typically includes strategy instruction, opportunities to observe others demonstrating the strategies, using the skills as others observe, receiving feedback and participating in discussion and reflection on teaching practices (Desimone, 2009). Instructional coaches can play an important role in the active learning process by collaborating with teachers to support their implementation of new strategies and encourage self-reflection regarding classroom practices (Knight, 2009).

In Project Core, this professional development is packaged in a series of modules for self-directed or facilitated use. The interactive modules (Table 10–3) deliver key content and employ activities and interaction or self-reflection to support application and use. Coaches or facilitators are supported with step-by-step facilitator guides and video-based content delivery. In both formats, teachers are encouraged to get started using the Universal Core vocabulary from the

first module, with the expectation that they can refine and improve their implementation of key practices as they work through the remaining modules.

As teachers and related classroom staff begin using the Universal Core vocabulary and complete the professional development modules, coaches (often SLPs) support teachers in reflecting on their practice using a series of self-reflection and observation guides. The items on the General Self-Reflection and Observation Guide are listed in Table 10–4. The complete guide, as well as guides that apply to specific instructional routines, are also available on the project website (http://www.project-core.com/instructional-planning-and-reflection/).

Table 10–3. Project Core Professional Development Modules (http://project-core.com/professional-development-modules/)

Module Title and Recommended Order	Description
1. Project Core Overview	This module provides an overview of the development of the Project Core implementation model with an emphasis on classroom teachers and staff.
2. Universal Core Vocabulary	This module provides an introduction to the Universal Core vocabulary, the various formats available for free download, and examples of the flexibility offered for teaching and learning the use of the Universal Core vocabulary across natural contexts.
3. Beginning Communicators	This module provides an introduction to the many ways that beginning communicators express themselves, and it describes strategies for identifying and honoring all early forms of communication, while making meaningful connections to symbols in the Universal Core vocabulary.
4. Aided Language Input	This module provides an overview of how to use aided language input strategies to show students what is possible and encourage their use of graphic symbols.
5. Supporting Individual Access to the Universal Core	This module focuses on access considerations for students with SCD and a range of physical, sensory, and cognitive needs, It then provides an overview of tools available for identifying suitable Universal Core vocabulary formats.

Table 10–3. *continued*

Module Title and Recommended Order	Description
6. Teaching Communication During Daily Routines and Activities	This module provides an overview and case examples illustrating how to teach the Universal Core vocabulary during common routines across the school day (e.g., arrival/departure, meals, transitions).
7. Teaching Communication During Academic Instruction	This module provides an overview and case examples illustrating how to support interaction and teach communication during common academic routines across the school day.
8. Shared Reading	This module provides an overview and case examples illustrating how to teach communication during shared reading lessons.
9. Predictable Chart Writing	This module provides an overview and case examples illustrating strategies for teaching communication during predictable chart writing lessons.
10. Alphabet Knowledge and Phonological Awareness	This module provides an overview and case examples illustrating strategies for teaching communication while teaching lessons focused on alphabet knowledge and phonological awareness.
11. Independent Reading	This module provides an overview and case examples illustrating how to teach communication while students engage in independent reading and exploration of books.
12. Independent Writing	This module provides an overview and case examples illustrating how to teach communication while students engage in independent writing using the alphabet.

Table 10–4. Project Core General Self-Reflection and Observation Guide

Evidence	Consistently	Occasionally	Never	Comments & Examples
ALL students have access to their own personal communication system with core vocabulary.				
Adults recognize and respond to each student's efforts to communicate. *Example: Adult sees a student reaching for something and provides access to it.*				

continues

Table 10–4. *continued*

Evidence	Consistently	Occasionally	Never	Comments & Examples
Adults tell students very clearly what they did to communicate. *Example: Adult says, "I see you reaching. You want that."*				
Adults show students how to communicate using symbols. *Example: Adult points to the symbol for want while saying, "You could tell me, want."*				
Adults show students how to use core vocabulary using each student's personal communication system (or a system that is very similar).				
Adults encourage students to communicate in any way they can.				
Adults invite students to use their core vocabulary system, without requiring use. *Example: Adult says, "tell me" and gestures to the student's communication system.*				
Adults provide wait time for students to initiate and respond.				
Adults use strategies other than physical support (e.g., hand-over-hand) to encourage student communication.				

The intent of the self-reflection and observation forms is to support teachers in working toward the consistent implementation of the evidence-based practices that compose Project Core.

Observing and Documenting Communication Development

Although teachers work to reflect on their practices, and coaches observe and support their efforts, the adults work together to observe and document student progress. The primary tool to accomplish this is the Communication Matrix (Rowland, 2004, 2011; http://communicationmatrix .org). The Communication Matrix is a direct observational tool or behavioral inventory used to measure early communication behaviors, including those that occur before students begin to demonstrate symbolic communication understanding and use. The Communication Matrix includes a set of 24 yes/no questions that are dispersed across four major communication purposes (refuse, obtain, interact socially, and provide or seek information). Each yes response is then further defined using nine categories of communication behaviors (body movements, early sounds, facial expressions, visual behaviors, simple gestures, conventional gestures and vocalizations, concrete symbols, abstract symbols, and language) that occur at seven levels of communication complexity (pre-intentional behavior, intentional behavior, unconventional communication, conventional communication, concrete symbols, abstract symbols, and language). The Communication Matrix was originally designed for parents, which means that teachers and teams with little background knowledge regarding early communication can successfully use the tool.

In addition to the Communication Matrix, teachers and teams are encouraged to track the frequency of student initiations using the Universal Core vocabulary and other conventional means of communication including gestures, vocalizations, and concrete symbols. The goal with Project Core is to improve communication across all forms, not just through the use of the Universal Core vocabulary.

■ Hillside Developmental Center: A Project Core Development Site

The Hillside Developmental Center was an important partner in the development of Project Core. Like many students with SCD, most students at Hillside Developmental Center struggle to meet their communication needs. In fact, many do not have any symbolic communication skills. Students at Hillside are educated in classrooms of 5 to 8 students in grade-level bands at the elementary ($n = 4$), middle ($n = 2$), and high school levels ($n = 4$). Each classroom has a teacher, a full-time assistant, and access to a floating assistant to support personal care needs. A team of three full-time SLPs provides direct and indirect services to students throughout the school. Other full-time (i.e., physical therapy, occupational therapy, nursing) and itinerant (i.e., teacher of the deaf and hard of hearing, teacher of the blind and visually impaired) related service professionals provide services as dictated by student Individualized Education Programs (IEPs).

Nine of the ten teachers and about half of the students in the school-aged program (i.e., grades K–12) participated in Project Core, the symbolic communication implementation model described in this chapter. The 39 student participants were 5 to 21 years of age and eligible for special education under a range of IDEA categories (Table 10–5).

All of the students had complex communication needs and little, if any, symbolic communication skills as indicated by an overall average level of communication below five (uses concrete symbols) on the seven-point communication complexity scale that is part of the Communication Matrix (Rowland, 2011; Table 10–6). The SLPs had been working diligently to implement a variety of communication interventions and supports, but there was limited carry over in the classroom. In spite of this history of limited carry-over, the teachers throughout the school recognized the need to improve their students' communication skills and eagerly consented to participate in the project when asked.

Through two years of participation, teachers, teaching assistants, SLPs, and other faculty (e.g., physical education teacher, art teacher) at Hillside Developmental Center completed early versions of the professional development modules that are now available on the project website (Table 10–7). The SLPs continued to provide direct and indirect speech and language services, but they placed a greater emphasis on supporting

Table 10–5. Student Demographics (*n* = 39)

Race	White	17 (44%)
	Black	12 (31%)
	Hispanic	4 (10%)
	Asian	4 (10%)
	Multiracial	1 (3%)
	American Indian or Alaskan Native	1 (3%)
Gender	Male	26 (67%)
	Female	13 (33%)
IDEA Eligibility	Multiple Disabilities	20 (51%)
	Intellectual Disability	11 (28%)
	Development Disability	7 (18%)
	Other Health Impairment	1 (3%)
Grade band	K–5	16 (41%)
	6–8	7 (18%)
	9–12	16 (41%)

Table 10–6. Communication Matrix (Rowland, 2004, 2011) Profiles at Pretest (*n* = 39)

	Fall Year 1
Average Level of Communication Complexity	
Refuse	2.72
Obtain	2.85
Social	2.28
Overall Highest Level of Communication Across Purposes	3.72
Total Number of Students Able to Provide or Seek Information*	9 (23%)
Total Number of Students With Symbolic Communication for Any Purpose	11 (28%)

*Note: This scale on the Communication Matrix requires communication at Level IV (Conventional Communication) or higher.

use of the Universal Core vocabulary in the classroom.

The students who were able to point to the symbols on the 36-location Universal Core vocabulary display had fairly consistent access to their own copy of the display from early in the project. Teams had more difficulty providing access to students who needed other formats of the Universal Core vocabulary (i.e., partner-assisted scanning or eye-pointing), but across classrooms, teachers, and other classroom staff began looking for and attributing meaning to all behaviors that could have communicative intent. Most adults also started demonstrating the use of at least some symbols from the Universal Core vocabulary by pointing to or showing students symbols that matched their spoken words. At the end of the first year of implementing Project Core, the school as a whole was implementing the evidence-based practices imperfectly, but they were moving in the right direction.

As one teacher said, "It [core vocabulary] just flows with the whole day now. It isn't like I will use it now and not use it now . . . I use it all the time." More importantly, students were communicating in more sophisticated ways, across multiple purposes, as demonstrated via the Communication Matrix (Table 10–8).

In the following year, the school continued to participate in Project Core and the emphasis during professional development sessions focused on helping teams integrate communication intervention across the school day, during instructional and noninstructional routines. There was a particular focus on helping adults learn to use aided language input for purposes other than directing student behavior. Specifically, adults throughout the school had picked up the habit of

Table 10–7. Topics Addressed During Professional Development Sessions

Session	Topic(s) Covered	Current Online Modules That Address the Content
1	• Overview of participatory action research and development project • Overview of teaching principles: aided language input, core vocabulary, naturalistic teaching	Module 1: Project Core Overview
2	• Early forms of communication • The Communication Matrix • Importance of personal access to an AAC system with core vocabulary • Aided language input • Universal Core vocabulary formats • Example lesson incorporating Universal Core vocabulary into literacy instruction	Module 3: Beginning Communicators Module 4: Aided Language Input Module 5: Supporting Individual Access to the Universal Core
3	• Review of Universal Core vocabulary formats and importance of all students having personal access to an AAC system • Example lessons incorporating Universal Core vocabulary into common activities, including: art, mealtime, and reading	Module 2: Universal Core Vocabulary

4	• Incorporating the Universal Core vocabulary into literacy instruction
	  ▫ Shared reading
	  ▫ Predictable chart writing
		Module 7: Teaching Communication During Academic Instruction

5	• Review of participatory action research and development goals • Facilitated exchange of examples of specific ways teachers used the Universal Core vocabulary in their classrooms	Module 1: Project Core Overview
6	• Use of core vocabulary during daily routines (teaching assistants and preschool teachers only)	Module 6: Teaching Communication During Daily Activities and Routines
7	• Attributing meaning • Encouraging versus requiring communication • Modeling communication versus managing behaviors • Ways to support communication of yes and no • Partner-assisted scanning	Module 3: Beginning Communicators Module 4: Aided Language Input Module 5: Supporting Individual Access to the Universal Core

Table 10–7. *continued*

Session	Topic(s) Covered	*Current Online Modules That Address the Content*
8	▪ Incorporating the Universal Core vocabulary into literacy instruction ▫ Shared reading ▫ Predictable chart writing ▫ Independent writing	Module 8: Shared Reading Module 9: Predictable Chart Writing Module 12: Independent Writing

Table 10–8. Communication Matrix Profiles at the Beginning and End of Year 1 (*n* = 39)

	Fall Year 1	*Spring Year 1*
Average Level of Communication Complexity*		
Refuse	2.72	3.28
Obtain	2.85	3.79
Social	2.28	3.44
Overall Highest Level of Communication Across Purposes	3.72	4.56
Total Number of Students Able to Provide or Seek Information**	9 (23%)	16 (41%)
Total Number of Students With Symbolic Communication for Any Purpose	11 (28%)	22 (56%)

*Maximum score is 7.
**Must have conventional communication (level 4 or higher) on the Communication Matrix.

pointing to symbols on the Universal Core vocabulary to direct and correct student behaviors, supplementing their verbal reprimands for messages such as *"STOP" or "DO NOT"* with the use of graphic symbols. This habit devalued the Universal Core vocabulary as a student's tool for personal expression. There was also an emphasis on helping adults use aided language input with the personal versions of the Universal Core vocabulary provided for each student rather than using single symbols pulled from a classroom display. Specifically, classroom teachers had begun to remove individual symbols that were attached with Velcro to a poster-sized version of the 36-location Universal Core vocabulary. They would hold up just one or two symbols rather than drawing student attention to the symbols in the location where they exist on their system. Observing these applications was important as it helped the team identify ways to help adults implement practices with higher levels of fidelity. It also guided the development of implementation supports that discouraged the use of communication boards with individual symbols attached with Velcro. Instead, adults were taught to provide aided language input by pointing to symbols in their permanent location on the Universal Core vocabulary displays that matched students' personal systems. It also led to revisions of professional development modules to ensure they explicitly described the need to demonstrate the use of the Universal Core vocabulary as a means of personal expression for students rather than behavioral control.

As adults continued to improve their ability to attribute meaning and honor all forms of communication, use aided language input, and teach symbolic communication in naturally occurring routines throughout the school day, students had increased access to personal versions of the Universal Core vocabulary. They also continued to make progress in their overall level of symbolic communication across purposes. A total of 33 of the original 39 students were still at the school at the end of two years of participation. These students were slightly below the average for the original group of 39 at the beginning of the project, but were slightly above the group of 39 at the end of year one and continued to make growth through year two (Table 10–9).

Hillside Developmental Center continues to work to ensure that all students have successful access to classroom-based symbolic communication instruction. One important indicator of the generalized impact of this focus has been the school's performance on the state's required end-of-grade test in English language arts. All of the students participate in the state's alternate assessment based on alternate achievement standards because of their significant cognitive disabilities. They are required to complete the assessment in English language arts in grades 3 through 8 and again in grade 10. From the begin-

Table 10–9. Communication Matrix Profiles Across Two Years (*n* = 33)

	Fall Year 1	Spring Year 1	Spring Year 2
Average Level of Communication Complexity			
Refuse	2.64	3.33	3.33
Obtain	2.88	3.82	4.48
Social	2.15	3.42	3.48
Overall Highest Level of Communication Across Purposes	3.73	4.58	4.88
Total number of students able to Provide or Seek Information*	7 (21%)	13 (39%)	15 (45%)
Total Number of Students with Symbolic Communication for Any Purpose	10 (30%)	18 (55%)	21 (64%)

*Must have conventional communication (level 4 or higher) on the Communication Matrix.

ning of the project, the principal at Hillside attached little importance to this test because he knew that his students lacked the symbolic skills required to receive and give information on any type of performance-based assessment. More than once he said, "We don't pay much attention because it doesn't tell us much." But his view changed as the students improved their symbolic communication and their performance on the state assessment improved markedly.

In the spring prior to participating in Project Core, 94.1% of the students with SCD who completed the state assessment performed at the lowest possible level. On the four-point scale reported by the state, no students performed at levels 3 or 4, the two levels deemed to indicate "proficiency." After one year of participation in Project Core, during which no specific attention was given to the state standards or preparation for the alternate assessment, 58.3% of the students performed at the lowest level, and 12.5% performed at level 3. The trend continued after a second year of participation with only 44.4% performing at the lowest level. As displayed in Table 10–10, the emphasis on symbolic communication development through Project Core not only improved the targeted communication skills but also led to generalized improvements in academic performance as measured by the state's end-of-grade test in reading.

■ Moving Toward More Robust Solutions

It is the intent of the Project Core implementation model to increase student symbolic communication skills in a way that supports their initial learning and grows with them as they begin to communicate in increasingly complex ways across purposes, partners, and contexts. The Universal Core vocabulary provides a freely available (i.e., open-source), flexible set of words to start this journey. As students begin using the Universal Core vocabulary to initiate and respond, teams are encouraged to move toward more robust communication solutions. In Project Core, this is accomplished through partnerships with the developers and distributors of speech generating devices and apps. A variety of developers and distributors have created supports to help students and teams move from the available open-source Universal Core vocabulary formats to innovative Universal Core vocabulary designs for their systems. These supports

Table 10–10. Performance on the State Alternate Assessment Based on Alternate Achievement Standards in English Language Arts (Reading) Across Three Years

	Level 1	*Level 2*	*Level 3*	*Level 4*	*Proficient*
Year Prior to Participating in Project Core	94.1%	5.9%			
End of Year 1	58.3%	29.2%	12.5%		12.5%
End of Year 2	44.4%	40.0%	12.0%	3.6%	15.6%

range from documents that describe where the Universal Core vocabulary is located in various apps and SGDs to specific sets of dynamic pages that feature the Universal Core vocabulary. These solutions are available on the Project Core website (http://www.project-core.com/app-and-sgd-product-keys/).

Regardless of which app or SGD a student uses, students in classrooms implementing Project Core should have access to at least the 36 words included in the Universal Core vocabulary. Many communication apps and SGDs offer these core words as part of their robust vocabulary options, but the organization of the vocabulary varies across systems. As such, a simple key to support access to the Universal Core vocabulary across devices is available for download from the Project Core website (http://www.project-core.com/key). When a word is not available or the organization does not support efficient access to each word, teams are encouraged to add the word(s) or revise the organization to make the 36 Universal Core vocabulary words more readily available.

■ A Charge to Raise the Floor With a Universal Solution for All

Too many students with SCD and complex communication needs do not have access to aided AAC (Erickson & Geist, 2016), or the speech and language services they require to learn to use aided AAC (ASHA, 2018). This chapter describes an implementation model, Project Core, that was designed to address this challenge. The model provides classroom teachers and teams with the materials, professional development, assessment, self-reflection, and coaching the supports they need to successfully teach symbolic communication to their students with SCD and complex communication needs. Helping classroom teachers focus on communication instruction throughout the school day dramatically increases opportunities for learning among a group of students who find it challenging to learn (Kleinert et al., 2009; Nash et al., 2015). Teacher-mediated intervention does not diminish the important role of SLPs. Rather, it serves to maximize SLPs' positive impact on communication development by reducing the time they spend reviewing basic evidence-based approaches with teachers and teams and increasing the time they have to focus on improving or refining the practices and working directly with students.

Individual teachers, teams, schools, and school systems that choose to implement Project Core will find a full array of resources and supports, including manuals for coaches and administrators that lay out all of the components of the model across a school year. All of the components of the implementation model are open source, which means SLPs and others can use them as they would like to support their colleagues in their efforts to support early symbolic communication development for students with SCD and complex communication needs. As a complete package, Project Core provides everything that is needed to universally provide access to early symbolic communication instruction and dramatically increase the number of students with SCD and complex communication needs who have access to a flexible means of symbolic communication.

Acknowledgments. This document was produced in part under U.S. Department of Education, Office of Special Education Programs Grant No. H327S140017.

The views expressed herein do not necessarily represent the positions or policies of the Department of Education. No official endorsement by the U.S. Department of Education of any product, commodity, service, or enterprise mentioned in this publication is intended or should be inferred. Project Officer, Terry Jackson.

■ References

Adamson, L., Romski, M. A., Deffebach, K., & Sevcik, R. (1992). Symbol vocabulary and the focus of conversations: Augmenting language development for youth with mental retardation. *Journal of Speech and Hearing Research, 35,* 1333–1343. https://doi.org/10.1044/jshr.3506.1333

American Association of Intellectual and Developmental Disabilities. (2017). *Definition of intellectual disability.* Retrieved from http://aaidd.org/intellectual-disability/definition#.WdpE5ROPKYU

American Speech-Language-Hearing Association. (2018). *2018 Schools survey. Survey summary report: Numbers and types of responses, SLPs.* Retrieved from https://www.asha.org/uploadedFiles/2018-Schools-Survey-Summary-Report.pdf

Balandin, S., & Iacono, T. (1998). Crews, wusses, and whoppas: Core and fringe vocabularies of Australian meal-break conversations in the workplace. *Augmentative and Alternative Communication, 15,* 95–109. https://doi.org/10.1080/07434619912331278605

Banajee, M., Dicarlo, C., & Stricklin, S. B. (2003). Core vocabulary determination for toddlers. *Augmentative and Alternative Communication, 19,* 67–73. https://doi.org/10.1080/0743461031000112034

Beukelman, D. R., Jones, R. S., & Rowan, M. (1989). Frequency of word usage by nondisabled peers in integrated preschool classrooms. *Augmentative and Alternative Communication, 5,* 243–248. https://doi.org/10.1080/07434618912331275296

Beukelman, D. R., McGinnis, J., & Morrow, D. (1991). Vocabulary selection in augmentative and alternative communication. *Augmentative and Alternative Communication, 7,* 171–185. https://doi.org/10.1080/07434619112331275883

Beukelman, D. R., & Mirenda, P. (2013). *Augmentative and alternative communication: Supporting children & adults with complex communication needs* (4th ed.). Brookes.

Beukelman, D. R., Yorkston, K. M., Poblete, M., & Naranjo, C. (1984). Frequency of word occurrence in communication samples produced by adult communication aid users. *Journal of Speech and Hearing Disorders, 49,* 360–367. https://doi.org/10.1044/jshd.4904.360

Binger, C., & Kent-Walsh, J. (2012). Selecting skills to teach communication partners: Where do I start? *Perspectives on Augmentative and Alternative Communication, 21*(4), 127–135. https://doi.org/10.1044/aac21.4.127

Binger, C., Kent-Walsh, J., Ewing, C., & Taylor, S. (2010). Teaching educational assistants to facilitate the multisymbol message productions of young students who require augmentative and alternative communication. *American Journal of Speech-Language Pathology, 19,* 108–120. https://doi.org/10.1044/1058-0360(2009/09-0015

Boenisch, J., & Soto, G. (2015). The oral core vocabulary of typically developing English-speaking school-aged children: Implications for AAC practice. *Augmentative and Alternative Communication, 31,* 77–84. https://doi.org/10.3109/07434618.2014.1001521

Brandel, J., & Loeb, D. (2011). Program intensity and service delivery models in schools: SLP survey results. *Language, Speech, and Hearing Services in Schools, 42,* 461–490. https://doi.org/10.1044/0161-1461(2011/10-0019

Brady, N. C., Thiemann-Bourque, K., Fleming K., & Mathews, K. (2013). Predicting language outcomes for children learning augmentative and alternative communication: Child and environmental factors. *Journal of Speech, Language, and Hearing Research, 56,* 1595–1612. https://doi.org/10.1044/1092-4388

Cafiero, J. M. (2001). The effect of an augmentative communication intervention on the communication, behavior, and academic program of an adolescent with autism. *Focus on Autism and Other Developmental Disabilities, 16,* 179–189. https://doi.org/10.1177/108835760101600306

Cameto, R., Bergland, F., Knokey, A.-M., Nagle, K. M., Sanford, C., Kalb, S. C., . . . Ortega, M., & National Center for Special Education Research (ED). (2010). *Teacher perspectives of school-level implementation of alternate assessments for students with significant cognitive disabilities.* A Report from the National Study on Alternate Assessments [NCSER 2010-3007]. https://doi.org/10.1037/e599852011-001

Center for Medicare and Medicaid Services. (2017). *Local coverage determination (LCD): Speech generating devices (SGD).* Retrieved from https://www.cms.gov/medicare-coverage-database

Clendon, S. A., & Anderson, K. (2016). Syntax and morphology in aided language development. In M. Smith, & J. Murray (Eds.) *The silent partner? Language, interaction, and aided communication* (pp. 119–140). J & R Press

Clendon, S. A., & Erickson, K. (2008). The vocabulary of beginning writers: Implications for children with complex communication needs. *Augmentative and Alternative Communication, 24,* 281–293. https://doi.org/0.1080/07434610802463999

Copeland, S. R., Keefe, E. B., Calhoon, A. J., Tanner, W., & Park, S. (2011). Preparing teachers to provide literacy instruction to all students: Faculty experiences and perceptions. *Research and Practice for Persons with Severe Disabilities, 36,* 126–141. https://doi.org/10.2511/027494481180082449

Costigan, A., & Light, J. (2010). A review of preservice training in augmentative and alternative communication for speech-language pathologists, special education teachers, and occupational therapists. *Assistive Technology, 22,* 200–212. https://doi.org/10.1080/10400435.2010.492774

Cowan, R. J. & Allen, K. D. (2007). Using naturalistic procedures to enhance learning in individuals with autism: A focus on generalized teaching within the school setting. *Psychology in the Schools, 44*(7), 701–715. https://doi.org/10.1002/pits.20259

Cress, C. J., Arens, K. B., & Zajicek, A. K. (2007). Comparison of engagement patterns of young children with developmental disabilities between structured and free play. *Education and Training in Developmental Disabilities, 42*(2), 152–164. https://www.jstor.org/journal/eductraidevedisa

Cross, R., Erickson, K., Geist, L., & Hatch, P. (in press). Vocabulary selection. In L. Lloyd & D. Fuller (Eds.), *Principles and practices in augmentative and alternative communication.* Slack Publishing.

Deckers, S. R. J. M., Van Zaalen, Y., Van Balkom, H., & Verhoeven, L. (2017). Core vocabulary of young children with Down syndrome. *Augmentative and Alternative Communication, 33,* 77–86, https://doi.org/10.1080/07434618.2017.1293730

Desimone, L. (2009). Improving impact studies of teachers' professional development: Toward better conceptualizations and measures. *Educational Researcher, 38,* 181–199. https://doi.org/10.3102/0013189X08331140

Dodd, J. L., & Gorey, M. (2013). AAC intervention as an immersion model. *Communication Disorders Quarterly, 35,* 103–107. https://doi.org/10.1177/1525740113504242

Dolch, E. W. (1955). *Methods in Reading.* Garrard Press.

Drager, K., Postal, V., Carrolus, L., Castellano, M., Gagliano, C., & Glynn, J., (2006). The effect of aided language modeling on symbol comprehension and production in two preschoolers with autism. *American Journal of Speech-language Pathology, 15,* 112–125. https://doi.org/10.1044/1058-0360(2006/012)

Dynamic Learning Maps Consortium. (2016). *2014–2015 Technical manual. Integrated model.* Lawrence, KS: University of Kansas, Center for Educational Testing and Evaluation. Retrieved from http://dynamiclearning maps.org/sites/default/files/documents/publication/Technical_Manual_IM_2014-15.pdf

Erickson, K., & Geist, L. (2016). The profiles of students with significant cognitive disabilities and complex communication needs. *Augmentative and Alternative Communication, 32,* 187–197. https://doi.org/10.1080/07434618.2016.1213312

Erickson, K., & Koppenhaver, D. (2020). *Comprehensive literacy for all: Teaching students with significant disabilities to read and write.* Brookes.

Fixsen, D., Blasé, K., Metz, A., & Van Dyke, M. (2013). Statewide implementation of evidence-based programs. *Council for Exceptional Children, 79,* 213–230. https://doi.org/10.1177/001440291307900206

Frost, L., & Bondy, A. (2002). *The Picture Exchange Communication System training manual* (2nd ed.). Pyramid Educational Products.

Ganz, J., Earles-Vollrath, T., Heath, A., Parker, R., Rispoli, M., & Duran, J. (2012). A meta-analysis of single case research studies on aided augmentative and alternative communication systems with individuals with autism spectrum disorder. *Journal of Autism Developmental Disorder, 42,* 60–74. https://doi.org/10.1007/s10803-011-1212-2

Holyfield, C., Drager, K., Kremkow, J., & Light, J. (2017). Systematic review of AAC intervention research for adolescents and adults with autism spectrum disorder. *Augmentative and Alternative Communication, 33,* 201–212. https://doi.org/10.1080/07434618.2017.1370495

Kent-Walsh, J., Murza, K., Malani, M., & Binger, C. (2015). Effects of communication partner instruction on the communication of individuals using AAC: A meta-analysis. *Augmentative and Alternative Communication, 31,* 271–284. https://doi.org/10.3109/07434618.2015.1052153

Kleinert, H. L., Browder, D. M., & Towles-Reeves, E. A. (2009). Models of cognition for students with significant cognitive disabilities: Implications for assessment. *Review of Educational Research, 79,* 301–326. https://doi.org/10.3102/0034654308326160

Knight, J. (2009). Instructional coaching. In J. Knight (Ed.), *Coaching: Approaches and perspectives.* Corwin Press.

Leko, M., & Brownell, M. (2009). Crafting quality professional development for special educators: What school leaders should know. *Teaching Exceptional Children, 42,* 64–70. https://doi.org/10.1177/004005990904200106

Light, J. (2016). *Designing effective AAC systems for young children with complex communication needs to support communication development.* Paper presented at the Biennial meeting of the International Society for Augmentative and Alternative Communication, Toronto, Canada. Retrieved from https://rerc-aac.psu.edu/wp-content/uploads/2016/08/ISAAC-2016-Designing-AAC-systems-HO-B_W1.pdf

Light, J., Wilkinson, K., Thiessen, A., Beukelman, D., & Fager, S. (2019). Designing effective AAC displays for individuals with developmental or acquired disabilities: State of the science and future research directions, *Augmentative and Alternative Communication, 35*(1), 42-55. https://doi.org/10.1080/07434618.2018.1558283

Marvin, C. A., Beukelman, D. R., & Bilyeu, D. (1994). Vocabulary-use patterns in preschool children: Effects of context and time sampling. *Augmentative and Alternative Communication, 10,* 224–236. https://doi.org/10.1080/07434619412331276930

McLean, J., & McLean, L. (1999). *How children learn language: A guide for professionals in early childhood and special education.* Singular Publishing.

Nash, B., Clark, A. K., & Karvonen, M. (2015). *First contact: A census report on the characteristics of students eligible to take alternate assessments* (Technical Report No. 15–02). University of Kansas, Center for Educational Testing and Evaluation.

National Center for Education Statistics. (2019). *Back to school basics.* Washington, DC. Retrieved from https://nces.ed.gov/fastfacts/display.asp?id=372#PK12_enrollment

North Carolina State Board of Education. (2014). *Policies governing services for children with disabilities.* Retrieved from http://ec.ncpublicschools.gov/policies/nc-policies-governing-services-for-children-with-disabilities/policies-children-disabilities.pdf

Office of Special Education Programs. (2005). *Alternate assessment standards for students with the most significant cognitive disabilities: Non-regulatory guidance.* U.S. Department of Education. Retrieved from https://www2.ed.gov/policy/elsec/guid/altguidance.doc

Olswang, L. B., & Prelock, P. A. (2015). Bridging the gap between research and practice: Implementation science. *Journal of Speech, Language, and Hearing Research, 58*(6), S1818–S1826. https://doi.org/10.1044/2015_JSLHR-L-14-0305

O'Neill, T., Light, J., & Pope, L. (2018). Effects of intervention that include aided augmentative and alternative communication input on the communication of individuals with complex communication needs: A meta-analysis. *Journal of Speech, Language, and Hearing Research, 61*, 1743–1765. https://doi.org/10.1044/2018_JSLHR-L-17-0132

Pindiprolu, S. (2012). A review of naturalistic interventions with young children with autism. *The Journal of International Association of Special Education, 12*, 69–78. https://www.iase.org/publications.htm

Plante, E., & Gómez, R. L. (2018). Learning without trying: The clinical relevance of statistical learning. *Language, Speech, and Hearing Services in Schools, 49*, 710–722. https://doi.org10.1044/2018_LSHSS-STLT1-17-0131

Quick, N., Erickson, K., & Mccright, J. (2019). The most frequently used words: Comparing child-directed speech and young children's speech to inform vocabulary selection for aided input. *Augmentative and Alternative Communication, 35*, 120–131. https://doi.org/10.1080/07434618.2019.1576225

Reichle, J. (1997). Communication intervention with persons who have severe disabilities. *The Journal of Special Education,*

31, 110–134. https://doi.org/10.1177/002246699703100110

Romski, M. A., & Sevcik, R. A. (1993). Language comprehension: Considerations for augmentative and alternative communication. *Augmentative and Alternative Communication, 9*, 281–285. https://doi.org/10.1080/07434619312331276701

Romski, M. A., & Sevcik, R. A. (1996). *Breaking the speech barrier: Language development through augmented means.* Brookes.

Romski, M. A., & Sevcik, R. A. (2005). Augmentative communication and early intervention: Myths and realities. *Infants & Young Children, 18*, 174–185. https://doi.org/10.1097/00001163-200507000-00002

Romski, M. A., Sevcik, R. A., Adamson, L. B., Cheslock, M., Smith, A., Barker, R. M., & Bakeman, R. (2010). Randomized comparison of augmented and nonaugmented language interventions for toddlers with developmental delays and their parents. *Journal of Speech, Language, and Hearing Research, 53*, 350–364. https://doi.org/10.1044/1092-4388(2009/08-0156)

Romski, M.A., Sevcik, R. A., Barton-Hulsey, A., & Whitmore, A. S. (2015). Early intervention and AAC: What a difference 30 years makes. *Augmentative and Alternative Communication, 31*, 181–202. https://doi.org/10.3109/07434618.2015.1064163

Rowland, C. (2004, 2011). *Communication Matrix* [Assessment instrument]. Retrieved from http://communicationmatrix.org

Schlosser, R., & Lee, D. (2000) Promoting generalization and maintenance in augmentative and alternative communication: A meta-analysis of 20 years of effectiveness research. *Augmentative and Alternative Communication, 16*, 208–226. https://doi.org/10.1080/07434610012331279074

Schlosser, R. W., & Sigafoos, J. (2002). Selecting graphic symbols for an initial request lexicon: Integrative review. *Augmentative and Alternative Communication, 18*, 102–123. https://doi.org/10.1080/07434610212331281201

Senner, J., & Baud, M. (2017). The use of an eight-step instructional model to train school staff in partner-augmented input. *Communication Disorders Quarterly, 38*, 89–95. https://doi.org/10.1177/1525740116651251

Sennott, S., Light, J., & McNaughton, D. (2016). AAC modeling intervention research review. *Research and Practice for Persons with Severe Disabilities, 41*, 101–115. https://doi.org/10.1177/1540796916638822

Sevcik, R. A., Barton-Hulsey, A., Romski, M., & Fonseca, A. H. (2018). Visual-graphic symbol acquisition in school age children with developmental and language delays. *Augmentative and Alternative Communication, 34*, 265–275. https://doi.org/10.1080/07434618.2018.1522547

Shire, S., & Jones, N. (2014). Communication partners supporting children with complex communication needs who use AAC: A systematic review. *Communications Disorders Quarterly, 37*, 3–15. https://doi.org/10.1177/1525740114558254

Showers, B., & Joyce, B. (1996). The evolution of peer coaching. *Educational Leadership, 53*(6), 12–16. Retrieved from http://www.ascd.org/publications/educational-leadership/mar96/vol53/num06/The-Evolution-of-Peer-Coaching.aspx

Sigafoos, J., & Reichle, J. (1992). Comparing explicit to generalized requesting in an augmentative communication mode. *Journal of Developmental and Physical Disabilities, 4*, 167–188. https://doi.org/10.1007/BF01046398

Smith, A., Barker, R. M., Barton-Hulsey, A., Romski, M., & Sevcik, R. (2016). Augmented language interventions for children with severe disabilities. In R. A. Sevcik & M. Romski (Eds.), *Communication interventions for individuals with severe disabilities* (pp. 123–146). Brookes.

Snell, M. E., Brady, N., McLean, L., Ogletree, B. T., Siegel, E., Sylvester, L., . . . Sevcik, R. (2010). Twenty years of communication intervention research with individuals who have severe intellectual and developmental disabilities. *American Journal on Intellectual and Developmental Disabilities, 115*, 364–380. https://doi.org/10.1352/1944-7558-115-5.364

Snell, M. E., Chen, L. Y., & Hoover, K. (2006). Teaching augmentative and alternative communication to students with severe disabilities: A review of intervention research 1997–2003. *Research & Practice for Persons with Severe Disabilities, 31*, 203–214. https://doi.org/10.1177/154079690603100301

Snodgrass, M. R., Stoner, J. B., & Angell, M. E. (2013). Teaching conceptually referenced core vocabulary for initial augmentative and alternative communication. *Augmentative and Alternative Communication, 29*, 322–333. https://doi.org/10.3109/07434618.2013.848932

Stephenson, J. (2009). Iconicity in the development of picture skills: Typical development and implications for individuals with severe intellectual disabilities. *Augmentative and Alternative Communication, 23*, 187-201. https://doi.org/10.1080/07434610903031133

Thistle, J., & Wilkinson, K. M. (2009). The effects of color cues on typically developing preschoolers' speed of locating a target line drawing: Implications for AAC display design. *American Journal of Speech-Language Pathology, 18*, 231-240. https://doi.org/10.1044/1058-0360(2009/08-0029)

Thurlow, M., & Wu, Y.C. (2016). *2013-2014 APR snapshot #12: AA-AAS participation and performance.* University of Minnesota, National Center on Educational Outcomes. Retrieved from https://nceo.info/Resources/publications/APRsnapshot/brief12/index.html

Tomasello, M. (2003). *Constructing a language: A usage-based theory of language acquisition.* Harvard University Press.

Trembath, D., Balandin, S., & Togher, L. (2007). Vocabulary selection for Australian children who use augmentative and alternative communication. *Journal of Intellectual & Developmental Disability, 32*, 291–301. https://doi.org/10.1080/13668250701689298

U.S. Department of Education. (2012). *National Center for Education Statistics, Schools and Staffing Survey (SASS), "Public School Data File," 2011-2012.* Retrieved from https://nces.ed.gov/surveys/sass/tables_list.asp#2012

Van Tatenhove, G. M. (2009). Building language competence with students using AAC devices: Six challenges. *SIG 12 Perspectives on Augmentative and Alternative Communication, 18,* 38–47. https://doi.org/10.1044/aac18.2.38

van Tilborg, A., & Deckers, S. R. J. M. (2016). Vocabulary selection in AAC: Application of core vocabulary in atypical populations. *Perspectives of the ASHA Special Interest Groups SIG 12, 1,* 125–138. https://doi.org/10.1044/persp1.SIG12.125

von Tetzchner, S. (2015). The semiotics of aided language development. *Cognitive Development, 36,* 180–190. https://doi.org/ 10.10 16/j.cogdev.2015.09.009

Wilkinson, K. M., & Coombs, B. (2010). Preliminary exploration of the effect of background color on the speed and accuracy of search for an aided symbol target by typically developing preschoolers. *Early Childhood Services, 4,* 171–183. Retrieved from https://escholarship.umassmed.edu/health policy_pp/137

Wilkinson, K. M., & Snell, J. (2011). Facilitating children's ability to distinguish symbols for emotions: The effects of background color cues and spatial arrangement of symbols on accuracy and speed of search. *American Journal of Speech-Language Pathology, 20,* 288–301. https://doi.org/10.1044/ 1058-0360(2011/10-0065)

Woods, J., Kashinath, S., & Goldstein, H. (2004). Effects of embedding caregiver-implemented teaching strategies in daily routines on children's communication outcomes. *Journal of Early Intervention, 26,* 175–193. https://doi.org/10.1177/1053815 10402600302

Worah, S., McNaughton, D., Light, J., & Benedek-Wood, E. (2015). A comparison of two approaches for representing AAC vocabulary for young children. *International Journal of Speech-Language Pathology, 17,* 1–10. https://doi.org/10.3109/17549507.2014.9 87817

Yoder, P. J., Kaiser, A. P., & Alpert, C. L. (1991). An exploratory study of the interactions between language teaching methods and child characteristics. *Journal of Speech and Hearing Research, 34,* 155–167. https://doi.org/10.1044/jshr.3401.155

Yoder, P., McCathren, R., Warren, S., & Watson, A. (2001). Important distinctions in measuring maternal responses to communication in prelinguistic children with disabilities. *Communication Disorders Quarterly, 22,* 135–147. https://doi.org/10.1177/1525740 10102200303

Implementing the Visual Immersion System™ in a Classroom for Children with Autism Spectrum Disorder: Challenges and Solutions

Ralf W. Schlosser, Howard C. Shane, Anna A. Allen, Christina Yu, Amanda M. O'Brien, Jackie Cullen, Andrea Benz, Lindsay O'Neil, Laurel Chiesa, and Lisa Miori-Dinneen

Recently, the Centers for Disease Control and Prevention updated their prevalence data; now one in 54 children aged eight years meets criteria for a diagnosis of Autism Spectrum Disorder (ASD), which occurs across ethnic, racial and socioeconomic groups (Maenner et al., 2020). Children with ASD experience deficits in social communication (American Psychological Association, 2017) and some children also experience marked difficulties with, or an absence of, spoken language (Mirenda & Iacono, 2009). It is estimated that between 25% and 30% of children with ASD present with little or no functional speech even after years of intervention (Rose, Trembath, Keen, & Paynter, 2016; Tager-Flusberg & Kasari, 2013). Although often understudied, many children with ASD tend to have difficulties

with receptive language as well (Dada et al., 2020; Mechling & Hunnicutt, 2011). Finally, children with ASD may also experience difficulties with executive functioning, such as following the steps of a task or transitioning between activities and settings (e.g., Quill, 1997).

Visual supports have the potential to help alleviate difficulties with receptive language, expressive language, and executive functioning (Quill, 1997). As an umbrella term, visual supports include a variety of visuals that target a range of behavioral and language outcomes (Rutherford, Baxter, Grayson, Johnston, & O'Hare, 2019). That being said, what is considered a visual support is sometimes unclear and the boundaries of the construct are often ill-defined as documented by Rutherford and colleagues. We classify visual supports as either aided (i.e., involving something external to the body) or unaided (i.e., involving nothing but the body) in the pursuit of a variety of learner outcomes. Aided visual supports include low-tech, static two-dimensional representations (e.g., photograph, graphic symbol, paper-based activity schedule), or three-dimensional object proxies. They also include high-tech dynamic (video or animated symbols) presentations, dedicated devices (e.g., speech-generating devices [SGDs]) and repurposed general consumer-level technologies (e.g., iPad®, smartwatches). Unaided visual supports involve gestures, manual signs, fingerspelling, all of which can be produced by the learner or communication partner without any external aide.

Visual supports are generally considered efficacious and effective for individuals with ASD, as documented by various systematic reviews (Arthur-Kelly, Sigafoos, Green, Mathisen, & Arthur-Kelly, 2009; Banda & Grimmett, 2008; Bellini & Akullian, 2007; Knight, Sartini, & Spriggs, 2015; Lequia, Machalicek, & Rispoli, 2012; National Autism Center, 2015; Steinbrenner et al., 2020). Upon closer inspection, however, it is apparent that the range in type of visual supports, as well as potential outcomes in the cited reviews is not reflective of visual supports as an umbrella term. Until recently, the breadth of visual support strategies and potential outcomes had not been considered within a unifying assessment and intervention approach.

The Visual Immersion System™ (VIS™) is an assessment and intervention approach aimed at improving expressive and receptive communication and language proficiency, as well as executive functioning for individuals with moderate-to-severe ASD. The principles of the

VIS™ are contained in a clinical textbook (Shane et al., 2014). The VIS™ features three modes of instruction: the (a) Visual Instructional Mode (VIM), Visual Organizational Mode (VOM), and the Visual Expressive Mode (VEM). Within the VIM, visual supports are used in conjunction with speech or as an alternative to speech to aid comprehension. Within the VOM, visual supports are used to represent the organization of an activity, routine, script, or schedule. Finally, within the VEM, visual supports aid expressive communication by either supplementing or replacing natural speech.

The VIS™ leverages: (a) the processing strengths of individuals with ASD in the visual modality (Althaus, de Sonneville, Minderaa, Hensen, & Til, 1996; Ashwin et al., 2009; Shah & Frith, 1993; Thaut, 1987); (b) the benefits of the visual modality for learning (Mesibov, Schopler, & Hearsey, 1994); and (c) the proclivity and preference of individuals with ASD for electronic screen media (Charlop-Christy, Le, & Freeman, 2000; Shane & Albert, 2008; Shane et al., 2012; Sherer, 2000). Strategies within the VIM (e.g., video modeling, dynamic scene cues) are grounded in social learning theory (Bandura, 1997), the constructs of augmented input (e.g., Allen, Schlosser, Shane, & Brock, 2017), and alternative input (e.g., Peterson, Bondy, Vincent, & Finnegan, 1995). Augmented input supplements spoken language with visual supports to glean information, whereas alternative input allows children to bypass spoken language altogether. Strategies within the VOM offer individuals with ASD a sustained referent, whereas spoken language is ephemeral (Hogdon, 1995). Strategies within the VEM are those often associated with augmentative and alternative communication (AAC) systems and modalities such as speech-output technologies (Schlosser & Koul, 2015) and nonelectronic communication boards. The visual supports utilized in the VIS™ are created, stored, and accessed using a wide variety of tools that may be low-tech (e.g., paper-based) or high-tech (e.g., iPad, smart-speakers) in nature (Shane et al., 2012).

Instruction within the VIS™ is focused on seven operations that include six pragmatic functions, as well as instructions affecting organization/transitions. The pragmatic functions that are possibly targeted are as follows: protesting, requesting, directive-following, commenting, questions, and social pragmatics. In order to achieve acquisition, generalization, and maintenance, recipients of the VIS™ are preferably immersed in a visually rich language-learning environment

analogous to environments experienced by individuals who are deaf and hard of hearing who are learning sign language (Adamo-Villani, Carpenter, & Arns, 2006) and immersive daycare and preschools for children who are learning a second language (Cummins, 1998).

Many visual supports and instructional methods used as part of the VIS™ enjoy varying degrees of empirical support. These include animated graphic symbols, augmented input, miniature linguistic systems (aka matrix training), scene cues (i.e., line drawings, photographs, or full-motion video clips that portraying relevant concepts and their relationships in context) (Schlosser et al., 2013, p. 133), smart speakers, smartwatches, speech-output technologies, video modeling, and visual schedules (Table 11–1).

Table 11–1. Research-Based Visual Supports and Instructional Methods Used as Part of the VIS™

Visual Supports/ Instructional Method	Studies
Animated graphic symbols	Harmon et al., 2014; Schlosser, Brock, Koul, Shane, & Flynn, 2019; Schlosser et al., 2012, 2014
Augmented input	Allen, Schlosser, Brock, & Shane, 2017; Biggs, Carter, & Gilson 2018; Sennott, Light, & McNaughton, 2016
Miniature linguistic training	Nigam, Schlosser, & Lloyd, 2006
Scene cues	Dauphin, Kinney, Stromer, & Koegel 2004; Mechling & Gustafson 2008; Pierce & Schreibman 1994; Remner, Baker, Karter, Kearns, & Shane, 2016; Schlosser et al., 2013
Smartspeakers	Allen, Shane, & Schlosser, 2018; Yu et al., 2018
Smartwatches	O'Brien et al., 2016; O'Brien, Schlosser, Yu, Allen, & Shane, 2020; O'Brien et al., submitted; Schlosser et al., 2017
Speech-output technologies	Schlosser & Koul, 2015
Video modeling	Bellini & Akullian, 2007; Hong et al., 2016
Visual schedules	Knight, Sartini, & Spriggs, 2015; Watanabe & Sturmey, 2003

Until recently, the effectiveness of the VIS™ as a treatment package had not been studied. However, a recent exploratory study examined the effectiveness and social validity of a coaching-based intervention involving the VIS™ and an interdisciplinary school team supporting an elementary school classroom for children with moderate-to-severe ASD over the course of an entire school year (Schlosser et al., 2020). The study evaluated the effects a coaching intervention had on child outcomes and school team outcomes. Child outcomes pertained to one of the six communicative functions plus organization targeted by the VIS™ whereas staff outcomes related to self-efficacy in implementing the VIS™ as well as treatment acceptability by relevant stakeholders. The students improved significantly from pre- to posttest. Likewise, staff self-efficacy scores improved and the VIS™ was perceived as an acceptable treatment. Focus group results (with relevant stakeholder groups) corroborated treatment acceptability and self-efficacy data. As such, this study offers preliminary evidence for the effectiveness and social validity of this coaching-based intervention for implementing the VIS™ in a self-contained classroom serving children with ASD.

Drawing from our experiences in implementing a coaching-based intervention study involving the VIS™ in a classroom for children with ASD, as well as our collective clinical experiences in supporting children with moderate-to-severe ASD, the purpose of this chapter is to (a) identify challenges in implementation, and (b) propose solutions for these challenges. To conclude the chapter, a vignette will illustrate an actual example of how one challenge identified was addressed.

■ Challenges in Implementing the VIS™

Translated into a classroom setting, the VIS™ teaching space is replete with low- and hi-tech options that enable the efficient delivery of visual information. Although most classroom settings for students with ASD apply some level of visual supports and include some level of technology, in a VIS™-powered classroom the fundamental underpinnings of instruction requires unprecedented reliance on visual supports that are delivered by a multitude of media platforms. Accordingly, the establishment of a VIS™-powered classroom with its specific approach to instruction requires both a full understanding of its underlying principles, but also the practical obstacles posed by adopting a full complement of visual supports and various technologies.

As is the case for any assessment and treatment package with relevance to school settings, there are implementation challenges with the VIS™. For the purposes of this chapter, we selected four main challenges for further consideration: (a) recognizing the VIS™ as a language accommodation, (b) understanding how to implement the VIS™ as an overlay function, (c) how to take advantage of teachable moments, and (d) how to monitor progress.

Challenge: Recognizing the VIS™ as a Language Accommodation

What makes the VIS™ a unique approach to learning is the idea that it is not just an assortment of visual supports applied to improve temporal understanding (e.g., when invoked as a visual schedule) or used to enhance expressive communication (e.g., when summoned as an AAC tool). Instead, the VIS should be viewed as a supplementary language meant to improve overall comprehension (and expression) (Shane et al., 2014). As such, the application of the VIS™ in the classroom should give rise to a set of visual supports that clarify, for example, how a directive is to be followed, or how the day is to be organized, and so on. Perhaps the most fitting analogy is offered by Shane et al. (2014) suggesting that the systematic application of visual supports should be thought of as a language (and an accommodation) with a purpose not unlike that of sign language. In this comparison, although the student with moderate-to-severe ASD is able to hear spoken language, they generally experience deficits in the understanding of spoken language. The student who is deaf or hard-of-hearing, on the other hand, would also experience difficulty understanding if sign language, as an accommodation, was not available. In both cases the accommodation leads to improved comprehension.

The special educator described a situation in which a student was not able to tolerate a change in routine at the beginning of the project period, " . . . how he was unable to deal with change in his transition waiting for the bus that broke down." Relatedly, one of the SLPs noted "you know, sometimes there's that confusion, and we'd see some behavioral outbursts," seemingly related to a lack of predictability of events as they unfold.

Challenge: Understanding How to Implement the VIS as an Overlay Function

The VIS™ is not an academic curriculum, per se. Rather, it serves as an educational accommodation meant to clarify lessons relating to academic, daily living and life skills, classroom directives, and classroom and individual schedules. As an example, transitioning from an individual matching and sorting lesson to a group lesson in a different area of the classroom, the instructor may use static or dynamic scene cues to make the path and the destination clear rather than relying on spoken instruction alone. As a matter of technology, that visual cue might be presented by the instructor through a high-tech system (e.g., a tablet, smartwatch) or with low-tech supports (e.g., laminated paper-based symbol). Similarly, when an activity involves multiple steps, visual supports that logically define those segments are provided. These supports generally appear in the form of text, graphic symbols, photographs, or video cue (such as video models or dynamic scene cues).

The challenge to the instructor responsible for providing the necessary visual supports is twofold. First, the logical steps that define the activity must be identified, particularly within teachable moments. The second challenge pertains to the creation of the content itself. The idea of task analysis or breaking a skill into smaller, more manageable components is generally not foreign to most educators. However, the responsibility of determining how to best represent any task with suitable visual supports that enhance meaning requires an appreciation of how low- and hi-tech can be applied in a constructive and creative manner. The special educator who received coaching in our year-long classroom-based intervention described the challenge this way:

Typically, classroom teachers provide the special education teacher the specific content which is being taught in each content area. It is the job of the special education teacher to alter the lesson content so that the child with special needs gains purposeful meaning from the differentiated lesson material. . . . Modification strategies of cutting out confusing language, decreasing the amount of work, or decreasing the actual content are typically not enough to assist the student in truly learning the new concepts. . . . Teachers need to begin to see that simply cutting back expectations for the child with autism will not work in helping them to learn new concepts.

Challenge: How Do You Take Advantage of Spontaneous Teaching Opportunities?

Teachable moments may be described as opportunities that arise for student learning due to a learner's excitement and interest in a given topic (Ayers, 1989). Typically, when an educator capitalizes on a teachable moment, there is a deviation from the original outlined lesson plan so that the educator may provide additional knowledge related to an aspect of the lesson that unexpectedly captured a learner's interest. In this opportune instance, an educator has the chance to provide various exemplars or to offer novel information to further educate the learner. These teachable moments are not just confined to a classroom, but may also take place almost anywhere such as on the playground, in the cafeteria, on a field trip, or even in the hallways.

In a typical general education classroom, capitalizing on a teachable moment may involve asking additional questions or having an open discussion. In a special education classroom, particularly in a classroom supporting students with ASD, modifications may need to be made due to considerations of attention, memory, comprehension, cognitive-linguistic skills, and so forth. Many children with ASD also demonstrate difficulty comprehending auditory input (Peterson et al., 1995). Using visual supports as a learning modality not only aligns with this population's interest in electronic media, but also their visual processing strengths, as reviewed earlier. Current literature, and our clinical observations, have supported the positive impact of visuals in enhancing communication, learning, and behaviors in this population.

In many cases, capitalizing on "teachable moments," or spontaneous teaching opportunities in the special education classroom becomes difficult, whether it is due to the challenges associated with quickly accessing pre-existing materials, quickly creating new materials or adapting existing materials. One of SLPs receiving coaching provided an illustration of this challenge:

"You know, just the other day I was blowing bubbles with Student 1 and Student 2 came over and obviously had an interest and I was like oh he doesn't have a way of asking and I was like that's not good. This kid has no way of requesting that he wants to play too."

Additional challenges may include modifying the curriculum to meet the needs of individual learners within a classroom and recognizing when to capitalize on a teachable moment.

Challenge: How to Monitor Progress?

Progress monitoring in schools serving students with ASD is typically done via the Individualized Education Plan (IEP), which demands repeated evaluation of goals and objectives during a given school year. In this particular research project, our interest was in monitoring the student and (some staff) outcomes of the coaching intervention in VIS™ implementation as part of a research study. Although individual student progress was certainly of interest, we also wanted to understand whether the students as a group made improvements as a result of the intervention. Hence, the challenge was to either (a) identify a method that could address both measurement needs or (b) select two distinct methods that tackle individual and group outcomes separately but in a complementary fashion. Another consideration was to develop feasible measures for monitoring student progress (without imposing an undue burden) that could be carried out by the school team rather than the researchers. In part, this challenge stemmed from the physical distance between the school site and the researchers. Also, it was intended to create buy-in and develop ownership among the school team. Furthermore, the progress monitoring needed to yield objective information that allowed for data-based assessments as to the effectiveness of the coaching intervention. Finally, the progress monitoring method chosen needed to be able to accommodate the breadth of VIS-related outcomes.

■ Evidence-Based Solutions From Research or Practice or Well-Reasoned, Possibly More Speculative Solutions

Solutions for Recognizing the VIS™ as a Language Accommodation

The VIS™ is meant to function not merely as a sporadically applied set of symbols and other visual supports, but rather as a language accommodation applied throughout the day. This is paramount to its successful implementation within a classroom environment. In view of that, learners should be immersed in a visually symbol-rich classroom whereby spoken language instruction is supplemented by corresponding visual linguistic content (Shane & Weiss-Kapp, 2008; Shane et al., 2014)—analogous to the environments created for learners who are deaf and hard-of-hearing learners who acquire a second language (Adamo-Villani et al., 2006; Cummins, 1998). Second, such visual input is meant to support both comprehension and expression. Returning to the example of the student who found it difficult to adjust to a change in routine while transitioning to the bus, the special educator noted the following change by the end of the school year: " . . . how he was unable to deal with change in his transition waiting for the bus that broke down. He would not have been able to do that in September or even through mid-year. So, that's remarkable progress with transitioning." One of the SLP describes how the use of video modeling (that could be extended to dynamic scene cues) has helped with the earlier noted challenge of managing behavioral outbursts:

"I think it's, yeah I would say the same thing. I think there's a different state of calmness where I think a lot of the students understand, okay now I know what you mean. Now I know what I'm supposed to do. You know, sometimes there's that confusion and we'd see some behavioral outbursts and you'd show them a video, like, okay now I know what I'm supposed to do. So I think, you know, not all the time, but I think it has helped a lot in general in that area."

The special educator also noted how video modeling helped with comprehension: "Just even for them walking down the—making a video [model, added by author] of them on a good day walking from place to place and then on a bad day and going here's the video, it calms him right down and he's able to."

Third, unlike approaches where requesting is the predominant communication function (e.g., Picture Exchange Communication System; Bondy & Frost, 2001), the VIS also focuses on the additional communicative functions of protesting and refusal, directives, questions, commenting and social pragmatics.

Solutions for Implementing the VIS as an Overlay Function

The special educator offered the following solution to the earlier-noted challenge of making the curriculum accessible to students with ASD:

VIS principles are an integral component within any modified lesson because it provides the student with visual consistency and helps to promote true understanding of the material. For example if the special education teacher selects one goal from the unit about "turtles," then he/she determines how to address this goal visually so that the student can relate the topic to concepts that are directly related and meaningful to his/her own life. So it is not only important to just decrease the amount of objectives or cut out confusing information, but it is most important to decide HOW to present the information in a way that the students can visualize and make connections to the material. Creating topic displays on the student's AAC device to teach them all about turtles, all about things that are "green" and how to comment on or request green objects, all will provide a visual structure for the students. Creating static or dynamic scene cues to help the student follow directions using different kinds of turtles is an excellent way to work on following directions and learning about the various species of turtles. Building the lesson visually, instead of the old style of cutting down the lesson, is a much more effective way to help children with ASD gain concepts from the typical classroom curriculum. These children require additions not subtractions to their differentiated instruction. Using VIS strategies will promote learning and help the students generalize the concepts in meaningful ways. So, they might only learn a few selected attributes about a turtle, but they will learn how to sort green objects, comment on green objects, follow directions with different-sized turtles. They might learn how to follow a dynamic scene cue to work on walking to a different place and "Get" or "Pick up" pictures of "where" turtles live. If similar VIS principals are utilized for all classroom content that requires modifications, then the student will develop a solid ability to learn visually and this learning will only enhance the content they are able to obtain within each new unit of study. Children with ASD thrive when they are presented with material in ways so that their brains can take in the information, process it, and demonstrate the knowledge. Using the VIS as an overlay to curriculum modifications is necessary to help these students 'see' what they are learning.

It is recognized that creating visual materials for every lesson is an arduous task. That said, the outcome of such an effort will result in far more effective lessons for a visual learner. It has been the experience of teams creating visually-based lessons that building a large and functional warehouse of visual supports over time not only provides a set of materials that will greatly aid in a student's ability to derive meaning from each lesson, but will also, in due course, reduce the time needed to create suitable materials. Suggested strategies for building such a library of visual supplements include:

- Assign, create, and identify visual support materials as an essential and necessary part of Educational Assistant's (EA's) responsibilities. This statement underscores the importance of EAs as integral members of the academic team entrusted with carrying out the VIS™ in a classroom setting. In addition to supporting and utilizing the VIS™ strategies across all school environments, EAs should take on some responsibility for creating tactical videos, images, and various displays, which will reflect present and future lessons.

- Encourage parent participation (assistance). Collaborating with parents and caregivers to assist with creating videos, collecting photographs and other forms of media, and will help expand your school's VIS™ media library. In addition, their participation gives the parents a clearer understanding of the critical importance of using visual content to teach communication and language concepts to their children. For instance, a parent might create a series of static scene cues related to community and daily living activities that will both enhance the library and also entice and clarify for them how certain materials can benefit their child (e.g., brushing teeth, skiing, etc.).

- Assemble a library of symbol-based lessons over time. Each school that adopts the VIS™ approach is encouraged to assemble lessons and materials that are personalized for their students within their own settings. From the outset, the team should prepare materials and lessons that can be reused and reorganized.

Solutions for Taking Advantage of Teachable Moments

Given our knowledge of the impact that a visually-based curriculum can have on this population in enhancing communication, learning, and behaviors, we propose that visual supports can be introduced "in the moment" or "just in time" (JIT) to further enhance teachable moments. This section will focus on the use of the JIT construct and capitalizing on the visual predilection of individuals with ASD to better capitalize on teachable moments. Teachable moments arise when communication partners observe, recognize, and interpret the spontaneously occurring interactions (here, in the classroom) (Schlosser et al., 2016). The earlier quote of the SLP describing the challenge of taking advantage of teachable moments actually offers an exquisite demonstration of how a teachable moment arises, and therefore is repeated here for purposes of deconstruction: "You know, just the other day I was blowing bubbles with Student 1 and Student 2 came over [*observing*] and obviously had an interest [*recognizing & interpreting*] and I was like oh he doesn't have a way of asking and I was like that's not good [*recognizing*]." This kid has no way of requesting that he wants to play too [*interpreting*]. Now, that a teachable moment has emerged, JIT solutions become possible: "We were always checking before, what do you think of this topic display? Does it include . . . now we're just quickly making one, you know, even sometimes on the spot if the student, you know, if the need arises. So sometimes, even we went over to his iPad and added a bunch."

Although the JIT construct is a logical solution to further optimize teachable moments, the plethora of JIT-related mobile technologies can be quite overwhelming, and educators are left to determine the most appropriate JIT solution. The proliferation of technological advances has led to a fundamental shift in the availability and use of mobile technologies to support individuals with little or no functional speech (McNaughton & Light, 2013; Shane et al., 2012). The wide range of features of mobile technologies

offers educators novel capabilities to provide opportune supports to these individuals (O'Brien et al., 2017). These JIT supports can be used in a variety of ways to capitalize on "teachable moments." For instance, if a child with ASD is standing too close to a peer, a mentor may send a discrete text that is received on a Smartwatch to support social pragmatic skills, without interrupting natural interactions between peers. Additional proposed JIT supports and applications to teachable moments in the classroom are offered in Figure 11–1.

However, educators are also now being faced with the task of selecting the most appropriate JIT technology to support a wide range of learners. We propose a four-step decision-making process to make a clinically sound decisions when selecting JIT supports for learners with ASD: (a) identify the intended purpose, (b) identify required JIT features, (c) apply identified features to available technologies and compare and contrast features, and (d) participate in a data-based trial (Figure 11–2).

JIT Feature Matching Checklist

The new prospects that are offered with the burgeoning availability of mobile technologies offers educators a wide spectrum of avenues to provide learners with accessing educational materials and enhancing teachable moments. At the same time, the vast array of features and technologies available may result in a "one JIT fits all model" versus identifying the features necessary for a specific individual. As such, we propose selecting the most appropriate JIT support should be a feature match between learners' strengths and areas of needs within the JIT taxonomy. In a seminar presented at the ASHA

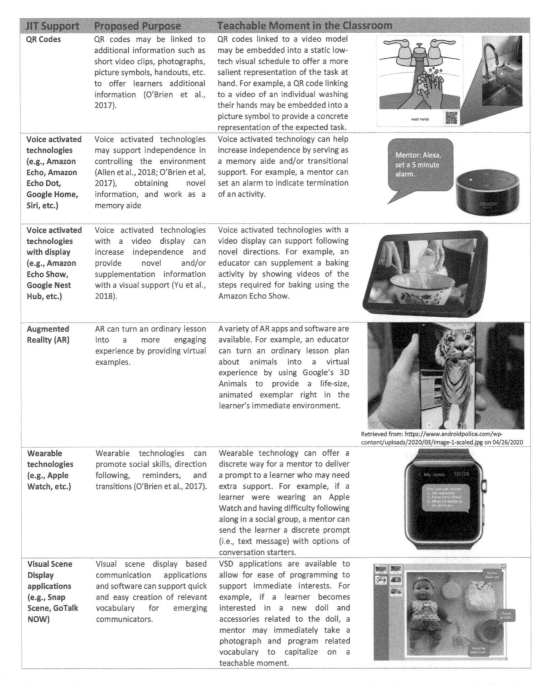

JIT Support	Proposed Purpose	Teachable Moment in the Classroom
QR Codes	QR codes may be linked to additional information such as short video clips, photographs, picture symbols, handouts, etc. to offer learners additional information (O'Brien et al., 2017).	QR codes linked to a video model may be embedded into a static low-tech visual schedule to offer a more salient representation of the task at hand. For example, a QR code linking to a video of an individual washing their hands may be embedded into a picture symbol to provide a concrete representation of the expected task.
Voice activated technologies (e.g., Amazon Echo, Amazon Echo Dot, Google Home, Siri, etc.)	Voice activated technologies may support independence in controlling the environment (Allen et al., 2018; O'Brien et al, 2017), obtaining novel information, and work as a memory aide	Voice activated technology can help increase independence by serving as a memory aide and/or transitional support. For example, a mentor can set an alarm to indicate termination of an activity.
Voice activated technologies with display (e.g., Amazon Echo Show, Google Nest Hub, etc.)	Voice activated technologies with a video display can increase independence and provide novel and/or supplementation information with a visual support (Yu et al., 2018).	Voice activated technologies with a video display can support following novel directions. For example, an educator can supplement a baking activity by showing videos of the steps required for baking using the Amazon Echo Show.
Augmented Reality (AR)	AR can turn an ordinary lesson into a more engaging experience by providing virtual examples.	A variety of AR apps and software are available. For example, an educator can turn an ordinary lesson plan about animals into a virtual experience by using Google's 3D Animals to provide a life-size, animated exemplar right in the learner's immediate environment. Retrieved from: https://www.androidpolice.com/wp-content/uploads/2020/03/image-1-scaled.jpg on 04/26/2020
Wearable technologies (e.g., Apple Watch, etc.)	Wearable technologies can promote social skills, direction following, reminders, and transitions (O'Brien et al., 2017).	Wearable technology can offer a discrete way for a mentor to deliver a prompt to a learner who may need extra support. For example, if a learner were wearing an Apple Watch and having difficulty following along in a social group, a mentor can send the learner a discrete prompt (i.e., text message) with options of conversation starters.
Visual Scene Display applications (e.g., Snap Scene, GoTalk NOW)	Visual scene display based communication applications and software can support quick and easy creation of relevant vocabulary for emerging communicators.	VSD applications are available to allow for ease of programming to support immediate interests. For example, if a learner becomes interested in a new doll and accessories related to the doll, a mentor may immediately take a photograph and program related vocabulary to capitalize on a teachable moment.

Figure 11–1. Proposed JIT supports and applications to "teachable moments" in the classroom.

convention, Shane and Costello (1994) defined feature matching as "a systematic process by which a person's strengths and current and future needs are matched to available tools and strategies." Schlosser et al. (2016) proposed an organizational

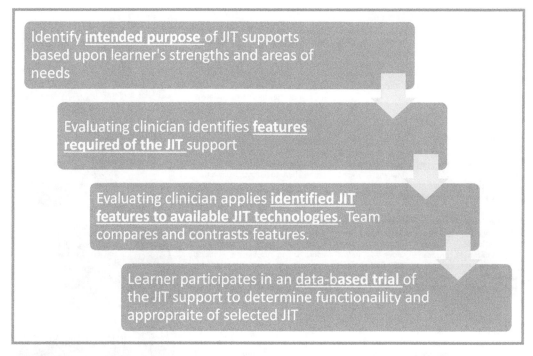

Figure 11–2. Processes to make an informed, clinical decision on an appropriate JIT support.

taxonomy in order to classify four domains for JIT supports: (a) intended purpose, (b) modality, (c) source, and (d) delivery method. We have combined aspects of both of these two frameworks and created a decision-making process in order for an evaluator to select a JIT support based upon needs of a learner (Tables 11–2 and 11–3). Individuals who conduct the evaluation and determine the JIT support should be well versed in AAC and/or Assistive Technology.

Given that technological advances occur continuously, it would be impossible to list all of the features that may be available within a JIT support; there may be features that do not currently exist. Instead, we provide a clinical framework and decision-making considerations for a clinician in order to make the most appropriate JIT recommendation as shown in

Tables 11–2 and 11–3. This chart provides four domains to consider when completing a JIT assessment related to a learner with ASD and their strengths and areas of need:

■ Learner domain: This includes medical history and sensory behaviors that may affect selecting various JIT supports. For example, the clinician needs to take into consideration if a learner has tactile sensitivities and cannot tolerate certain textiles, wearables, and so forth. This may affect the learner's ability to tolerate wearable technologies and may pose further evaluation and/or necessitate further supports to introduce (e.g., social story to demonstrate step-by-step instructions on how to introduce wearable technology).

Table 11–2. Clinical Features of a Learner's Strengths and Areas of Needs to Consider When Selecting a JIT Support

Domain	Considerations for Feature Matching
Learner	Medical: • Hearing (e.g., hearing loss) • Vision (e.g., acuity, corrective lenses, etc.) • Gross Motor (e.g., access, positioning, etc.) • Fine Motor (e.g., operational skills, access, etc.) • Behaviors (e.g., maladaptive, self-stimulatory, etc.) Sensory: • Vision sensitivities (e.g., light tolerance, color, etc.) • Auditory sensitivities (e.g., loudness, tones, etc.) • Tactile sensitivities (e.g., texture, heat, etc.)
Cognitive-Linguistic	Receptive Language: • Level of symbolic representation (e.g., photographs, videos, picture symbols, text, speech, etc.) • Comprehension of spoken language (e.g., directions, various parts of speech) Expressive Language: • Use of unaided expressive language modalities (e.g., speech, signs, gestures, etc.) • Use of aided expressive language modalities (e.g., low-tech, mid-tech, high-tech AAC) Speech Production: • Speech intelligibility • Mean length of utterance Cognitive: • Attention • Memory • Executive functioning
Environmental	• Environments for intended use (e.g., home, school, community, multiple locations, etc.) • Connectivity capabilities (e.g., Wi-Fi, Bluetooth, airdrop, cloud-based, etc.) • Finances and funding sources • Training and ongoing technical support
Communication Partner(s)	• Previous experience with technology • Previous experience with AAC/AT • Circle of communication partners and mentors (e.g., family members, school team, etc.) • Variability and consistency of communication partners and mentors

Table 11–3. Clinical Features of JIT Supports Based Upon JIT Taxonomy by Schlosser et al. (2016)

JIT Domain	Features of JIT
Intended Purpose	Receptive • Prompts • Reminders • Teaching novel vocabulary and concepts • Teaching novel play skills Expressive • Conversation starters • Communication breakdown supports Organizational/Behavioral • Rewards • Encouragement • Generalization of skill(s) across settings • Increasing independence • Safety
Modality	Auditory ("Earcons") • Speech • Digitized speech • Synthesized speech • Nonlinguistic environmental sounds (e.g., tones, ring, buzz) Visual ("Eyecons") • Light • Photographs • Videos • Static graphic symbols • Animated graphic symbols • Orthography Vibrotactile ("Vibrons") • Vibration
Source	Self-initiated • Direct selection with device navigation (e.g., navigating to folder of categorically relevant photographic prompts) • Direct selection without device navigation (e.g., preset page or schedule) Automated • Time-based • Pattern/frequency of use-based • Location-based (e.g., GPS)

Table 11–3. *continued*

JIT Domain	Features of JIT
Source *continued*	Mentor generated (adapted from Blackstone, 1999) • Inner circle (e.g., parents/guardians, spouse, siblings, children and grandchildren, etc.) • Secondary circle (e.g., good friends, etc.) • Tertiary circle (e.g., neighbors, colleagues and acquaintances, etc.) • Quaternary circle (e.g., service providers such as teachers, speech-language pathologists, occupational therapists, physical therapists, instructional aides, etc.) • Outer circle (e.g., unfamiliar communication partners)
Method for Delivery	On-the-fly • Face-to-Face • Wireless transmission • Telepractice Preprogrammed • Time-based • Location-based

■ Cognitive-linguistic domain: This includes receptive language, expressive language, speech production, and cognitive skills that may affect selecting various JIT supports. For example, if a learner's level of symbolic representation is at the photograph level (and they do not yet comprehend graphic symbols or attach meaning to orthography), a clinician may rule out technologies that do not offer a touch-screen display and/or allow the delivery of photographs and video supports.

■ Environmental domain: This includes areas in which the JIT is intended to be used, technical requirements, and funding sources that may affect ruling-in/ruling-out JIT supports. For example, the clinician will need to take into consideration the school's Wi-Fi connectivity, and speed and cellular service availability if the school is the primary environment the JIT will be used.

■ Communication partner domain: This includes the stakeholders who the learner will be interacting with, as well as, the stakeholders who may be supporting JIT use and their previous experience with technologies. For example, a clinician may need to take into consideration the most familiar platform to a wider spread of individuals depending on the number of individuals supporting the learner.

Another reported challenge in capitalizing on spontaneous teaching opportunities, particularly with individuals with ASD, is the ability to quickly create materials and program vocabulary to enhance AAC supports. Families and professionals reported difficulty in programming, creating, and implementing AAC supports due primarily to a lack of time (Yu et al., 2019), resulting in infrequent vocabulary updates (Light, McNaughton, & Caron, 2019). In addition to using JIT supports as rewards, prompts, reminders, vocabulary instruction, and conversation starters, the JIT construct may be applied to vocabulary programming in AAC devices (Light et al., 2019). As previously noted, advances in technology offers a host of possibilities to enhance language learning and AAC interventions. In this instance, hand-held devices, global positioning system, cameras, and object recognition are all features that may support JIT programming and material creation (O'Brien et al., 2017).

Light et al. (2019) suggested that JIT programming of visual scene displays (VSD) may be particularly advantageous for individuals with intellectual and developmental disabilities who do not yet have functional speech. VSDs "portray events, people, actions, objects and activities against the backgrounds in which they occur or exist" (Blackstone, Light, Beukelman, & Shane, 2004, p. 3) and as such, may be especially beneficial to improve communication for those with ASD as it provides contextual support, in comparison to traditional grid displays where symbols are separated (Shane, 2006). VSDs also seem promising in terms of time constraints, as previous research indicates adults who are unfamiliar with VSD applications are able to program vocabulary quickly (Caron, Light, Davidoff, & Drager, 2017; Caron, Light, & Drager, 2016). In addition, JIT program-

ming allows for quick access not only to relevant vocabulary, but also motivating and engaging contexts. Holyfield and colleagues (2019) proposed six steps in JIT programming for beginning communicators in order to capitalize on spontaneous learning opportunities: (a) contextualize the interaction, (b) capture engaging moments, (c) map vocabulary, (d) model immediately, (e) respond accordingly, and (f) revisit repeatedly. In practice, using these proposed steps, a mentor may capitalize on a teachable moment by following the child's lead and quickly programming a VSD with associated relevant vocabulary within a VSD communication application.

Solutions for Monitoring Progress

Goal Attainment Scaling (GAS) (Kiresuk, Smith, & Cardillo, 1994) was chosen as the primary method for monitoring student progress as a way for goals to be specific, measurable, achievable, relevant, and time-based (SMART). GAS is a technique for evaluating *individual progress* toward goals (Kiresuk et al., 1994; Oren & Ogletree, 2000; Ruble, McGrew, & Toland, 2012; Schlosser, 2004), meeting one of our more critical challenges. Unlike goals one might typically find in IEPs or treatment plans in speech-language pathology, GAS features a gradation of goal attainment, ranging from −2 (worst expected outcome) to +2 (best expected outcome) at the lower and upper end, with the following attainment levels in between: −1 (worse than expected outcome), 0 (expected outcome), and +1 (better than expected outcome) (see Appendix A in Schlosser et al., 2020, for an example). As a result of this gradation, it is possible to track subtle progress increasing the likelihood that the measure is sensitive to changes. Contrast this with traditional goals (e.g., "at least 80% correct across three consecutive sessions"), which are either met or they are not. Because the underlying definition of what constitutes a particular level (e.g., the "expected outcome") is flexible, this technique makes personalized goal-setting achievable.

Additionally, because the anchors of the 5-point scale (e.g., "expected outcome," "better than expected outcome," etc.) are consistent across goals and individuals, GAS enables the aggregation across goals and individuals. Hence, the GAS technique meets our second critical challenge related to progress monitoring. That is, as a result of this feature we were able to determine the effectiveness of the coaching intervention for the classroom as a whole in addition to each individual learner. By doing so, one of the seven students was identified as a non-responder to the intervention leading to a discussion of potential reasons for this and paving the way for adaptation going forward.

School teams supporting students with ASD are accustomed to goal-setting and evaluating attainment of goals (e.g., Wilczynski, Menousek, Hunter, & Mudgal, 2007). For that reason alone, GAS seemed to be a good fit. During the first two years of the three-year project, the GAS goals developed were separate from students' respective IEP goals and any overlap that did occur was not by design. Therefore, this required work by the school team in addition to their usual IEP-related activities both in terms of data collection, instructional time, and reporting (in Year 1, a complicating factor was the fact that the IEP goals in place had been written by another school team). Gradually, however, the school team and the administration gained a greater understanding of and appreciation for the value of GAS. This set the stage for an alignment of the GAS goals with the IEP goals in the third year, minimizing the earlier imposed additional work burden. As one of the SLPs put it so eloquently, "in the third year of research, the GAS and IEP goals were aligned more purposefully which streamlined both systems of progress measurement and data collection." One surprising positive side-effect occurred in terms of the infusion of GAS levels into IEP goals, although there was slight disagreement between the two SLPs to which degree this did occur:

"Yes, the SLPs were able to infuse the gradation of GAS attainment levels into the IEP goals and present levels of performance section of the IEP. Description of the type of VIS cue (e.g., DSC, SSC, language elements, etc.) and level of verbal/gestural prompting was added to make IEP goals and progress reporting more measurable and descriptive"
—(SLP1).

"I would say yes to a certain extent. IEP goals are not developed with the same extensive levels as GAS goals but we tried our best to reflect GAS levels in our objectives"
—(SLP2).

In our experience, the collaborative development of goal matrices helped with creating buy-in. Here, the school team and the research team jointly developed the goals with the research team providing constructive feedback iteratively as drafts of goals emerged. In all likelihood, this made the goals a focal point for team energies (e.g., Evans, Oakey, Almdahl, & Davoren, 1999; Schlosser, 2004; Smith, 1994).

The challenge of yielding objective outcome measurement in practice-based school settings is certainly a formidable one. In order to make the GAS matrices objectively measurable, the researcher team developed drafts of operational definitions that were then reviewed and eventually approved by the school team. On a superficial level, any GAS matrices invoke the perception that they are objec-

tive due to the use of numeric anchors for each level of attainment. That assumption, however, is tedious to uphold if the underlying performance demanded by each level is not operationally defined. Table 11–4 provides an example of a GAS matrix along with the underlying definition.

School teams that are not part of research projects should be in a good position to develop level-specific operational definitions on their own given their training in data-based teaching, and exposure to some research methods in the SLP preservice curriculum.

Table 11–4. Example of GAS Matrix With Underlying Definitions

Brian (pseudonym) will follow novel 2-step directives containing simple verbs in 4/5 trials.	
+2	Brian will follow novel 2-step directives, given a verbal cue only.
+1	Brian will follow novel 2-step directives, given a verbal cue with one repetition.
0	Brian will follow novel 2-step directives, given a written cue only.
−1	Brian will follow novel 2-step directives, given a static scene cue with a written cue.
−2	Brian will follow novel 2-step directives, given a dynamic scene cue with a written cue.

Correct response: A response is considered correct if Brian completes the novel 2-step directive within 10 s of the appropriate cue. A response would be incorrect if he completes only 1 step of the directive, does not respond at all, completes the steps in reverse order, or takes longer than 10 s to respond.

Baseline testing: Present 5 trials with appropriate objects/figurines/props at each of the above levels of (visual) support beginning with +2. Record correct responses at each level. Please note that the 2-step directive is novel (i.e., previously untrained). If the student gets 3 or fewer correct at a given level, do not go on the next level.

Initial performance level: the highest level at which 4/5 directives are completed successfully

Suggested instructional procedures: Follow the prompt hierarchy allowing for 0-s delay (errorless learning) to follow the directives. Combine with time delay as instruction progresses. Possibly include written directive below or above static scene cue and gradually fade out the static scene cue.

■ Enhancing Directive-Following Via JIT Supports on a Smartwatch: A Vignette

Wearable technology is a promising and discrete medium through which to provide visual, auditory, and haptic JIT intervention to individuals with ASD. The visual augmentation of spoken directives (i.e., via static or dynamic scene cues) is one strategy for improving directive-following for some children with ASD (Schlosser et al., 2013). These scene cues can be transmitted in a timely manner to a smartwatch worn by learners with ASD (O'Brien, Schlosser, Yu et al., 2020). This vignette illustrates the evaluation process described earlier and the intervention protocol used to systematically introduce a smartwatch intervention to support directive- following for a child with ASD.

Sophie is a happy and hard-working 9-year-old girl with an ASD diagnosis. She participates in a VIS-powered special education classroom with daily opportunities for integration in a general education classroom. She receives support from a one-to-one Educational Assistant (EA). Each week, Sophie receives speech-language therapy, occupational therapy, and physical therapy at school.

Assessment

Expressively, Sophie uses limited speech (1 to 3 word spoken utterances) to request preferred items (e.g., "want swing," "bathroom") and to comment ("blue iPad"). Sophie scores below the 1st percentile on the Expressive Vocabulary Test, Third Edition. Socially, Sophie benefits from adult support to initiate interactions with peers. Sophie uses both low-tech (i.e., paper-based supports) and high-tech AAC (i.e., GoTalk NOW application) strategies to expand her communicative functions and length of utterances. She benefits from the use of customized topic displays to support language expansion. Receptively, Sophie demonstrates difficulty following spoken directives and is prompt-dependent on her mentors. As such, Sophie frequently requires prompting to complete a given directive and the EA assigned to her remains nearby throughout the school day. Sophie scores below the 1st percentile on the Peabody Picture Vocabulary Test, Fourth Edition. Sophie benefits from visual supports (e.g., photographs and written text) to follow directives. During transitions, she relies on a paper-based written schedule presented by communication partners to support her directive-following.

Regarding literacy skills, Sophie decodes and reads with comprehension at the second-grade level. She fluently reads short sentences with comprehension and matches pictures to the sentences that they represent. She answers who, what, and where questions related to 2 to 3 sentence texts, given a single picture prompt.

Based on a conversation with Sophie's school team (teacher, SLP, EA), and Sophie's communication profile described above, the following clinical goal was identified for Sophie: Sophie will: (a) in-crease her independent directive following across three settings, and (b) demonstrate reduced dependence on her EA as measured by increased distance from her EA. An AAC-based JIT assessment, using the previously described JIT Feature Matching Checklist, was used to identify the best strategy by which to support Sophie's acquisition of this goal. The following features were identified as relevant (Table 11–5).

Table 11–5. Feature Matching Assessment, Completed by SLP, to Support the Selection of the Most Appropriate JIT-Based Technology for Julia

Domain	Considerations for Feature Matching
Learner	Medical: ☐ Hearing (e.g., hearing loss) ☐ Vision (e.g., acuity, corrective lenses, etc.) ☐ Gross Motor (e.g., access, positioning, etc.) ☐ Fine Motor (e.g., operational skills, access, etc.) ☒ Behaviors (e.g., maladaptive, self-stimulatory, etc.) Sensory: ☐ Vision sensitivities (e.g., light tolerance, color, etc.) ☒ Auditory sensitivities (e.g., loudness, tones, etc.) ☐ Tactile sensitivities (e.g., texture, heat, etc.)
Cognitive-Linguistic	Receptive Language: ☒ Level of symbolic representation (e.g., photographs, videos, picture symbols, text, speech, etc.) **Reads short sentences with comprehension, Uses visual schedules (text and picture-based) for daily routines** ☒ Comprehension of spoken language (e.g., directives, various parts of speech) **Difficulty following two-step spoken directives** Expressive Language: ☒ Use of unaided expressive language modalities (e.g., speech, signs, gestures, etc.) **Uses speech (1 to 3-word utterances) for requesting and commenting** ☒ Use of aided expressive language modalities (e.g., low-tech, mid-tech, high-tech AAC) **Uses topic displays on GoTalk NOW to expand language** Speech Production: ☐ Speech intelligibility ☐ Mean length of utterance Cognitive: ☐ Attention ☐ Memory ☒ Executive functioning
Environmental	☒ Environments for intended use (e.g., home, school, community, multiple locations, etc.) **School (special education classroom, general education classroom, hallway)** ☒ Connectivity capabilities (e.g., Wi-Fi, Bluetooth, airdrop, cloud-based, etc.) **Wi-Fi available at school, slower when sending larger files (e.g., photographs, videos)** ☒ Finances and funding sources **Funding is available from the school** ☒ Training and ongoing technical support **Technology specialist support available at school**

Table 11–5. *continued*

Domain	Considerations for Feature Matching
Communication Partner(s)	☒ Previous experience with technology **Experience primarily with Apple devices** ☒ Previous experience with AAC/AT **Experience with VIS-based technology (e.g., communication applications on an iPad, receptive language supports on an iPad, preliminary experience with an Apple Watch)** ☒ Circle of communication partners and mentors (e.g., family members, school team, etc.) ☒ Variability and consistency of communication partners and mentors **Consistent 1:1 classroom aide**

JIT Domain	Features of JIT
Intended Purpose	Receptive ☐ Prompts ☐ Reminders ☒ Directives. **Demonstrates difficulty with two-step directives, prompt-dependence on communication partners** ☐ Teaching novel vocabulary and concepts ☐ Teaching novel play skills Expressive ☐ Communicative function support (e.g., request, protest, comment) ☐ Conversation starters ☐ Communication breakdown supports Organizational/Behavioral ☐ Rewards ☐ Encouragement ☒ Generalization of skill(s) across settings ☒ Increasing independence ☐ Safety
Modality	Auditory ("Earcons") ☐ Speech ☐ Digitized speech ☐ Synthesized speech ☒ Nonlinguistic environmental sounds (e.g., tones, ring, buzz)

continues

Table 11–5. *continued*

JIT Domain	Features of JIT
Modality *continued*	Visual ("Eyecons") ☐ Light ☐ Photographs ☐ Videos ☐ Static graphic symbols ☐ Animated graphic symbols ☒ Orthography Vibrotactile ("Vibrons") ☒ Vibration
Source	Self-initiated ☐ Direct selection without device navigation (e.g., pre-set page or schedule) ☐ Direct selection with device navigation (e.g., navigating to folder of categorically relevant photographic prompts) Automated ☐ Time-based ☐ Pattern/frequency of use-based ☐ Location-based (e.g., GPS) Mentor generated (adapted from Blackstone, 1999) ☐ Inner circle (e.g., parents/guardians, spouse, siblings, children and grandchildren, etc.) ☐ Secondary circle (e.g., good friends, etc.) ☐ Tertiary circle (e.g., neighbors, colleagues & acquaintances, etc.) ☒ Quaternary circle (e.g., service providers such as teachers, speech-language pathologists, occupational therapists, physical therapists, instructional aides, etc.) **1:1 classroom aide to provide JIT directives** ☐ Outer circle (e.g., unfamiliar communication partners)
Method for Delivery	On-the-fly ☐ Face-to-Face ☒ Wireless transmission ☐ Telepractice Preprogrammed ☐ Time-based ☐ Location-based

Based on the AAC-JIT feature match, Sophie's team decided to trial a smartwatch with capacity for sending text-based directives. Sophie's team chose to use an Apple Watch® based on the team's familiarity with Apple products, its wearability, and the range of applications available for future organizational support, as well as prior feasibility studies related to using an Apple Watch® for JIT supports (O'Brien et al., 2016; Schlosser et al., 2017). Sophie's EA was identified as the source of the directives, and the messages were sent wirelessly over a Wi-Fi connection.

Data-Based Trial

Sophie participated in a two-week data-based trial of the smartwatch intervention (for a complete write-up of the study see O'Brien, Schlosser, Shane, et al., submitted). Sophie's EA texted three JIT directives to her in each of three different settings, the general education classroom, the special education classroom, and the hallway. The nine unique directives were identified by Sophie's teacher and SLPs as directives that she had previously demonstrated difficulty completing independently when given a spoken and written schedule (e.g., "Get your paper and put it in your mailbox").

To prevent possible novelty effects from wearing a new watch during baseline and intervention, Sophie wore the Apple Watch® before the start of intervention (Schlosser, 2003). When it was time in Sophie's schedule to follow a given directive (e.g., snack time), the EA used the messages application to send the directive to be followed to the Apple Watch® (e.g., "Get your snack and eat it"). The EA did not instruct Sophie on how to look at, or respond to, the watch during baseline.

She collected data on how many directives Sophie followed before intervention.

During intervention, the EA instructed Sophie how to look at and respond to the directive received on the watch. If Sophie looked at the watch and followed the directive within 10 s, her response was considered correct. If she did not, her response was marked as incorrect and the EA provided gestural, spoken (e.g., "Check your watch," "You do it"), and physical prompts (e.g., tilting the watch to show the message) to instruct her on how to look at the directive on the watch. After Sophie looked at the watch, if she did not follow the directive after an additional 10 s, the EA provided spoken (e.g., "You do it," "Ride bike to the green line and stop") and gestural (e.g., pointing) prompts to support her completion of the directive. The EA began by providing the directives from 5 feet away, and gradually increased her distance in 2-feet increments until she was 9 feet away. At the end of the intervention, two school-based SLPs, the classroom teacher, and the EA completed a 10-item treatment acceptability survey, the modified Treatment Evaluation Inventory–Short Form (TEI–SF) (Kelley, Heffer, Gresham, & Elliott, 1989).

Results

Throughout the trial, Sophie tolerated wearing the watch, and the auditory and haptic prompts provided by the watch. Sophie generally appeared to understand intuitively that she should look at her watch upon receiving an auditory and haptic prompt during baseline. Sophie demonstrated improvements in directive-following from baseline to intervention across the three settings. She also began to demonstrate so-called anticipatory responses (Slamecka, 1977); that is, in two settings she began to complete the successive directive before receiving the text-based directive, suggesting a paired association between the two successive tasks. The EA successfully increased her distance from Sophie to 9 feet. The SLPs and the special education teacher involved in this trial rated the intervention as more than moderately acceptable, with greatest agreement that the intervention was successful in providing directives from a distance.

Discussion

Sophie demonstrated improvements in her directive-following after receiving the smartwatch intervention. Further, the use of a smartwatch permitted discrete provision of support and an increase in the distance between Sophie and her EA. This intervention may result in improved independence through remote support and the acquisition of anticipatory responses as well as improved independence as perceived by peers and others. Based on Sophie's successful trial with the Apple Watch®, continued use of the smartwatch intervention is recommended. Sophie's team should consider increasing the number of directives, settings, and distance from the mentor to continue to reduce her prompt dependence and increase her independence.

■ Summary and Conclusions

The Visual Immersion System™ is an assessment and treatment package for individuals with moderate-to-severe ASD who require supports in language, communication, and organization/executive function. Based on our collective experiences gained from a three-year project with a coaching-based intervention supporting a school team in the implementation of the VIS™ in an elementary school classroom, we discussed four everyday challenges and presented solutions that proved viable throughout this journey. The vignette of Sophie illustrated the challenge of providing just-in-time supports along with how a solution was approached. It is our hope that readers will benefit from the problem-solving and decision-making processes shared in this chapter.

Acknowledgments. We would like to thank the parents and legal guardians of the children who participated over the course of the three-year project. Likewise, we are indebted to the educational assistants who provided much of the frontline support to the students. Finally, we express our appreciation to the administrative leadership of the Fayetteville-Manlius school district for being so supportive of the effort.

■ References

Adamo-Villani, N., Carpenter, E., & Arns, L. (2006). An immersive virtual environment for learning sign language mathematics. In *Proceeding SIGGRAPH 06' Educators Program, Article # 20*, ACM. https://doi.org/10.1145/1179295.1179316.

Allen, A. A., Schlosser, R. W., Brock, K. L., & Shane, H. C. (2017). The effectiveness of aided augmented input techniques for persons with developmental disabilities: A systematic review. *Augmentative and Alternative Communication, 33*, 149–159.

Allen, A., Shane, H. C., & Schlosser, R. W. (2018). The Echo™ as a speaker-independent speech recognition device for children with autism: An exploratory study. *Advances in Neurodevelopmental Disorders, 2*(1), 69–74. https://doi.org/10.1007/s41252-017-0041-5

Althaus, M., de Sonneville, L. M., Minderaa, R. B., Hensen, L. G., & Til, R. B. (1996). Information processing and aspects of visual attention in children with the DSM-III-R diagnosis "pervasive developmental disorder not otherwise specified (PDDNOS).: II. Sustained attention. *Child Neuropsychology, 2*, 30-38. https://doi.org/10.1080/09297049608401348

Arthur-Kelly, M., Sigafoos, J., Green, V., Mathisen, B., & Arthur- Kelly, R. (2009). Issues in the use of visual supports to promote communication in individuals with autism spectrum disorder. *Disability and Rehabilitation, 31*, 1474–1486. https://doi.org/10.1080/09638280802590629

Ashwin, E., Ashwin, C., Rhydderch, D., Howells, J., & Baron-Cohen, S. (2009). Eagle-eyed visual acuity: An experimental investigation of enhanced perception in autism. *Biological Psychiatry, 65*(1), 17–21.

Ayers, W. (1989). *The good preschool teacher.* Teachers College Press.

Banda, D. R., & Grimmett, D. (2008). Enhancing social and transition behaviors of persons with autism through activity schedules: A review. *Education and Training in Developmental Disabilities, 43*, 324–333. Retrieved from https://www.jstor.org/stable/23879794

Bandura, A. (1977). *Social learning theory.* Prentice-Hall.

Bellini, S., & Akullian, J. (2007). A meta-analysis of video modeling and video self-modeling interventions for children and adolescents with autism spectrum disorders. *Exceptional Children, 73*(3), 264–287.

Biggs, E. E., Carter, E. W., & Gilson, C. B. (2018). Systematic review of interventions involving aided AAC modeling for children with complex communication needs. *American Journal on Intellectual and Developmental Disabilities, 123*(5), 443–473. https://doi.org/10.1352/1944-7558-123.5.443

Blackstone, S. (1999). Clinical news: communication partners. *Augmentative Communication News, 12*(1–2), 2–3. https://www.augcominc.com/newsletters/newsletter_22.pdf

Blackstone, S., Light, J., Beukelman, D., & Shane, H. (2004). Visual scene displays. *Augmentative Communication News, 16*(2), 1–5.

Bondy, A., & Frost, L. (2001). Picture Exchange Communication System. *Behavior Modification, 25*, 725–744.

Caron, J., Light, J., Davidoff, B. E., & Drager, K. D. (2017). Comparison of the effects of mobile technology AAC apps on programming visual scene displays. *Augmentative and Alternative Communication, 33*, 239–248.

Caron, J., Light, J., & Drager, K. (2016). Operational demands of AAC mobile technology applications on programming vocabulary and engagement during professional and child interactions. *Augmentative and Alternative Communication, 32*, 12–24.

Charlop-Christy, M. H., Le, L., & Freeman, K. A. (2000). A comparison of video modeling with in vivo modeling for teaching children with autism. *Journal of Autism and Developmental Disorders, 30*, 537–552. https://doi.org/10.1023/a:1005635326276

Cummins, J. (1998). Immersion education for the millennium: What have we learned from 30 years of research on second language immersion? In M. R. Childs & R. M. Bostwick (Eds.), *Learning through two languages: Research and practice. Second Katoh Gakuen International Symposium on Immersion and Bilingual Education* (pp. 34–47). Katoh Gakuen, Japan.

Dada, S., Flores, C., Bastable, K., & Schlosser, R. W. (2020). The effects of augmentative and alternative communication interventions on the receptive language skills of children with developmental disabilities: A scoping review. *International Journal of Speech-Language Pathology.* Advance online publication. https://doi.org/10.1080/17549507.2020.1797165

Dauphin, M., Kinney, E. M., Stromer, R., & Koegel, R. L. (2004). Using video-enhanced activity schedules and matrix training to teach sociodramatic play to a child with autism. *Journal of Positive Behavior Interventions, 6*(4), 238–250.

Evans, D. J., Oakey, S., Almdahl, S., & Davoren, B. (1999). Goal attainment scaling in a geriatric day hospital. Team and program benefits. *Canadian Family Physician, 45,* 954–960. https://doi.org/10.1111/j.1532-5415.1992 .tb02105.x

Harmon, A., Schlosser, R. W., Gygi, B., Shane, H. C., Kong, Y.-Y., Book, L., . . . Hearn, E. (2014). The effects of environmental sounds on the naming of animated AAC graphic symbols. *Augmentative and Alternative Communication, 30,* 298–313. https://doi .org/10.3109/07434618.2014.966206

Hogdon, L. (1995). *Visual strategies for improving communication.* Quirk Roberts.

Holyfield, C., Caron, J., & Light, J. (2019) Programing AAC just-in-time for beginning communicators: The process. *Augmentative and Alternative Communication, 35,* 309–318. https://doi.org/10.1080/07434618 .2019.1686538

Hong, E. R., Ganz, J. B., Mason, R., Morin, K., Davis, J. L., Ninci, J., . . . Gilliland, W. D. (2016). The effects of video modeling in teaching functional living skills to persons with ASD: A meta-analysis of single-case studies. *Research in Developmental Disabilities, 57,* 158–169. https://doi.org/10.1016/ j.ridd.2016.07.001

Kelley, M. L., Heffer, R. W., Gresham, F. M., & Elliott, S. N. (1989). Development of a modified Treatment Evaluation Inventory. *Journal of Psychopathology and Behavioral Assessment, 11*(3), 235–247. https://doi.org/ 10.1007/BF00960495

Kiresuk, T. J., Smith, A., Cardillo, J. E. (1994). *Goal attainment scaling: Applications, theory, and measurement.* Psychology Press.

Knight, V., Sartini, E., & Spriggs, A. D. (2015). Evaluating visual activity schedules as evidence-based practice for individuals with autism spectrum disorders. *Journal of Autism and Developmental Disorders, 45,* 157–178. https://doi.org/10.1007/s10803-014-2201-z

Lequia, J., Machalicek, W., & Rispoli, M. J. (2012). Effects of activity schedules on challenging behavior exhibited in children with autism spectrum disorders: A systematic review. *Research in Autism Spectrum Disorder, 6,* 480–492. https://doi.org/10.1016/j .rasd.2011.07.008

Light, J., McNaughton, D., & Caron, J. (2019). New and emerging AAC technology supports for children with complex communication needs and their communication partners: State of the science and future research directions. *Augmentative and Alternative Communication, 35,* 26–41. https:// doi.org/10.1080/07434618.2018.1557251

Maenner, M. J., Shaw, K. A., Baio, J., Washington, A., Patrick, M., DiRienzo, M., . . . Dietz, P. M. (2020). Prevalence of Autism Spectrum Disorder among children aged 8 years—Autism and Developmental Disabilities Monitoring Network, 11 Sites, United States, 2016. MMWR Surveill Summ, 69 (No. SS-4), 1–12. https://doi.org/10.15585/ mmwr.ss6904a1external_icon.

McNaughton, D., & Light, J. (2013). The iPad and mobile technology revolution: Benefits and challenges for individuals who require augmentative and alternative communication. *Augmentative and Alternative Communication, 29,* 107–116. https://doi.org/ 10.3109/07434618.2013.784930

Mechling, L. C., & Hunnicutt, J. R. (2011). Computer-based video self-modeling to teach receptive understanding of prepositions by students with intellectual disabilities. *Education and Training in Autism and Developmental Disabilities, 46,* 369-385.

Mesibov, G. B., Schopler, E. & Hearsey, K. A. (1994). Structured teaching. In E. Schopler & G. B. Mesibov (Eds.), *Behavioral issues in autism* (pp. 195–207). Plenum Press.

Mirenda, P., & Iacono, T. (2009). *Autism Spectrum Disorders and AAC.* Brookes.

National Autism Center. (2015). *National standards project, Phase 2.* Randolph, MA.

Nigam, R., Schlosser, R. W., & Lloyd, L. L. (2006). Concomitant use of the matrix strategy and the mand-model procedure in teaching graphic symbol combinations. *Augmentative and Alternative Communication, 22*(3), 160–177. https://doi.org/10.1080/ 07434610600650052

O'Brien, A., O'Brien, M., Schlosser, R. W., Yu, C., Allen, A. A., Flynn, S., . . . Shane, H. C. (2017). Repurposing consumer products as a gateway to just-in-time communication. *Seminars in Speech and Language, 38,* 297–312. https://doi.org/10.1055/s-0037-1604 277.

O'Brien, A., Schlosser, R. W., Shane, H. C., Abramson, J., Allen, A., Yu, C., & Dimery, K. (2016). Just-in-time visual supports for children with Autism via the Apple Watch: A pilot feasibility study. *Journal of Autism and Developmental Disorders, 46*(12), 3818–3823. https://doi.org/10.1007/s108 03-016-2891-5

O'Brien, A., Schlosser, R. W., Shane, H. C., Yu, C., Allen, A. A., Cullen, J., . . . O'Neil, L. (submitted). *Providing visual supports via a smartwatch to a child with Autism Spectrum Disorder: An exploratory study.*

O'Brien, A., Schlosser, R. W., Yu, C., Allen, A. A., & Shane, H. (2020). Repurposing a smartwatch to support individuals with Autism Spectrum Disorder: Sensory and operational considerations. *Journal of Special Education Technology.* https://doi.org/ 10.1177/0162643420904001

Oren, T., & Ogletree, B. T. (2000). Program evaluation in classrooms for students with autism: Student outcomes and program processes. *Focus on Autism and Other Developmental Disabilities, 15,* 170–175. https://doi.org/10.1177/108835760001500308

Peterson, S., Bondy, A., Vincent, Y., & Finnegan, C. (1995). Effects of altering communicative input for students with autism and no speech: Two case studies. *Augmentative and Alternative Communication, 11*(2), 93–100. https://doi.org/10.1080/07434619 512331277189

Pierce, K. L., & Schreibman, L. (1994). Teaching daily living skills to children with autism in unsupervised settings through pictorial self-management. *Journal of Applied Behavior Analysis, 27*(3), 471–481. https:// doi.org/10.1901/jaba.1994.27-471

Quill, K. A. (1997). Instructional considerations for young children with autism: The rationale for visually cued instruction.

Journal of Autism and Developmental Disorders, 27(6), 697-714. https://doi.org/10 .1023/A:1025806900162

Remner, R., Baker, M., Karter, C., Kearns, K., & Shane, H. (2016). Use of augmented input to improve understanding of spoken directives by children with moderate to severe Autism Spectrum Disorder. *eHearsay, 6*(3), 4–10. https://www.ohioslha.org/wp-content/uploads/2016/10/eHearsay2016-Autism.pdf

Rose, V., Trembath, D., Keen, D., & Paynter, J. (2016). The proportion of minimally verbal children with autism spectrum disorder in a community-based early intervention programme. *Journal of Intellectual Disabilities Research, 60*(5), 464-477. https://doi.org/ 10.1111/jir.12284

Ruble, L. McGrew, J. H., & Toland, M. D. (2012). Goal attainment scaling as an outcome measure in randomized controlled trials of psychosocial interventions in autism. *Journal of Autism and Developmental Disorders, 42*(9), 1974–1983.

Rutherford, M., Baxter, J., Grayson, A., Johnston, L., & O'Hare, A. (2019). Visual supports at home and in the community for individuals with autism spectrum disorders: A scoping review. *Autism, 24*(2), 447-469. https://doi.org/10.1177/ 1362361319871756

Schlosser, R. W. (2003). *The efficacy of augmentative and alternative communication: Toward evidence-based practice.* Academic Press.

Schlosser, R. W. (2004). Goal attainment scaling as a clinical measurement technique in communication disorders: A critical review. *Journal of Communication Disorders, 37*(3), 217–239. https://doi.org/10.1016/j.jcomdis .2003.09.003

Schlosser, R. W., Brock, K., Koul, R., Shane, H. C., & Flynn, S. (2019). Do animations facilitate understanding of graphic symbols representing verbs in children with autism spectrum disorder? *Journal of Speech, Language, and Hearing Research, 62*(4), 965–978. https://doi.org/10.1044/2018_JSL HR-L-18-0243

Schlosser, R. W., & Koul, R. (2015). Speech output technologies in interventions for individuals with Autism Spectrum Disorders: A scoping review. *Augmentative and Alternative Communication, 31*(4), 285–309. https://doi.org/10.3109/07434618.2015.1063689

Schlosser, R. W., Koul, R., Shane, H., Sorce, J., Brock, K., Harmon, A., . . . Hearn, E. (2014). Effects of animation on naming and identification across two graphic symbol sets representing verbs and prepositions. *Journal of Speech, Language, and Hearing Research, 57*(5), 1779–1791. https://doi.org/10.1044/2014_JSLHR-L-13-0193

Schlosser, R. W., Laubscher, E., Sorce, J., Koul, R., Flynn, S., Hotz, L., . . . Shane, H. (2013). Implementing directives that involve prepositions with children with autism: A comparison of spoken cues with two types of augmented input. *Augmentative and Alternative Communication, 29*, 132–145. https://doi.org/10.3109/07434618.2013.784928

Schlosser, R. W., O'Brien, A., Yu, C., Abramson, J., Allen, A., Flynn, S., & Shane, H. C. (2017). Repurposing everyday technologies to provide just-in-time visual supports to children with intellectual disability and autism: A pilot feasibility study with the Apple Watch®. *International Journal of Developmental Disabilities, 63*(4), 221–227. https://doi.org/10.1080/20473869.2017.1305138

Schlosser, R. W., Shane, H. C., Allen, A., Abramson, J., Laubscher, E., & Dimery, K. (2016). Just-in-time supports in augmentative and alternative communication. *Journal of Physical and Developmental Disabilities, 28*(1), 177–193. https://doi.org/10.1007/s10882-015-9452-2

Schlosser, R. W., Shane, H. C., Allen, A., Benz, A., Cullen, J., Chiesa, L., Miori-Dineen, L., Koul, R., & Pasupathy, R. (2020). *Coaching a school team to implement the Visual Immersion System™ in a classroom for children with Autism Spectrum Disorder: A mixed methods proof-of-concept study.* https://doi.org/10.1007/s41252-020-00176-5.

Schlosser, R. W., Shane, H., Sorce, J., Koul, R., Bloomfield, E., Debrowski, L., . . . Neff, A. (2012). Animation of graphic symbols representing verbs and prepositions: Effects on transparency, name agreement, and identification. *Journal of Speech, Language, and Hearing Research, 55*, 342–358. https://doi.org/10.1044/1092-4388(2011/10-0164)

Sennott, S. C., Light, J. C., & McNaughton, D. (2016). AAC modeling intervention research review. *Research and Practice for Persons with Severe Disabilities, 41*(2), 101–115.

Shah, A., & Frith, U. (1993). Why do autistic individuals show superior performance on the block design task? *Journal of Child Psychology and Psychiatry, 34*(8), 1351–1364.

Shane, H. C. (2006). Using visual scene displays to improve communication and communication instruction in persons with autism spectrum disorders. *Perspectives on Augmentative and Alternative Communication, 15*, 8–13. https://doi.org/10.1044/aac15.1.8

Shane, H., & Costello, J. (1994). *Augmentative communication assessment and the feature matching process.* Miniseminar presented at the annual convention of the American Speech-Language-Hearing-Association, New Orleans, LA.

Shane, H. C., & Albert, P. D. (2008). Electronic screen media for persons with autism spectrum disorders: Results of a survey. *Journal of Autism and Developmental Disorders, 38*(8), 1228-1235. https://doi.org/10.1007/s10803-007-0527-5

Shane, H. C., Laubscher, E., Schlosser, R. W., Fadie, H. L., Sorce, J. F., Abramson, J. S., . . . Corley, K. (2014). *Enhancing communication for individuals with autism: A guide to the Visual Immersion System.* Brookes.

Shane, H. C., Laubscher, E. H., Schlosser, R. W., Flynn, S., Sorce, J. F., & Abramson, J. (2012). Applying technology to visually support language and communication in individuals with autism spectrum disorders. *Journal of Autism and Developmental Disorders, 42*, 1228–1235. https://doi.org/10.1007/s10803-011-1304-z

Shane, H. C., & Weiss-Kapp, S. (2008). *Visual language in autism*. Plural Publishing.

Slamecka, N. J. (1977). A case for response-produced cues in serial learning. *Journal of Experimental Psychology: Human Learning and Memory, 3*, 222–232. https://doi.org/10.1037/0278-7393.3.2.222

Smith, A. (1994). Introduction and overview. In T. Kiresuk, A. Smith, & J. Cardillo (Eds.), *Goal attainment scaling: Applications, theory, and measurement* (pp. 1–14). Erlbaum.

Steinbrenner, J. R., Hume, K., Odom, S. L., Morin, K. L., Nowell, S. W., Tomaszewski, B. . . . Savage, M. N. (2020). *Evidence-based practices for children, youth, and young adults with Autism*. The University of North Carolina at Chapel Hill, Frank Porter Graham Child Development Institute, National Clearinghouse on Autism Evidence and Practice Review Team.

Tager-Flusberg, H., & Kasari, C. (2013). Minimally verbal school-aged children with autism: The neglected end of the spectrum. *Autism Research, 6*(6), 468-478. https://doi.org/10.1002/aur.1329

Thaut, M. H. (1987). Visual versus auditory (musical) stimulus preferences in autistic children: A pilot study. *Journal of Autism and Developmental Disorders, 17*(3), 425–432.

Watanabe, M., & Sturmey, P. (2003). The effect of choice making opportunities during activity schedules on task engagement of adults with autism. *Journal of Autism and Developmental Disorders, 33*, 535–538.

Wilczynski, S. M., Menousek, K., Hunter, M., & Mudgal, D. (2007). Individualized education programs for youth with Autism Spectrum Disorders. *Psychology in Schools, 44*, 653–666. https://doi.org/10.1002/pits.20255

Yu, C., Shane, H. C., O'Brien, A. M., Schlosser, R. W., Abramson, J., Allen, A., Flynn, S. (2019, November). *Predictors of successful implementation of recommendations for children with moderate to severe autism spectrum disorder*. Poster presented at the annual convention of the American Speech-Language Hearing Association (ASHA), Orlando, FL.

Yu, C., Shane, H. C., Schlosser, R. W., O'Brien, A., Allen, A. A., Abramson, J., & Flynn, S. (2018). An exploratory study of speech-language pathologists using the Echo Show™ to deliver visual content. *Advances in Neurodevelopmental Disorders, 2*(3), 286–292. https://doi.org/10.1007/s41252-018-0075-3

12

Fostering Communication About Emotions: Aided Augmentative and Alternative Communication Challenges and Solutions

Krista M. Wilkinson, Ji Young Na, Gabriela A. Rangel-Rodriguez, and Dawn J. Sowers

■ Introduction

This chapter will discuss the importance of including vocabulary to talk about emotions using aided forms of augmentative and alternative communication (AAC), in ways that are consistent with family preferences. We describe the theoretical and practical reasons for this effort, review some of the challenges of communicating about emotions using AAC, and offer a means to address these challenges. We also provide detailed case examples of how to solicit family preferences about how they communicate about emotions as well as strategies for supporting families to encourage communication via AAC. These approaches are illustrated by descriptive case examples from our laboratories.

Brief Overview of Augmentative and Alternative Communication

As reviewed in Beukelman and Light (2020), many people with complex communication needs (CCN) benefit from augmentative and alternative communication (AAC) technologies and associated interventions. AAC includes both "unaided" forms of communication, such as gesture and signs, as well as "aided" forms in which an external aid is used to communicate. These aided types of AAC include low technology books or boards containing symbols as well as high-technology speech generating devices and mobile technologies such as tablets. Both low and high-tech aided AAC systems provide individuals who have difficulty using natural speech a way to communicate a range of functions, including their basic wants and needs as well as sharing information, expressing internal emotions and beliefs, promoting social closeness, and other important functions. Aided AAC systems for children are usually developed around pictures or symbols to access meaningful vocabulary. In terms of its design, vocabulary typically is presented within a traditional row-column grid display or, more recently, within a visual scene display (VSD) (cf. Light, Wilkinson, Theissen, Beukelman, & Fager, 2019). Grid displays are made up of rows and columns of vocabulary with each word/phrase occupying one cell. In contrast, VSDs arrange vocabulary within a familiar schema, represented by a real-life photograph or, more recently video (with video visual scene displays; see, for instance, O'Neill, Light, & McNaughton, 2017; use of visual VSDs is detailed in Chapter 5, this volume). VSDs provide semantic context for the child to retrieve the vocabulary needed and have been successful especially for early communicators (Drager et al., 2019; Holyfield, Caron, Drager, & Light, 2019). Targeted vocabulary is selected based on the child's current interests and environments and immediate as well as future needs.

Relation of the Development of Language and Emotional Competencies

As Na, Wilkinson, Blackstone, Karny, and Stifter (2016) and Saarni (1999) have noted, the umbrella term "emotional competencies" (or emotional competence) is often considered primarily to the ability to manage one's own emotions during periods of heightened emotional arousal. However, this term also includes several other fundamental abilities, including

a child's ability to (a) be aware of and able to identify one's own and others' emotions; (b) label those emotions, discuss the reasons for those emotions, and develop independence in managing their responses to those emotions; and (c) engage in communication about those emotions within individual and group relationships. A child's development of culturally appropriate emotional competencies has far-reaching implications for a variety of developmental outcomes, including (among others): (a) the fundamental readiness to learn; (b) use of conventional communication forms rather than challenging behaviors; (c) engagement in individual and peer group relationships; and (d) as adolescents and adults, successful participation in self-advocacy, vocational, and community participation (Aro, Laakso, Määttä, Tolvanen, & Poikkeus, 2014; Buckley, Storino, & Saarni, 2003; Trentacosta & Izard, 2007). For instance, a child who is highly stressed, or even over- or under-aroused (overexcited or sleepy) will have difficulty learning in the classroom setting; individuals who cannot identify and respond to their own emotions or those of others appropriately may find it difficult to make or maintain friendships or enter into peer groups successfully; individuals who are still learning self-regulation skills may find it challenging to engage in vocational activities.

In typical development, caregivers' spoken input and general guidance are primary avenues by which children are exposed to culturally accepted means of identifying, labeling, reasoning about, and responding appropriately to emotions and emotional situations. Although largely correlational in nature, research suggests a relation between the development of language/linguistic skills and the development of behaviors associated with emotional competencies (such as using emotion terms/labels, emotional regulation; Beck, Kumschick, Eid, & Klann-Delius, 2011; Kubicek & Emde, 2012; Roben, Cole, & Armstrong, 2013; Vallotton & Ayoub, 2011; see Na et al., 2016, for detailed consideration). This idea of language both scaffolding and being scaffolded by other cognitive processes has a direct basis in the socio-cultural theories of Vygotsky (1986) in which social interactions with a "more-able" caregiver is considered to be a primary mechanism for development.

Little direct research has examined the relation of development of language and emotional competencies in individuals with intellectual disabilities (ID). However, there are a number of reasons to believe that this relationship is critical for individuals who have communication and language disabilities, including those with ID. First, the logic of Vygotsky's (1986) theory most likely applies for children with developmental disabilities. The role of caregiver modelling and scaffolding of language as a means to label, discuss, and reason about emotions is equally (if not more) important for children who struggle to learn these skills as they are for children with typical development (cf. Warren & Yoder, 1998). Second, research suggests that similar to children with typical development, correlational relationships between language and emotional competencies occur in individuals with general language delays or language impairment (Fujiki, Brinton, & Clarke, 2002; Fujiki, Spackman, Brinton, & Hall, 2004). Finally, it is well established that many unconventional or challenging behaviors (such as inappropriate behavior, aggression, or property destruction) serve communicative functions, and that provision of conventional forms of communication can replace these challenging behaviors (Mirenda & Brown, 2007;

Reichle & Johnston, 1993; see Wilkinson & Reichle, 2009). Although this latter research does not typically address development of emotional competencies, it reinforces the notion that language can be a means to promote skills related to emotional competencies (for instance, use of an alternative communication form than the challenging behavior) in individuals with ID.

Challenge: Communicating About Emotions With an AAC System

Emotional expression is multimodal, meaning that emotions can be expressed through a wide range of means. An individual can express emotion through posture, facial expression, gesture, speech, intonation, writing (including both formal text and informal emojis), and, when designed well, through AAC. Yet Blackstone and Wilkins (2009) have argued that children with CCN can experience difficulty in communication and emotional development. These challenges may result from a variety of barriers, from factors intrinsic to the child (difficulty expressing emotion due to physical, motor, or intellectual disabilities; difficulty with social interactions more generally) to factors related to the communication partner (difficulty interpreting a child's expression of emotion; low awareness of the need to address emotional development) and/or external or attitude barriers such as myths about emotional development in individuals with CCN or technology limitations (Blackstone & Wilkins, 2009; Na et al., 2016). The presence of these barriers means that children with CCN may have restricted opportunities to learn to communicate about their emotions using conventional means.

This observation by Blackstone and Wilkins (2009) is supported by emerging data from our own laboratories. For instance, the third author has interviewed 24 families with children with CCN from Sweden, India, Mexico, the United States, and Spain, in Spanish and in English, using an interview tool that is discussed in detail later in this chapter. A consistent theme in these interviews is that emotional expression is particularly challenging for persons with CCN whose idiosyncratic body-based modes of expression (posture, facial expression, etc.) are difficult to interpret. Parents of children with CCN comment on their inability to determine why their children are frustrated, or why they engage in other behaviors. One parent noted, "*Sometimes, I don't know why my child feels/behaves like that.*" Another parent reported that "*Although her Dad and I explain things to her, she suddenly cries seemingly for no reason, or worse, makes a tremendous tantrum.*" One parent of a 5-year old noted:

With her intellectual deficiency and lack of language, it is difficult to identify her emotions. Sometimes her mood is very flat, and yet, I know her feelings are there, like when sometimes her brother gets more attention, and she isolates herself and feels sad. Or when she once watched a scene of "The Ugly Duckling" and cried silently. Or when she gets angry if we try to give her some new food. Or when she gets happy when we go to the park. But on other occasions, I have not been able to identify her crying, anger, or laughs, and that generates a lot of frustration and anxiety for me.

As illustrated by these observations, individuals may engage in challenging or unconventional behaviors when they experience communication limitations, including difficulties in expressing or understanding emotional situations. AAC can play a role in the development of skills that help individuals with CCN regulate their behavior. For instance, a number of clinical research efforts have focused on identifying the function of challenging behavior and then finding a replacement behavior (using AAC) that serves the same function, while being equally efficient and effective as the original behavior (Mirenda & Brown, 2007; Reichle & Johnston, 1993). An example of this would be when AAC is used to replace an aggressive act that serves as an escape behavior with an AAC message that requests a break. Another evidence-based means for supporting individuals with CCN in understanding potential emotional situations are social stories (Gray & Garand, 1993). Social stories follow a specific structure that break situations down via task analysis into their critical parts, allowing individuals with CCN to anticipate upcoming events and scaffold their behavior within those events. An example of this might be a social story that promotes appropriate behavior for entering a peer group at recess that would include an introduction to the topic ("In third period there is recess"), the perspective of the individual using the social story ("I want to play with friends at recess"), a body that provides detail ("I will watch my friends. I will approach my friends. I will ask if I can play"), and a conclusion with possible outcomes ("When it is my turn, I will join the game"). Social stories are generated through careful observations of individuals who might use them as well as from detailed information gathered from the individual, caregivers, and other sources.

Although both of these strategies have been demonstrated to be effective at promoting specific desired behaviors, we propose that there is value in adding vocabulary that allows for discussion of the emotions themselves, as well as the antecedent events/experiences leading to the emotions (the reason for the emotion), and the functional strategies that could be used to manage the emotions (the response strategies). Adding this vocabulary to AAC systems, and aiding parents in using it to discuss emotions with their children, could offer families a means to respond to the challenges highlighted in the following quote from the family of Sophie.

> *When she is happy, everyone is happy, and we expressed, "Wow! That's great, fun, and exciting!" But when she is sad, angry, and cries, we are sometimes annoyed and say: "Oh my god, she is going to start again." Generally, we ask her what's going on? But she doesn't have a way to answer to us. So, we try to calm her down and tell her: "you must not cry" "no one has done anything to you, so stop being angry" "your teddy bear is leaving, he gets sad when you cry, so he is going away." Then, she continues crying, and sometimes I hug or squeeze her, take her to her room, bathe her, go to take a walk around the street, or cuddle her. We try to use some technique to respond to what is happening and try to control her.*

This quote illustrates that parents find it challenging not just to interpret their child's emotion-related behaviors and the reasons behind them, but also to come up with ways to respond to that behavior given that, as the parents note, "she doesn't have a way to answer to us." In this chapter, we argue that it is critical to empower the individual with CCN to begin to comprehend, express, and internalize the communication strategies that might promote independent emotional competencies.

Responding to the Challenge: AAC System Design and the EDEC Instrument

Na et al. (2016) argued that AAC systems should include vocabulary to allow for three specific types of communication regarding emotions: (1) a variety of labels for emotions, beyond common labels such as "happy" or "angry"; (2) a means to validate and discuss the reasons underlying the emotion; and (3) a means to strategize possible responses to the emotion.

Rationale for This Approach

Providing a variety of emotion labels allows the child to cultivate an awareness of the diversity of their own emotional states as well as the states of others around them. Yet simply having labels for the emotion does not provide an opportunity for rich discussion about the reasons for or the responses to the emotions. A child who is crying may have a range of reasons for that behavior; perhaps someone teased them, or perhaps they are frustrated for some reason, or feeling left out of a group, or perhaps they are hot and overtired. Each of those reasons is quite different from one another, and different types of language need to be available to talk about the different causes. Another critical step is to allow the child to consider the possible responses to the emotion, which will themselves vary depending on the underlying reason. For instance, the response when the child is crying due to being overly hot will be different than the response for that child who is feeling left out. Na et al. (2016) offered a detailed model of AAC designs that could incorporate these; a simpler form of a display that would have these different types of language symbols is presented in Figure 12–1.

As Na et al. (2016, also Na, Liang, & Wilkinson, 2018) noted, if AAC systems do not contain diverse vocabulary to engage in these discussions, then children with CCN will not have access either to the scaffolding that would occur via augmented input from communication partners or to the means to express themselves via AAC regarding their emotions. Thus, the theorized scaffolding mechanisms that likely promote the development of both language and emotional competencies in children learning to speak will be unavailable to children using AAC unless the system is specifically designed to include relevant language. In addition to the provision of the three important types of vocabulary, the discussions about emotions must be moderated and scaffolded by caregivers before expecting the child to begin to express them independently. Just as caregivers provide oral models for children learning to speak ("Oh, you look happy! [label] Is that because your friend just gave you a teddy bear? [reason] Let's go thank your friend" [response]), adults should provide aided input in their dis-

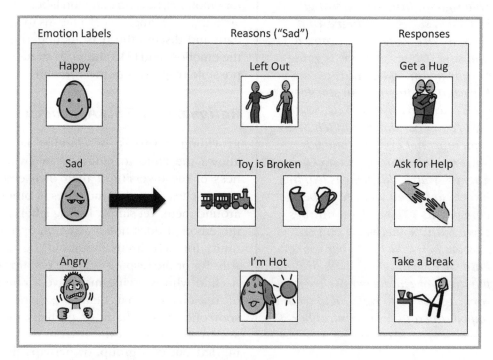

Figure 12–1. Simple communication board with vocabulary related to labels, reasons, and responses.

cussions of emotions with children who are using AAC.

Not only does this promote support for the child's comprehension of the AAC symbols, it provides the child an opportunity to internalize the language and, in turn, begins to use it independently and for their own self-regulation (Vygotsky, 1986). In addition, as Na et al. (2016) noted, these scaffolded discussions should not be initiated during moments of heightened emotional states; the midst of a tantrum is not the ideal time to initiate this type of discussion. Rather, caregivers might use preferred activities to discuss emotions. For example, a family may enjoy watching television together. This would be an ideal time to discuss emotions, reasons, and potential responses of the characters in the show, as well as their own and family members' emotions about the show. Depending on the family's preferences, this same scenario could be applied to book reading, dinner conversation, or other engaging activities.

The EDEC: Soliciting Family Preferences for Communication About Emotions

An important consideration in designing AAC to promote conversations about emotions is the recognition that the process of learning to respond to and conversing about emotions is highly family- and culture-specific. Substantial literature indicates that although the experience of emotions is universal, specific responses to those experiences is the product of socialization within and across cultures (for instance, see Cole, Bruschi, & Tamang, 2002; Cole, Tamang, & Shrestha, 2006; Cole & Tan, 2015; Raval V., Martini, & Raval P. 2007; Raval V., Martini, & Raval P. 2010; Raver, 2004). Preferences regarding conversations with children about the experience of and response to emotions will, therefore, vary within and across families and cultures. Designing an AAC system that includes culturally and linguistically appropriate vocabulary for conversation about emotions cannot use a "one-size fits all" approach (Na et al., 2018). Even the selection of the types of symbols to be included in the AAC may warrant careful consideration (Na et al., 2018).

For this reason, Na et al. (2018) developed an instrument to solicit family preferences about such conversations that could guide decision making about AAC in this area. This instrument, called the Early Development of Emotional Competencies (EDEC), solicits information from parents and/or professionals about how children currently understand and express emotions, what the family (or professional) preferences are concerning emotional expression and conversations about emotions, and the family's (or professional's) current methods for conversing about emotions with their children. As the instructions note, the EDEC has two goals: (a) to raise awareness of the importance of communication about emotions, in family and culturally sensitive ways, and (b) to guide intervention decisions that allow AAC to support communication in ways that are consistent with family preferences. The EDEC consists of two main sections, one with 10 prompts to solicit information about the child's temperament and behavior, and another with 14 prompts to solicit information about the child's communication and family dynamics related to communication about emotions. This second section in particular solicits information in three key areas; (1) the child's current means of expressing or understanding emotions; (2) the events or experiences that may cause or trigger emotions; and (3) the ways in which communication partners respond to emotional expression and how they engage in prompting for the child to communicate emotions.

The EDEC was initially developed and field-tested with input from expert clinicians in the United States. After this, the EDEC underwent a rigorous 5-step process of translation, evaluation, and back-translation into two languages, Korean and Mandarin Chinese (the steps for translation were adapted from guidelines in Kang, Shin, & Song, 2010; see details of the steps in Na et al., 2018). Refinement of word selection, syntax, and examples within the EDEC occurred during this process, and the EDEC was evaluated by professionals within each language/cultural community to ensure acceptability of the content and language of the questions. The final step of back-translation was verification that the reverse-translated EDEC resulted in similar language/concepts as the original version. The tools in each of the three languages (English, Korean, and Chinese) are available for free download (https://figshare.com/articles/_/5643076). The instrument has also undergone the translation process for Spanish.

The final EDEC instruments in all languages were then field tested with 47 families that had children with typical development, and who were raising their children in the United States (families with children without disabilities were used for field testing in order to ensure the instrument itself was useful and culturally appropriate, before implementing it with families with a child with a disability). This field test included 10 English speakers from mainstream the United States, 10 Korean speakers, 10 Mandarin Chinese speakers, 10 Spanish speakers (from Mexico), and seven families from the Anishinaabe Native American community in Minnesota. These field tests revealed that the language of the instrument was acceptable to members of diverse linguistic/cultural communities and that detailed information about family-specific preferences regarding communication about emotions could be obtained (Wilkinson et al., 2018).

Summary: Designing AAC to Support Communication About Emotions

We argue that AAC system design should explicitly include language to communicate about emotions, with a particular emphasis on vocabulary for labeling diverse emotions, for discussing reasons for the emotions, and for strategizing a response to the emotion. Adding this type of language would allow clinicians to augment current evidence-based practices in replacing challenging behaviors as well as supporting appropriate behaviors via social stories. This language would also offer the individual with CCN the tools to begin to learn to independently identify and respond to different emotions. In the remainder of this chapter, we (1) discuss how the EDEC can be used for both purposes (raising awareness and guiding intervention decisions), across families of children with CCN from diverse linguistic and cultural communities; (2) review an intervention package that builds from the EDEC to aid parents in conversing with their children about emotions; (3) offer a detailed case study to illustrate the applications of the EDEC and the STEPS intervention; and (4) identify some other applications and future directions for research and practice in this area.

■ The EDEC Interview Tool

Raising Awareness of the Importance of Communication About Emotions

For many individuals, simply undergoing the EDEC interview can create awareness about the importance of starting to talk about emotions. The EDEC interview can also help families identify which strategies they might be comfortable using during these discussions. For instance, after the EDEC interview, parents reported the following comments:

> *I realized that I overlooked the importance of the feelings, even if they were there. . . . I think that feelings are something that should be explained or discussed*
> (Mateo's dad—3yo)
>
> *I realized that in the family we do not usually talk about our emotions. Everyone lives (the emotions) individually, and others interpret or assume what happens. From the interview, I am more aware of identifying my emotional changes and explaining it to Mateo.*
> (Mateo's mom—3yo)
>
> *I was impressed that I could discover more emotions that I thought my daughter feels. . . . I also realize that maybe I should pay more attention to emotions and "named" them to help my daughter and myself to differentiate them and know what to do when a specific emotion appears.*
> (Clara's mom—10yo)

> *I found the interview very interesting and I really think is nice the idea to learn how to help Ari to communicate and know how to differentiate the different emotions we can feel and know how to communicate them.*
> (Ari's mom—6yo)

These comments indicate that raising awareness of communication outcomes can be an important outcome of the interview. Future research should examine in closer detail the extent to which this effect holds across different families and also how such initial exposure to the awareness (the interview) affects long-term behavior by parents in communicating about emotions.

EDEC Guiding AAC Decision Making

In a quote provided earlier, Sophie's mother reported:

> *When she is happy, everyone is happy, and we expressed, "Wow! That's great, fun, and exciting!" But when she is sad, angry, and cries, we are sometimes annoyed and said, "Oh my god, she is going to start again." Generally, we ask her what's going on? But she doesn't have a way to answer us. So, we try to calm her down and tell her, "you must not cry" "no one has done anything to you, so stop being angry" "your teddy bear is leaving, he gets sad when you cry, so he is*

> *going away." Then, if she continues crying, sometimes I hug or squeeze her, take her to her room, bath her, go to take a walk around the street, or cuddle her. We try to use some technique to respond to what is happening and try to control her.*

With respect to how Sophie expresses emotions, the EDEC interview revealed that she is using her body, facial expressions, and vocalizations. Yet these methods of expression appear to be insufficient to communicate the reasons for Sophie's emotions, and what might help her to feel better. Moreover, it is possible that her frustration with communication is contributing to the challenging behavior she presents. An AAC system that provides Sophie and her family more conventional means to label these emotions, as well as to identify their causes or triggers is, therefore, the next critical step in AAC decision making. For example, Sophie may engage in behaviors that her family interprets as "angry" when in reality she has nothing to do. In this case, the behavior is reflecting the concept of "I'm bored," rather than actual anger. It may be important, once the EDEC is complete, to collaborate with a behavior specialist to conduct a functional analysis of Sophie's behaviors to clarify or verify the function of the behaviors (e.g., see Matson & Minshawi, 2007 for a review). Careful functional analysis can directly examine the antecedents and consequences that are triggering and maintaining Sophie's behavior, and to confirm or enrich the parent report from the EDEC.

Once the functions of Sophie's behaviors are established, (through the information obtained from the EDEC and, where necessary, direct functional analysis of Sophie's behavior), the AAC system can be set up to allow discussions of the reasons for the emotions themselves. Promoting discussion of the reasons for the behavior not only changes the parents' perceptions of that behavior, but also allows refinement of the communication partner's response. For example, if the reason for the behavior is boredom, then Sophie would benefit from having vocabulary to communicate, "I'm bored" (the emotion), perhaps caused by Sophie feeling that she has nothing to do (the cause). In this case, appropriate solutions might be and "I want to listen to music" or "I want to go outside" (potential solutions). Without such vocabulary, the challenging behavior is Sophie's only mode to communicate how she feels.

Na et al. (2016) suggested that an enjoyable and meaningful activity should be the initial context for introducing discussion of emotions, causes, and possible responses. This is in part because when a learning experience is associated with a pleasant emotion, people learn and consolidate the information received more effectively (Mora, 2013). In addition, any challenging situation can be tiring and stressful and may not be optimal for the participants (in this case, Sophie) to learn. We, therefore, suggest that conversations about emotions happen in low-stress natural situations (e.g., Na et al., 2018). For example, the parents reported that Sophie and her family enjoy watching videos while being interviewed with the EDEC. This daily activity provides an opportunity for Sophie's parents to start talking about emotions of the characters in the video, modeling the use of the AAC vocabulary for labeling the emotions and conversing about possible causes and responses. Finally, as Sophie develops, learns new skills, and enters new environments, the preliminary intervention plans that result from the EDEC information will require reevaluation and feedback to make changes and adaptations if needed.

The STEPS Intervention for Supporting Communication About Emotions

Children who have CCN often spend much of their time with parents and close caregivers. Therefore, training parents and caregivers of children with CCN is critical in communication development, including emotion-related conversations. Because the EDEC is designed to interview parents and professionals of children with CCN, a natural follow-up is to train those adults how to support their children's communication about emotions. The Strategies for Talking about Emotions as PartnerS (STEPS) instructional program was developed by Na and Wilkinson (2015) with this goal in mind.

Description of the STEPS Intervention

The STEPS instructional program was designed based on the recommendations in Na et al. (2016). The recommendations included the following three practical steps for parents/caregivers to follow during a conversation about emotions with a child who can be benefitted by using AAC. The three steps are: (1) Step 1: Providing and modeling labels for a variety of emotions; (2) Step 2: Validating and discussing emotions; (3) Step 3: Communicating about appropriate responses to emotions. The STEPS program instructs parents on how to discuss emotions at these three levels of emotion conversations. In

each level (label, reason, and solution), the parent initiates by asking the child an open-ended question about an emotion to discuss. For example, at the level of "labeling" of an emotion, the parents are recommended to ask, "How does the monkey feel here?" while reading a book about a monkey who has fallen from a tree. Then, the parent should wait at least 5 seconds to provide an opportunity for the child to respond to the question. The parent might need to wait longer until the child begins to answer, depending on their intellectual and/or physical profiles. Once the parent received a correct/incorrect or no response from the child after a certain period spent, the parent provides feedback with modelling of a correct labeling (e.g., "sad" for the monkey fallen from a tree). These three discussion strategies (i.e., ask, wait and respond) should be repeated for the three levels of emotion conversations suggested by Na et al. (2016). Figure 12–2 presents detailed guidance about how parents can follow these recommendations from the STEPS instructional program with some examples. The STEPS program also provides instructions for parents to design an emotion communication board, either as a separate page or as part of the child's current AAC system.

Na and Wilkinson (2017) conducted a single-subject study to evaluate the effectiveness of the STEPS instructional program with three parents of children with Down syndrome. The STEPS program can be used with anyone who can benefit from using visual aids for emotion conversations, including children with Down syndrome. The participating children were in the age range of 5:0 to 10:11, and had 50% speech intelligibility or less to an unfamiliar listener and previous or current exposure to aided AAC systems.

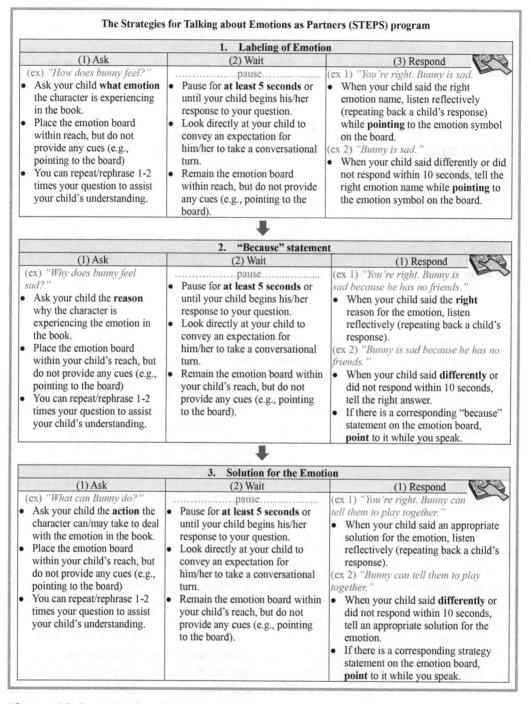

The Strategies for Talking about Emotions as Partners (STEPS) program

1. Labeling of Emotion		
(1) Ask	**(2) Wait**	**(3) Respond**
(ex) *"How does bunny feel?"* • Ask your child **what emotion** the character is experiencing in the book. • Place the emotion board within reach, but do not provide any cues (e.g., pointing to the board) • You can repeat/rephrase 1-2 times your question to assist your child's understanding.	...............pause............... • Pause for **at least 5 seconds** or until your child begins his/her response to your question. • Look directly at your child to convey an expectation for him/her to take a conversational turn. • Remain the emotion board within reach, but do not provide any cues (e.g., pointing to the board).	(ex 1) *"You're right. Bunny is sad.* • When your child said the right emotion name, listen reflectively (repeating back a child's response) while **pointing** to the emotion symbol on the board. (ex 2) *"Bunny is sad."* • When your child said differently or did not respond within 10 seconds, tell the right emotion name while **pointing** to the emotion symbol on the board.

2. "Because" statement		
(1) Ask	**(2) Wait**	**(1) Respond**
(ex) *"Why does bunny feel sad?"* • Ask your child the **reason** why the character is experiencing the emotion in the book. • Place the emotion board within your child's reach, but do not provide any cues (e.g., pointing to the board) • You can repeat/rephrase 1-2 times your question to assist your child's understanding.	...............pause............... • Pause for **at least 5 seconds** or until your child begins his/her response to your question. • Look directly at your child to convey an expectation for him/her to take a conversational turn. • Remain the emotion board within your child's reach, but do not provide any cues (e.g., pointing to the board).	(ex 1) *"You're right. Bunny is sad because he has no friends."* • When your child said the **right** reason for the emotion, listen reflectively (repeating back a child's response). (ex 2) *"Bunny is sad because he has no friends."* • When your child said **differently** or did not respond within 10 seconds, tell the right answer. • If there is a corresponding "because" statement on the emotion board, **point** to it while you speak.

3. Solution for the Emotion		
(1) Ask	**(2) Wait**	**(1) Respond**
(ex) *"What can Bunny do?"* • Ask your child the **action** the character can/may take to deal with the emotion in the book. • Place the emotion board within your child's reach, but do not provide any cues (e.g., pointing to the board) • You can repeat/rephrase 1-2 times your question to assist your child's understanding.	...............pause............... • Pause for **at least 5 seconds** or until your child begins his/her response to your question. • Look directly at your child to convey an expectation for him/her to take a conversational turn. • Remain the emotion board within your child's reach, but do not provide any cues (e.g., pointing to the board).	(ex 1) *"You're right. Bunny can tell them to play together."* • When your child said an appropriate solution for the emotion, listen reflectively (repeating back a child's response). (ex 2) *"Bunny can tell them to play together."* • When your child said **differently** or did not respond within 10 seconds, tell an appropriate solution for the emotion. • If there is a corresponding strategy statement on the emotion board, **point** to it while you speak.

Figure 12–2. STEPS handout for parents.

During the parent instruction phase, the parents were trained in the STEPS program as to how to talk about emotions in storybooks. Storybook reading was selected because it provides a rich context for language development and a naturalistic context for conversations about emotion. Moreover, it allowed for the discussion of emotions during a time in which the child was not in a state of heightened emotional arousal.

The results revealed an immediate effect of the STEPS instructional program. The parents were provided frequent opportunities to use each of the three elements of emotion communication using the parent-designed emotion communication boards. Their children also increased the number of emotion-related utterances through various communication modes, including intelligible words and selections on the emotion communication boards. Another positive change also occurred during the postinstruction phases on the parents' design of emotion communication boards. Whereas in the baseline phase parents included only labels for emotions, after STEPS intervention, all parents began to include multi-symbol expressions for each of the three levels (label, reasons, solution) of emotion communication on their emotion boards as trained.

Using Information From the EDEC to Guide Parent Instruction

Having some basic information about the parent's perception of the child's emotion expression and recognition skills is helpful to guide therapeutic decision making for intervention with each participant, particularly for parent instruction. Knowing how the parent might typically discuss emotions during shared book reading can be discussed during the instruction phase. Na (2015) conducted parent interviews using the EDEC tool during the screening phase and at the end of the study. During the pre-experiment EDEC interview,

all three parents reported that they rarely discuss the emotion labels and never talked about the reasons and solutions for the emotions during storybook reading.

Parent #1
I mean I have a background in education, so just the basics. In terms of how do you see a situation and you say, "how does the little boy feel," "how would that make him feel," "how would that make you feel"— just the basics though, ya know. In helping to identify the emotions.

Parent #2
Um. In the book. I would probably change the inflection of my voice. Like you know when your voice goes high up when they're happy or down when they're sad. Different voices for different people. We might look at the picture and ask questions like..., "Do you think they're happy/ sad?" Maybe a little bit of that. Like I said, we're more focused on the reading part so I think this is great to add another layer on it for him.

Parent #3
No. And, I would say to a degree of basic plot summary you know what's going on here, you know he has oranges. What do you think about that? Do you think that will help him? Oh, look at the ice cream flavors. But, we don't really get into kind of emotions of the characters.

Based on this background information gathered during the pre-experiment EDEC, the practitioner could discuss with each parent how they could enrich their conversations about emotions when they read storybook using the STEPS program.

During the postexperiment EDEC interview, two parents reported that they had a conversation about emotions during their shared book reading, and the other said that they sometimes did, depending on the book.

■ Case Study of EDEC and STEPS for AAC Design for a Child With CCN

In this section, we offer a detailed case of the use of the EDEC with Elvira, who is the mother of Laia, a 10-year-old child with CCN. We illustrate how the EDEC helped raise Elvira's awareness of the importance of communicating about emotions, in ways that are consistent with family preferences. We also illustrate how the results from the EDEC helped to guide decision-making about the AAC methods and vocabulary to add for the family. Finally, we discuss how the STEPS intervention helped the family feel comfortable integrating these discussions into their daily activities.

At the beginning of the assessment, Elvira was asked to express how she feels about talking about emotions with her daughter. Elvira responded:

Since my daughter was born and perhaps before, emotions have meant a lot in my life. I think emotions are a reflection of the deepest part of our being and speak about who we really are.

From my experience as a mother of a daughter with disabilities, emotions are a priority because I experience them in that different motherhood. Along this path, I have learned to recognize and name them. I felt them before, but I didn't know how to label them.

My daughter is 10 years old, and due to lack of oxygen, she had a brain injury when she was born. I have learned many things with her, one of them is to try to recognize and validate her emotions, a more difficult task than with my other children. However, I must confess that it is also a complex task to teach a regular child to express and name their emotions. In my case, I was taught that crying, getting angry, or any "negative"

emotion was not "good," and unconsciously you are transmitting those messages to your children. In situations as small as, for example, if she falls, "don't cry anymore, nothing happens . . . ," or if she loses in the game or something was taken away from her, "don't get mad, nothing happens, I'll get you another one."

The emotions of babies and young children are the only ones that are expressed day by day, and for that, they begin to use primary language such as cry, smile, or laugh. But as they grow, emotions become more complex, the language and speech begin, so they start little by little expressing their emotions or what they need. In my case, with my daughter, the process has been different. As a cause of the injury, her oral language was affected. Therefore, it has taken her more work to let me know how she feels.

A few years ago, she started using communication boards on the iPad or sign language. *That also helped her to say at least if she felt good or bad.*

Unfortunately, it is more complex for me to know her emotions and react to her discomforts. Before having some support such as emotional boards, it was easier to react by saying: "stop crying, don't smack, or don't swing anymore" (reactions generally used for discomfort or anger).

. . . I think it is essential to have and be able to understand her emotions and what she will be feeling, especially now that soon she will enter puberty. I know it is a difficult time because of all hormonal adjustments, and I would like to feel close to her to understand more how she feels, to have tools to communicate better, and that we can understand her own emotions about what she is living. Moreover, I know that I also need to integrate those own emotions and accept the reality of her growth.

I know it is not an easy task, but if we have tools that help us, we can feel better. That is why it is very important for me to learn to talk about emotions with my daughter.

During the EDEC Interview

During the interview, Elvira reported that Laia is an active, outgoing, optimistic, distractible, predictable, and charismatic girl, who sometimes is reserved with strangers. Elvira perceived her daughter as a self-confident girl who loves listening to storybooks.

Elvira commented that Laia, "*has difficulties in expressing her emotions*" properly. Elvira reported that Laia has a non-electronic communication aid (a printed book) that Laia rarely uses. Laia typically uses the board if an adult brings it and asks her to use it; however, even this type of prompted use is infrequent. At the time of the EDEC interview, this board contained seven symbols for emotions. Elvira also reported that at the time of the EDEC, Laia could pronounce some words like: happy, nervous, sad, and scared, but her speech lacked clarity and thus was difficult to understand. As Elvira underwent the interview, she identified that Laia expresses more than just "happiness." Laia also expresses what Elvira described as excitement and euphoria. Each of these was expressed in different ways; happiness was expressed by smiling and vocalizing, excitement by smiling and moving her body "like jumping," and euphoria by smiling, moving her body with more intensity, and shouting.

When asked about the possible triggers for emotions, Elvira identified certain situations, as illustrated in Table 12–1. Even though she could identify some causes, Elvira indicated: "*It's sometimes complicated to identify what caused her emotion, especially when they are negative.*"

In general, Laia's communication partners reported they only occasionally tried to get Laia to label her emotions; they did not tend to encourage it. Nevertheless, when Laia expresses some emotion, Elvira reported that she tries to understand how Laia feels and why. Elvira reported that she sometimes makes an effort to corroborate if she is right, asking, "*why do you feel like that?,*" "*do you feel angry because you can't go to play?*" When the answer is

Table 12–1. Perceptions of Elvira About Her Daughter Laia's Emotions Collected From the EDEC Interview

Causes That Can Trigger Emotions	Emotion	Expression
*meeting people she likes (friends, brothers, etc.)	Euphoria	*hugs strong *moves her body *shouts
*new or unknown situations	Fear/Anxiety	*pulls the clothes *repeats words or noises
*someone takes something from her	Anger	*flutters *slaps
*When things don't go her way	Sadness/Anger	*flutters *slaps *cries *difficult to answer how she feels or needs (even if someone asks her)
*Physical challenges	Frustration	
*When she has bathroom accidents	Nervousness	

yes, Elvira tries to give options verbally to make her feel better.

Elvira noted that she expresses all the emotions she feels in front of Laia, except for intense emotions of sadness and worry. Laia's Dad only feels comfortable expressing happiness in front of his daughter. However, Elvira remarked that neither parent talk consciously about feelings with Laia. In the EDEC interview, Elvira made comments about starting to be aware of the importance of talking about emotions, such as, *"maybe we should start labeling emotions more often."*

After the EDEC Interview

After the EDEC interview, the clinician asked Elvira to write about her perceptions, ideas, emotions, or reactions that appeared after the meeting. She wrote:

Although I knew that Laia had certain ways to express emotions, I realize that I don't have the necessary emotional training . . .

I felt a little frustrated because Laia does not have the traditional ways—as my other children do with their voice- of telling me she feels bad, something bothers her, or something doesn't like it. . . . I feel that in most of the occasions, when I scold her, Laia reacts without knowing what to do and react in ways that annoy me (for example, peeing). I wish I couldn't hurt her or put pressure on her . . .

I realized that I still have a lot to learn on this topic with my daughter, but, at the same time, I feel confident that little by little, we are getting to know each other.

> *. . . it made me more aware of my surroundings and what could affect her; she is very sensitive and perceives many more things than we as parents believe.*
>
> *I suddenly understood how important it is to know how we feel, validate it, and to know and express what to do with that emotion.*
>
> *I think I can be more aware of what causes me a specific feeling,* *and then know how I should handle it better. Subsequently, I can be conscious and aware of my daughter's emotions and help her to manage her negative emotions better, especially frustration.*
>
> *I believe it's a good time for us to have more communication and emotional tools for the next stage of development: adolescence.*

These comments support the first aim of the EDEC, that is, of raising Elvira's awareness about the relationship between emotional competence and language (Na et al., 2018). Moreover, it seems that Elvira was also more conscious about how she responds and what changes she can make to facilitate healthy communication about emotions.

The information from the EDEC also offers a range of potential guidance for structuring Laia's AAC system to promote more clear communication about emotions, which is the second aim of the EDEC. For instance, the family was uncomfortable with the shouting behaviors associated with euphoria, and reported that it was a challenge to respond to that behavior. This information can inform choices for AAC. It would be relevant to incorporate vocabulary such as *happy, excited,* and *euphoric,* either directly within Laia's existing AAC system or, if there are space constraints in the existing system, on a separate stand-alone page. The clinician could then work with Elvira to determine appropriate times and contexts for Elvira and Laia to take opportunities to talk about these feelings and to express them using more conventional symbols. Similarly, vocabulary could be added to discuss situations that are associated with behaviors of anger or sadness as well as to consider alternative means to respond to those emotions.

Post-EDEC Intervention

After the EDEC interview was complete, the clinician made observations from video recordings of a storybook reading activity between Elvira and Laia to understand their current general communication and especially the communication about emotions between them. The observations demonstrated that Laia enjoys the storybook activity, pays attention, and responds to some comments Elvira makes while reading. Elvira sometimes talks about the emotions of the book's characters and asks her, "How do you think -the character- feels?" Laia occasionally responds to these types of open-ended question, but other times she starts moving her body back and forth. Her most reliable response is when the question is asked in yes/no format ("Do you think the character is happy?").

The clinician met with Elvira to explain the current emotional and communicative competencies shown by Laia and suggested activities to foster communication about emotions. Storybook reading was recommended as an activity to foster communication about emotions, as Elvira reported that both she and Laia enjoyed reading books together. Elvira, together with the clinician, chose storybooks of interest to Laia that included opportunities to talk about emotions. The clinician instructed Elvira in the STEPS program so she could talk not only about the characters' emotions but also the causes of their feelings and the possible responses available to the character. The clinician then created communication boards according to the family's cultural and linguistic context.

Elvira reported that even though Laia uses speech, her verbal communication is not as spontaneous when expressing emotions, and her speech sometimes becomes unintelligible. Prior to intervention, Elvira and other communication partners rarely prompted her to use her AAC communication aid, both in general and to discuss emotions. Elvira received the STEPS instruction to model and encourage communication about emotions using aided AAC while reading a storybook. The clinician worked with Elvira to accomplish these objectives, facilitate AAC resources, and give feedback on their achievements.

Elvira noted that Laia started talking more about emotions in the storybook reading activity and communicated using her aided AAC system, gestures, vocalizations, facial expressions, and speech. She employed vocabulary to discuss characters' feelings, why they felt as they did, and what could they do when feeling an emotion. The communication boards and Elvira's communication support helped Laia to expand and grow more vocabulary about emotions, and she started expressing it verbally too. For instance,

her AAC symbol vocabulary grew from 7 symbols to 30 and is beginning to distinguish subtle emotions such as "afraid" versus "nervous." One video taken post-intervention shows Laia verbalizing and pointing to symbols to communicate: *"I'm in my house with my brothers and parents, and I feel (points in her board) HAPPY and EXCITED."* Importantly, little by little Elvira started using the aided AAC to talk about emotions in other daily situations, for example, how Elvira feels or how Laia's brothers might feel as well. These case observations parallel and reinforce the experimental findings reported in Na and Wilkinson (2017).

After the intervention, Elvira stated:

> *I have managed to identify and realize that something is happening with the emotions of Laia, and also mine. That has allowed me to be more aware at the moment when an emotion arises and to address it properly and with more serenity. The strategies suggested for Laia and me have helped me to understand the emotions, label them, and know how to solve and deal with them.*
>
> *Before the intervention, it was hard for me to identify some emotions in Laia, and of course, we did not have the means and supports so I could communicate with her fully. Although she has speech and articulates better, it is difficult to identify some of her emotions. Today I feel I have more tools to help my daughter recognize her emotions and at least identify that something is happening.*
>
> *Laia likes the storybook reading activity with the suggestions proposed*

in the sessions. She already identifies how the characters feel and spontaneously points out the icons of what those characters can do to face some situations.

I'm grateful for everything I've been learning and I feel great that I can give my daughter the tools she needed to know herself and feel valuable for what she feels and thinks.

Elvira reported gaining confidence and generalizing the strategies learned in other daily situations, including the ones where Laia presented heightened emotional arousal and challenging behaviors. Even though Laia needs more time to generalize what she has learned spontaneously, Elvira perceived that she has gained useful strategies that help her to give the support that Laia needs. If Elvira is calm and more confident, it will be easier to adapt to various situations. Future research should continue to study the impact of the STEPS intervention.

■ Other Potential Applications of the EDEC and STEPS Approaches

There are other possible ways that information from the EDEC interviews can benefit the child with CCN and the family. We describe a few of them here.

Checklist for Families and Professionals

A checklist version of the full EDEC tool has been developed based on clinicians'

feedback regarding the lengthy interview using the tool (Figure 12–3). The checklist version has the same sections as the original EDEC tool, but is intended as a "self-check" tool for parents to maintain the primary ideas in mind. Specifically, a parent and/or a teacher of a child with CCN can fill out by selecting one of the provided answer options (e.g., often, sometimes, rarely, never, not sure) for each question. The last few questions are open-ended designed to allow them to reflect the quality of their communication about emotions with their children who have CCN.

The checklist version of the EDEC tool offers at least two possible benefits. First, parents or teachers can report their observations on the child's emotion communication just by filling out the one-and-a-half-page checklist, rather than an hourlong EDEC interview. This is intended to let them repeat this process more often, and in turn monitor major and/or subtle changes regarding the child's emotion communication. In addition, parents or teachers could hang the checklist version of the EDEC on a wall (or refrigerator door) for ready daily access. Doing so could remind the parents and teachers to include different elements of emotion communication when discussing emotions with children who have CCN. For example, they might not only ask about the emotion name, but also check a child's access to emotion words/symbols. In addition, the few questions about adults' support for children's communication about emotions included in the checklist could help them to develop their own support strategies. Future research is necessary to evaluate the effectiveness of such strategies. Finally, another possible benefit of the checklist would be to allow parents and professionals to compare

- CHECKLIST -					
EARLY DEVELOPMENT OF EMOTIONAL COMPETENCE: A TOOL FOR CHILDREN WITH COMPLEX COMMUNICATION NEEDS (CCN)					
(Na, Wilkinson, Epstein, Rangel, Townsend, Thistle, Feldman, & Blackstone, 2014)					

BACKGROUND INFORMATION

Child's initials		Examiner's initials	
Date of Birth		Examiner's profession	
Nationality		Informant's initials	
Child's diagnosis		Informant's role	(e.g., parent, teacher)
Date of interview		Language for interview	

Section I: Child's Temperament	Yes	No	Not sure
1. Does {name} seem to enjoy being with **others**?			
2. Would you describe {name} as **affectionate**, in general?			
3. Would you describe {name} showing a strong **attachment** to others?			
4. Does {name} try to play with **peers**?			
5. How often does (name) show a **fear** of strangers?			
6. How often does (name) display **temper tantrums**?			
7. How often does (name) intentionally **hurt** themselves or other people?			
8. How often does (name) intentionally **damage** property?			

Section II: Child's Emotion Communication					
EMOTIONS	Often	Sometimes	Rarely	Never	Not sure
Affection/Love					
Anger					
Fear					
Joy/happiness					
Sadness					
Surprise					
Disgust					
Pride					
Adoration					
Amazement					
Cheerfulness					
Excitement					
Jealous/Envy					
Nervousness/ Anxiety					
Irritation/ Frustration					
Shame/ Embarrassment					

Emotion discussion					
1. How many signs, words or symbols are **available** on his/her system to **label** emotions?	< 6	6-10	11-20	20 <	50 <
2. How many signs, words, or other symbols does {name} **use** to **label** emotions?	< 6	6-10	11-20	20 <	50 <
3. How many signs, words, or other symbols does {name} **use** to **talk about** the related events?	< 6	6-10	11-20	20 <	50 <
4. Does {name} use these (signs, spoken words, and/or graphic symbols) in lots of different **settings**?	Often	Sometimes	Rarely	Never	Not sure
5. How often do you **try** to get {name} to label his/her own emotions using words, signs, or symbols?	Often	Sometimes	Rarely	Never	Not sure
6. How often does {name} **respond** to others emotions?	Often	Sometimes	Rarely	Never	Not sure
7. When {name} expresses emotion, in what ways do you **respond**?					

Figure 12–3. Brief EDEC checklist. *continues*

8. How does {name} **respond** when other people are expressing emotion?	
9. What kinds of emotions do you feel comfortable expressing **in front of** {name}?	
10. When you do **share** or talk about emotions with your child, what things do you say or do?	
11. How do you and your child "**gear up**" for difficult tasks and how do you "unwind" afterward?	
12. When you are reading **books** or watching **TV/movies**, do you talk about the emotions that the characters are experiencing?	

Figure 12–3. *continued*

their answers, as it might be that there are differences in interpretation of certain behaviors, or that one member has figured out a trigger that would be important to the other as well.

EDEC in Conjunction With Biomedical Signs

An additional application for the EDEC interviews is using the information to interpret the children's emotion/state-related biomedical signs. In case of children with severe and multiple disabilities who have very limited attention and responses to the presented stimuli, those biomedical signs such as heart rate, temperature, and the blood oxygen level may be used to figure out the children's physical, medical, and emotional status. Because each child has a different profile of those emotion/state-related biomedical signs for some reasons (e.g., medication status), having some basic information about a child's temperament and his/her communication about emotions and states from the EDEC interview will be helpful when analyzing those numbers.

As technology has advanced, it is possible to measure those biomedical signs daily. Using a smart watch with lights and sensors located on the back, it is possible to monitor a child's heart rate, temperature, and so forth. Lilly is a 10-year-old girl with severe and multiple developmental disabilities, along with cerebral palsy, who offers an example of how to use the collected information from the EDEC interview when analyzing those biomedical signs of a child with CCN. Table 12–2 presents the case, the information collected from the EDEC interview with Lilly's teacher, the biomedical signs measured during her intervention sessions, and possible plans for future interventions. As Table 12–2 illustrates, Lilly had some behaviors, such as facial expressions, that corresponded with certain emotions and from which her teacher created a personalized gesture/facial expression dictionary that attached to Lilly's wheelchair tray to help others interpret her medical and emotional status. However, the biomedical recording indicated that in some cases, Lilly's facial expressions did not match her arousal status measured via heart rate. The combination of the EDEC and the biomedical markers is, therefore, a potential solution.

Table 12–2. Case Example of Using EDEC Information for Biomedical Data Analysis

Case information	• **[Age & diagnosis]** Lilly is a 10-year-old girl who has severe and multiple developmental disabilities along with cerebral palsy. • **[Physical profile]** She is usually in her wheelchair at her school and can maintain her head upright less than one minute. She has frequent involuntary movements with her arms. • **[Communication]** She is nonverbal and rarely responds to other people or the presented with stimuli. She does not have previous or current experiences with any type of AAC.
Information collected from the EDEC interview with Lilly's teacher	• **[Temperament]** Lilly is a kind child. But her medical and emotional states are frequently up and down. • **[Emotion communication]** She sometimes smiles when she watches her favorite videos. It is difficult for her teachers to "read" her facial expressions and she is often absent of expressions. Her parents and teachers hope that others (e.g., other teachers and peers) could notice her emotion expressions better. • **[Lilly's gestural/facial expression dictionary]** Her teacher created a personalized gesture/facial expression dictionary and attached it to Lilly's wheelchair tray to help others interpret her medical and emotional status.
Biomedical signs during intervention sessions	• **[Intervention format]** Lilly receives a communication intervention with a speech-language pathologist once a week. The primary intervention goal is to interact with Lilly using various materials and improve her expressions in different modes of communication including facial expressions, vocalizations, gestures, and so forth. • **[Measurement techniques]** Lilly wore Samsung Galaxy smartwatch during each intervention session and the practitioner collected her heart rate and stress level data using the Samsung Health application, which is connected to the smartwatch via Bluetooth. Stress level was calculated by measuring the heart rate and the blood oxygen level. • **[Heart rate]** Throughout six intervention sessions, her heart rate was very high, ranging from 111 to 126 bpm compared to typical teenage girls (i.e., 70 to 87 bpm), although her facial expressions and vocalization was absent or calm in general. • **[Stress level]** Her stress level seemed to decrease across the intervention sessions having 94% during the first session and 11% during the last session, with ups and downs throughout six intervention sessions.
Possible plans for future interventions	• Lilly's facial expressions often do not match her actually arousal status. For example, although she is absent with facial expressions, her heart rate can be very high and she is actually very excited/stressed about something. • As Lilly's teacher reported during the EDEC interview, it is actually hard to "read" her facial expressions for this reason. • Therefore, having Lilly's current gestural/facial expression dictionary might not be enough to interpret her medical and emotional status. Monitoring her emotion and state-related biomedical signs during various daily activities is recommended.

▪ Final Considerations and Future Directions

We have introduced the theoretical and practical reasons for enriching AAC system design by adding vocabulary related to labeling, discussing, and strategizing responses to emotions that children with CCN might experience. We argue that without this kind of language, children with CCN will not have access to important avenues for learning emotional competencies and becoming independent in this regard. By doing so, challenging behaviors associated with frustration over inability to clearly express emotions will be mitigated.

Even though the EDEC tool offers a good starting point to solicit information from families or professionals, it is an interview where those individuals express their perceptions. It will be critical to also use the tool in conjunction with direct observational data. For instance, it would be possible to observe in situations where emotions could appear, or an interaction where parents could foster communication about emotions (like reading a storybook), and then explore the interaction between child and their communication partner. Observations could be videotaped with or without the presence of the clinician. For instance, the family might record themselves in a playful activity or while reading a storybook. The observational data permits the clinician to learn about the realities and challenges each child and his/her partners faces to talk about emotions.

It is also important to remember that the same circumstance can lead into different emotions depending on the person's perceptions (Lazarus, 1991a, 1991b; Scherer, 1997, 2004). It is, therefore, pos-sible to discuss how the same event can generate in one person a feeling of excitement but in another fear. For example, in one EDEC interview a mother expressed that her 7-year-old son Teo loves to go to the doctor and gets excited. Because of his medical needs, he visits the doctor often, and he is accustomed to syringes and injections. However, Teo's 9-year-old brother gets terrified of needles and does not like doctors. This situation could be a perfect opportunity to discuss the different feelings of the same circumstance. Considering the emotional triggers of oneself and others promotes self-consciousness, respect, and empathy.

The EDEC and STEPS intervention might also be an important source of information for generating social stories that can help prepare children for situations that might provoke anxiety. For instance, from the EDEC the clinician might learn that a child is nervous about going to the dentist and begins producing challenging behaviors as the appointment nears. With this information, the clinician might work with the parents to create a social story that includes discussion about the emotion ("nervous"), what parts of the dentist visit cause the emotion (perhaps the sound of the drill), and the possible responses the child might make, from bringing a comfort item to requesting a break. Clearly, future research is needed to determine the effectiveness of such strategies for helping children prepare and respond to such situations.

When suggesting activities in natural settings, clinicians must consider the interests and challenges of the individuals. Some families might have the habit of reading, but others might not. Other families might prefer to watch videos, or some kids might prefer role-playing, playing with puppets, or some might need activities with specific sensory stimulation. Children who have challenges in their attention span may need activities or storybooks that are short in length. Some children may be interested in e-storybooks because of the characters' movement, but this could be too much stimulation for others. Understanding children's interests will enhance all intervention decisions, and future research should examine how such personalization can occur most optimally and how it influences intervention outcomes.

In summary, emotional competency in individuals with CCN is integral to all aspects of development, from preparedness for learning to making and maintaining friendships to successful self-advocacy and vocational outcomes. As discussed in this chapter, developing emotional competency presents unique challenges to those who rely on AAC to communicate. Ideally, the early stages of AAC intervention will include an emotion component as a priority to aid in an individual's overall development and outcomes. The EDEC interview protocol and the STEPS intervention offer strategies for raising awareness of the importance of conversations about emotions with those who benefit from AAC. These two approaches offer guidance for families and interventionists to address this challenging topic. The next steps are to pursue clinical research that best scaffolds the development of emotional competencies for people with CCN.

■ References

Aro, T., Laakso, M.-L., Määttä, S., Tolvanen, A., & Poikkeus, A.-M. (2014). Associations between toddler-age communication and kindergarten-age self-regulatory skills. *Journal of Speech, Language, and Hearing Research, 57,* 1405–1417.

Beck, L., Kumschick, I. R., Eid, M., & Klann-Delius, G. (2011). Relationship between language competence and emotional competence in middle childhood. *Emotion, 12,* 503–515.

Beukelman, D. R., & Light, J. C. (2020). *Augmentative & alternative communication: Supporting children and adults with complex communication needs* (5th ed.). Brookes.

Blackstone, S., & Wilkins, D. P. (2009). Exploring the importance of emotional competence in children with complex communication needs. *SIG 12 Perspectives on Augmentative and Alternative Communication, 18,* 78–87.

Buckley, M., Storino, M., & Saarni, C. (2003). Promoting emotional competence in children and adolescents: Implications for school psychologists. *School Psychology Quarterly, 18,* 177–191.

Cole, P. M., Bruschi, C. J., & Tamang, B. L. (2002). Cultural differences in children's emotional reactions to difficult situations. *Child Development, 73*(3), 983-996.

Cole, P. M., Tamang, B. L., & Shrestha, S. (2006). Cultural variations in the socialization of young children's anger and shame. *Child Development, 77,* 1237–1251.

Cole, P. M., & Tan, P. Z. (2015). Emotion socialization from a cultural perspective. In J. E. Grusec & P. D. Hastings (Eds.), *Handbook of socialization: Theory and research* (pp. 499–519). Guilford Press.

Drager, K. D. R., Light, J., Currall, J., Muttiah, N., Smith, V., Kreis, D., . . . Wiscount, J. (2019). AAC technologies with visual scene displays and "just in time" programming and symbolic communication turns expressed by students with severe disability. *Journal of Intellectual & Developmental Disability, 44,* 321–336. https://doi.org/10.3109/13668250.2017.1326585

Fujiki, M., Brinton, B., & Clarke, D. (2002). Emotion regulation in children with specific language impairment. *Language, Speech, and Hearing Services in Schools, 33,* 102–111.

Fujiki, M., Spackman, M. P., Brinton, B., & Hall, A. (2004). The relationship of language and emotion regulation skills to reticence in children with specific language impairment. *Journal of Speech, Language, and Hearing Research, 47*, 637–646.

Gray, C. A., & Garand, J. D. (1993). Social stories: Improving responses of students with Autism with accurate social information. *Focus on Autistic Behavior, 8*(1), 1–10.

Holyfield, C., Caron, J. G., Drager, K., & Light, J. (2019). Effect of mobile technology featuring visual scene displays and "just-in-time" programming on the frequency, content, and function of communication turns by pre-adolescent and adolescent beginning communicators. *International Journal of Speech-Language Pathology, 21*, 201–211. https://doi.org/10.1080/17549507.2018.1441440

Kang, S. G., Shin, J. H., & Song, S. W. (2010). Reliability and validity of the Korean version of the Penn State Worry Questionnaire in primary school children. *Journal of Korean Medical Science, 25*(8), 1210–1216.

Kubicek, L. F., & Emde, R. N. (2012). Emotional expression and language: A longitudinal study of typically developing earlier and later talkers from 15 to 30 months. *Infant Mental Health Journal, 33*, 553–584.

Lazarus, R. S. (1991a). *Emotion and adaptation.* Oxford University Press.

Lazarus, R. S. (1991b). Progress on a cognitive-motivational-relational theory of emotion. *American Psychologist, 46*, 819–834.

Light, J., Wilkinson, K. M., Theissen, A., Beukelman, D., & Fager, S. (2019). Designing effective AAC displays for individuals with developmental or acquired disabilities: State of the science and future research directions. *Augmentative and Alternative Communication, 35*, 42–55.

Matson, J. L., & Minshawi, N. F. (2007). Functional assessment of challenging behavior: Toward a strategy for applied settings. *Research in Developmental Disabilities, 28*, 353–361.

Mirenda, P., & Brown, K. (2007). Supporting individuals with autism and problem behavior using AAC. *Perspectives on Augmentative and Alternative Communication, 16*, 26-31.

Mora, F. (2013). *Neuroeducación: Solo se puede aprender aquello que se ama.* Alianza.

Na, J. Y. (2015). *Communication about emotions using AAC during storybook reading: Effects of an instruction program for parents of children with Down syndrome* (Doctoral dissertation). Retrieved from Penn State Electronic Theses for Schreyer Honors College.

Na, J., & Wilkinson, K., (2017). Communication about emotions during storybook reading: Effects of an instruction program including visual communication supports for parents of children with Down syndrome. *International Journal of Speech-Language Pathology, 1-11.* https://doi.org/10.1080/17549507.2017.1356376

Na, J., Wilkinson, K. M., Blackstone, S., Karny, M., & Stifter, C. (2016). A synthesis of relevant literature on the early development of emotional competencies and communication about emotions in children with CCN and its implications for AAC design. *American Journal of Speech-Language Pathology, 25*, 441–452. https://doi.org/10.1044/2016_AJSLP-14-0124

Na, J., Wilkinson, K., & Liang, J. (2018). Early Development of Emotional Competence (EDEC) assessment tool for children with complex communication needs: Development and evidence. *American Journal of Speech-Language Pathology, 27*, 24–36. https://doi.org/10.1044/2017_AJSLP-16-0058

O'Neill, T., Light, J., & McNaughton, D. (2017). Videos with integrated AAC visual scene displays to enhance participation in community and vocational activities: Pilot case study with an adolescent with autism spectrum disorder. *Perspectives of the ASHA Special Interest Groups, 12*, 55–69. http://doi.org/10.1044/persp2.SIG12.55

Raval, V. V., Martini, T. S., & Raval, P. H. (2007). "Would others think it is ok to express my feelings?": Regulation of anger, sadness, and physical pain in Gujarati children in India. *Social Development, 16*(1), 79–105.

Raval, V. V., Martini, T. S., & Raval, P. H. (2010). Methods of, and reasons for, emotional expression and control in children with internalizing, externalizing, and somatic problems in urban India. *Social Development, 19*(1), 93–112.

Raver, C. C. (2004). Placing emotional self-regulation in sociocultural and socioeconomic contexts. *Child Development, 75,* 346–353.

Reichle, J., & Johnston, S. (1993). Replacing challenging behavior: The role of communication intervention. *Topics in Language Disorders, 13,* 61–76.

Roben, C. K., Cole, P. M., & Armstrong, L. M. (2013). Longitudinal relations among language skills, anger expression, and regulatory strategies in early childhood. *Child Development, 84,* 891–905.

Saarni, C. (1999). *The development of emotional competence.* Guilford.

Scherer, K. R. (1997). Profiles of emotion-antecedent appraisal: Testing theoretical predictions across cultures. *Cognition and Emotion, 11,* 113–150.

Scherer, K. R. (2004). Feelings integrate the central representation of appraisal-driven response organization in emotion. In A. S. R. Manstead, N. H. Frijda, & A. H. Fischer (Eds.), *Feelings and emotions: The Amsterdam symposium* (pp. 136–157). Cambridge University Press.

Trentacosta, C. J., & Izard, C. E. (2007). Kindergarten children's emotion competence as a predictor of their academic competence in first grade. *Emotion, 7,* 77–88.

Vallotton, C., & Ayoub, C. (2011). Use your words: The role of language in the development of toddlers' self-regulation. *Early Childhood Research Quarterly, 26,* 169–181.

Vygotsky, L. S. (1986). *Thought and language* (Rev. ed.). MIT Press.

Warren, S. F., & Yoder, P. (1998). Facilitating the transition from pre-intentional to intentional communication. In A. S. Wetherby, S. F. Warren, & J. Reichle (Eds.), *Transitions in prelinguistic communication.* Brookes.

Wilkinson, K. M., Na, J., Liang, J., Rangel-Rodriguez, G., Crawford, E., & Armendariz, K. (2018, November). *The EDEC Tool for American, Mandarin Chinese, Native American, Spanish, Korean, & Mexican American children.* One hour seminar presented at the annual conference of the American Speech-Language-Hearing Association, Boston, MA.

Wilkinson, K. M., & Reichle, J. (2009). The role of aided AAC in replacing unconventional communicative acts with more conventional ones. In P. Mirenda, T. Iacono, & J. Light (Eds.), *Autism spectrum disorders and AAC.* Brookes.

13

AAC and Multiculturalism: Incorporating Family Perspectives for Improved Outcomes

Mary Claire Wofford and Rachel Hoge

Among all individuals with communication disorders, those with complex communication needs (CCN) experience some of the most significant barriers to full participation in and beyond their communities. Speech-language pathologists (SLPs), families, and other stakeholders of people with CCN have the difficult charge of facilitating this group's communicative effectiveness in an increasingly fast-paced, technology-driven world where communication and connectivity is ever-evolving. Complicating this task, population mobility and societal globalization (Hyter, 2014) has led to a complex confluence of variables impacting speech and language services in today's world. SLPs see that their caseloads are increasingly representative of individuals who come from culturally or linguistically diverse (CLD) backgrounds in conjunction with demographic trends and the increased movement of people around the globe (Hyter & Salas-Provance, 2019).

This chapter seeks to illuminate certain variables that impact people with CCN who come from multicultural, multi-lingual, and nonmainstream backgrounds in the United States who collectively are referred to as CLD individuals and families. Though focused on U.S. dynamics, concepts discussed here apply to diverse settings where SLPs and their global counterparts practice. In particular this chapter will highlight challenges that SLPs and people with CCN face in making decisions about augmentative and alternative communication (AAC) use when CLD backgrounds are represented. Though representation of people with CCN from CLD backgrounds is still limited in the available evidence, evidence-based solutions for improving service delivery and considerations for serving CLD families that are rooted in the extant literature are available.

◼ Presentation of Challenges

There is no single challenge in the service of people with CCN who come from diverse backgrounds, but rather a series of challenges that caregivers, clients, and

SLPs face together. Families are often the primary advocates for their loved ones with CCN. Through the family's lens, SLPs can observe the different types of concerns related to AAC services experienced by majority- and minority-culture families. In the headings of subsequent sections, realistic quotes from families collected during clinical encounters give voice to the concerns of families.

Common issues in AAC services in majority groups are documented throughout the literature (e.g., social acceptability of AAC communication, capacity for learning, or device maintenance). When an individual does not have the same cultural or linguistic background as the majority culture and the school or health care system in which they seek services, complicated challenges can arise. In subsequent sections, the challenges voiced by SLPs and CLD families receiving AAC ser-

vices are discussed at distinct levels and appear summarized in Table 13–1. First are environmental issues that broadly govern education- and health-related trends. Second are challenges related to implementation of AAC systems with CLD families. Third, device-level features posing dynamic challenges as CLD groups increase in their use of technology-based support are discussed.

Environmental Challenges

"It can be difficult to dispel myths around AAC . . . and I find that the language barrier to be even more challenging when working with those myths."

—SLP

Table 13–1. Featured Challenges

Level of Challenge	Presentation of Challenge
Environmental	▪ Disparity in access to health care ▪ Lack of culturally and linguistically diverse providers ▪ Lack of availability of bilingual and bicultural services ▪ "Double-stigmatization" of individuals with disabilities and different cultural or linguistic background ▪ Prevalence of myths about dual language development ▪ Overrepresentation of young CLD children living in poverty
Implementation	▪ Client-provider mismatch in background ▪ Client-institution mismatch in value systems ▪ Lack of buy-in from CLD family partners
Communication Devices	▪ Ever-changing selection of devices ▪ Devices designed with majority-culture communication in mind ▪ Homogeneity in AAC iconography and prerecorded speech options ▪ Need for devices that support and reflect second language acquisition

Environmental-level challenges to AAC use in CLD groups are those that extend beyond the family unit and represent pervasive, systemic challenges in health care and education. Most importantly, there is evidence for ethnicity based disparity in access (Kaye, Yeager, & Reed, 2008; Lindsay & Tsybina, 2011). In the current structure of the U.S. health care system, people with CCN from CLD backgrounds and their families experience a systematic inaccessibility to AAC services (McNamara, 2018, p. 141). The Individuals with Disabilities Act (IDEA, 2004) governs the provision of services for people with CCN and provides guidance on services. The IDEA Part B and Part C Final Regulations (2004) mandate the use of the home language in evaluation, the right to an interpreter during an IEP meeting, and the use of assessment practices administered "in the form most likely to yield accurate information on what the child knows and can do academically, developmentally, and functionally" (IDEA, 2004, §300.304). These main tenets of practice with CLD groups are supported by numerous professional organizations in education and healthcare.

The American-Speech-Language-Hearing Association (ASHA) mandates culturally responsive service delivery for people with CCN through its Scope of Practice (2016) and the ASHA Code of Ethics (2016). ASHA Principles of Ethics I states that members have a responsibility "to hold paramount the welfare of persons they serve professionally" (ASHA, 2016, p. 4). Principle of Ethics I Rules A and B establish that all practice should be carried out competently and that referral and interprofessional collaboration are tools that practitioners might use. Importantly, Rule C states that, "Individuals shall not discriminate in the delivery of professional services or in the conduct of research and scholarly activities on the basis of race, ethnicity, sex, gender identity/gender expression, sexual orientation, age, religion, national origin, disability, culture, language, or dialect" (ASHA, 2016, p. 5). These guidelines are critical to any discussion of AAC services with CLD groups, because they demonstrate the fundamental need for SLPs to make collaborative partnerships with patients, clients, and their families irrespective of background with the patient's well-being in mind.

Despite government mandates, fully bilingual and bicultural services are not uniformly available or implemented across the United States. This is a major environmental challenge in AAC services. Central to this challenge is the simple fact that the availability of bilingual service providers in speech-language pathology and other disciplines fails to match demographic trends. Currently, approximately 64 million inhabitants speak a language other than English (U.S. Census, 2017). ASHA reported that approximately 80% of self-identifying bilingual service providers across the discipline (i.e., SLPs, audiologists, speech scientists) reported they were white, while 14% reported their race as Asian, 3% as Black or African-American, 2% as multi-racial, 1% as American Indian or Alaska Native, and fewer than 1% as Native Hawaiian/Pacific Islander (ASHA, 2018). One-third (42%) of ASHA bilingual service providers reported that they were of Hispanic or Latino descent. Of the ASHA practitioners who self-report to be bilingual service providers, the majority spoke Spanish (64%) and 81 total languages were represented, including sign languages. Although the number of CLD practitioners has increased, growth has not matched an increasingly diversifying population (National Center for Education

Statistics, 2018). By 2060, minority children enrolled within the public school system are expected to account for more than 60% of all students (U.S. Census, 2017).

Furthermore, the implementation of bilingual services is not uniform across the profession. In two surveys conducted with SLPs practicing in the United States, SLPs reported increasing knowledge and confidence in service of children with dual language backgrounds, as well as an increasing adherence to policies (Arias & Friberg, 2017; Caesar & Kohler, 2007). However, monolingual evaluations, lack of dynamic assessment, and overreliance on standardized measures were identified as persistent obstacles to best practice evaluation in bilingual service delivery (Arias & Friberg, 2017). Regarding implementation of bilingual service, another environmental challenge is the trend of CLD children being less likely to receive speech and language services overall (Morgan et al., 2017). Children with CLD backgrounds who also have severe disabilities are much less likely to receive bilingual support than those with mild-moderate disabilities (Marinova-Todd et al., 2016). Oftentimes, English-language ability is perceived to be a prerequisite for receiving any specialized disability service (Yu, 2013). For CLD families whose children with CCN are receiving AAC services, these observations are troubling. Schools or health centers serving greater numbers of CLD children may be under-resourced to provide bilingual and bicultural care. There is continued difficulty in response to trends toward cultural responsiveness and equity in health care resulting in deeply ingrained disparity in services received by CLD groups.

Another major environmental challenge has to do with perceptions of individuals with disabilities. Stigmatization of disabilities continues to be a major environmental challenge in society. For individuals coming from CLD backgrounds, those perceptions can be further complicated by compounding biases, such that family members and people with CCN may experience a "double-stigmatization" based on their disability and their cultural or linguistic background (Ripat & Woodgate, 2011). This is visibly evident when that individual uses augmentative and assistive technology. Alongside widely-adopted perceptions, there are also many unsubstantiated myths that exist and persist at the intersection of bilingualism and disabilities. A concern commonly expressed by non-English-speaking or bilingual caregivers and others is that home language use will hinder English language development (Yu, 2013), which is perceived to be critically necessary for any student's success. Also, commonly expressed are the notions that simplifying the linguistic input stream to include only one language is preferable for children with language learning difficulties and that bilingualism is an origin of developmental delays (Peña, 2016). These ideas and many other commonly heard myths conflict with current evidence on dual language development in children with and without developmental delays and communication difficulties (Hoff & Core, 2015; Kay-Raining Bird, Genesee, & Verhoeven, 2016). Unfortunately, these beliefs often prevail over current evidence for people with CCN from CLD backgrounds who are in systems where there is limited knowledge of that language or limited access to interpreters. The result is that services are provided monolingually or fail to take into consideration important family and community level variables. For

CLD people with CCN who are no longer in a developmental period of language learning, an acute loss of communication in any or either language can be falsely perceived as a cognitive deficit. This can disconnect and isolate the individual with CCN from community and impact quality of life.

A critical consideration and major challenge for SLPs working with CLD families on AAC options is the greater representation of young CLD children living in poverty (Koball & Jiang, 2018; Mindel & John, 2018). Less access to resources, including technology aids, educational materials, and basic school supplies in the home (Esping-Andersen et al., 2012) may prevent the implementation, carryover, and sustainability of both low-tech and high-tech AAC options. Low-income families are at risk for experiencing greater instability of the home environment, including evolving living and childcare scenarios, greater levels of chaos, more residents per household, or more transience in household residents (Mills-Koonce, Willoughby, Garrett-Peters, Wagner, & Vernon-Feagans, 2016). Caregivers who live in low-SES conditions with their child with CCN may not use the device because its financial cost represents an investment susceptible to breakage or loss. Caregivers stating, "The device is so expensive, and I can't stand the idea of breaking it" are expressing a valid concern about ownership of the device, particularly in contexts when long periods of negotiation and waiting preclude its implementation. Due to the inequity in health care, especially those of low-income backgrounds, these notions may disproportionately affect CLD families in receipt of AAC services (Marinova-Todd et al., 2016; Mindel & John, 2018).

Implementation Challenges

> "Is it going to hurt my child to learn or to continue learning their home language? When we add this device, will it be able to speak our language?"
>
> —Caregiver

A primary challenge faced by SLPs and stakeholders is effective implementation of AAC systems when the clinician and the family members of people with CCN are from different cultural or linguistic backgrounds. The mismatch in client and provider background, and its impact on service delivery, is evident across health professions (Castaño, Biever, González, & Anderson, 2007; Flores, 2005; Mazor, Hampers, Chande, & Krug, 2002; Suphanchaimat, Kantamaturpoj, Putthasri, & Prakongsai, 2015) and in speech-language pathology (Arias & Friberg, 2017; Pham, Kohnert, & Mann, 2011). Specialized skills and knowledge comprise the competencies required for SLPs to provide services in the area of AAC. SLPs' skills and knowledge and, therefore, their service delivery are largely centered on western perspectives and values. Among those values, individualism, equality, scientific discovery, social mobility, and optimism are preeminent ideals that govern how society and its systems function. These values are borne out in SLPs' implementation of services. To illustrate, mainstream caregivers living in the United States tend to value their own child's capacity to live independently as a measure of success, and as such, those priorities may be assumed for all families on an SLP's caseload. Nonmainstream groups may have different values and motivations, such as collectivism, respect, divine providence, personalism, fate, and realism (Roseberry-McKibbin, 2008). Caregivers from CLD backgrounds that espouse non-mainstream ideals may favor provision of lifelong support to their child with CCN over the majority-culture's notion of independence. Values affect not only communication style and content, but also caregiving practices, beliefs about the origin of disabilities, family roles, beliefs about scheduling appointments, and many other aspects of life (Huer, Parette, & Saenz, 2001; McCord & Soto, 2004). The degree to which a family is acculturated into the majority culture or to which the family maintains minority-culture practices may also dictate the choices a family makes surrounding their family member with CCN (Hyter & Salas-Provance, 2019).

Implementation challenges also include mismatches in cultural or ethnic background that may impact the interaction between schools, clinics, hospitals, or private practices and people with CCN and their families from CLD backgrounds. This is in part due to the values that underlie educational and health-related settings and systems, but is also due to linguistic differences. Language of intervention is one common point of contention in CLD families when making decisions about AAC services. For more commonly spoken languages in the United States (e.g., Spanish, French, Chinese), resources are more readily available in the form of speakers and language-specific knowledge resources (Mueller, Singer, & Carranza, 2006). For less commonly spoken languages, knowledge of cultural practices and linguistic expertise may be less widely disseminated. These implementation challenges often are addressed through interpreters. Use of an interpreter requires extended

time to gain background knowledge in the family's unique cultural practices. Extra time often is a valuable resource that practicing clinicians lack.

When implementation of services is flawed, CLD groups face high-stakes consequences. A systematic review revealed that parents who had limited English proficiency had poorer rates of access to insurance, access to medical services, and satisfaction in the care of their children with special health care needs (Ereniz-Wiemer, Sanders, Barr, & Mendoza, 2014). When these issues were not addressed in implementation of services, caregivers with limited English proficiency reported that they had poorer knowledge and self-efficacy in managing their child's special health care needs than English-speaking caregivers. Caregivers with limited English proficiency were less likely to report that their provider spent time teaching them to manage a child's health care condition and were less likely to report being treated as a partner in their child's care when compared to English-speaking caregivers.

In AAC services, the consequences of poor implementation can result in a dramatic impact on everyday communication with family members. When linguistic and cultural differences are ignored, AAC services do not have much promise of gaining traction in a CLD family. Critically, failure to acknowledge linguistic differences reduces buy-in from family partners involved in AAC service delivery and constitutes a major challenge in AAC service delivery. An AAC system that does not reflect languages spoken by a family likely will not get used by the family, because it does not reflect the home language environment. When homes are multicultural and multigenerational, it adds complexity to an AAC system's implementation. CLD families may occupy different physical spaces. An implementation challenge might include the need for AAC to be used in distinct settings from non-CLD families. Buy-in for use of a communication system may extend beyond typical expected stakeholders. These factors complicate an SLP's task to advocate for a culturally responsive communication system.

Device-Level Challenges

"She has to return to her settings to change between languages. It's not at all efficient, and it's not how we communicate."

—Caregiver

Many SLPs report that they struggle to find culturally appropriate AAC devices for CLD families. Device-level challenges are in constant flux with the changing landscape of technology. The speed with which technology changes is itself a challenge to implementing services, but more importantly, the selection of devices that provide CLD families with variety and customization options is still extremely limited. Most non-English options in AAC are provided in Spanish, which accounts for a majority of non-English-speakers, but does not capture lesser-spoken languages or groups. Majority-culture communication pervades device design and therefore messaging is culturally-loaded before a device ever reaches an individual. This is true for both high-tech options such as speech-generating devices and low-tech options such as communication boards. Communication style, lexical choice, sym-

bol choice, symbol interpretation, and pre-programmed messages are all created by AAC system developers who often exhibit majority-culture biases. A degree of customizability exists in almost every system, but the conceptualization of most AAC systems is rooted in a eurocentric view of language. This is evident at a phonological level in the homogeneity in SGD voice options and in orthographic writing systems. Writing systems that are depicted using a letter-based alphabet (e.g., English) are typologically different from those that use a logographic writing system (e.g., Chinese). This is a challenge for interventionists who wish to include icons from both languages in one device.

The homogeneity in racial, ethnic, and linguistic groups represented in AAC iconography and prerecorded speech options are a challenge. Trends show that AAC devices are increasingly designed with greater representation in visual depictions of race and ethnicity in icons and in diversity of voices available in SGDs. As efforts continue to improve customization options and culturally appropriate content, it is also critical for devices to reflect typical patterns of dual-language development. That is, people who use AAC should be able to use their devices to access both languages easily, as most bilingual speakers alternate language use. The alternating use of two languages is known as *code-switching* and is a typical process occurring in second language acquisition. Recognizing common features or settings where code-switching will occur and being able to represent languages alongside one another is an area of increasing need given population trends. Current AAC options for bilingual people who rely on AAC are limited and require development.

■ Evidence-Based Solutions

In consulting the evidence, three main solutions emerge that help to address challenges in AAC service delivery to people with CCN in CLD families. Subsequently these solutions and their applications for assessment and intervention are discussed and appear summarized in Table 13–2.

Develop Cultural Awareness and Competence

Given population trends, SLPs undoubtedly will encounter more and more CLD families in their practice. Culture-specific knowledge and skills will accumulate with greater exposure to cultural and ethnic groups. SLPs have a responsibility to inform themselves about those that they serve in holding paramount the well-being of their patient. They should look to evidence-based practices in the expanding literature base that addresses CLD families and their family members with CCN. Knowledge and skills can be gained from relevant continuing education and may extend to specialized training in AAC systems. Reflecting on cases benefits both families and practitioners and prevents stereotypical knowledge from prevailing in practice.

Although challenges surrounding broader cultural biases and stereotypes may seem too large to grapple with on a daily basis, SLPs' actions toward CLD families and people with CCN are critical

Table 13–2. Summary of Solutions

Solution	Suggestions
Develop cultural awareness and competence	• Examine own self first • Recognize own biases and check assumptions and stereotypes • Use tools for self-reflection • Employ a socio-cultural approach in assessment • Take a bilingual approach to intervention • Use culturally responsive tools and adaptations • Consider language of intervention
Work collaboratively	• Incorporate stakeholders' perspectives • Consult with other professionals in a team approach • Use an interpreter who can serve as a cultural and linguistic broker
Prioritize the family and their values	• Seek out client and family member perspectives • Using a family-centered model for all patients • Acknowledge diversity in family units • Collect information on skills in all languages spoken in the home • Prioritize language access in feature matching • Identify culturally congruent practices • Teach all caregivers about aided input

to their experiences in the broader world. Communication disabilities and linguistic racism are not always obvious. SLPs should examine themselves first. Recognizing one's own implicit and explicit biases and checking the assumptions and stereotypes that stem from those biases is only an initial step to serving CLD families with greater cultural responsivity. A follow-up step is examining how biases pertaining to CLD groups interact with those biases that deal with disability or poverty and how those biases are reinforced by school, hospital, or state policies and regulations. Once one's own biases are made clear, the individual practitioner's work is not over. Biases must be revisited over time as implementation of different cases underlines or undoes perceptions about communication, disability, and poverty. Practicing from an informed, culturally responsive, but adaptive viewpoint ensures higher quality of service delivered to CLD families, as well as greater knowledge, skill, and competence as a clinician.

Many tools are available that serve providers to inform themselves broadly in their practice. One tool is a checklist for personal reflection, policies and procedures, and service delivery to increase cultural competence of SLPs working with CLD populations (ASHA, 2010). Another available set of self-assessment tools was developed by Project Building Bridges, a program that prepares preservice SLPs to provide culturally and linguistically responsive services to school-age children with CCN (Solomon-Rice, Soto, & Robinson, 2018).

Assessment-Specific Solutions

Evaluating multilingual individuals poses unique challenges. However, evidence is available to inform assessment practices and result in more culturally responsive AAC service delivery. One recommendation to combat these challenges and minimize bias is to employ a socio-cultural approach. In short, this approach honors the interconnectedness of a person's cultural and social environment and their use of language (De Lamo White & Jin, 2011; Soto & Yu, 2014). By taking a socio-cultural approach to AAC assessment with CLD clients, the team explicitly acknowledges the value of cultural and linguistic diversity and its influence on a person's identity, communication abilities, and social relationships.

Implementation of this approach entails collecting data from various sources using a combination of methods such as ethnographic interviews and observations, participation inventories, language samples, evaluation of language processing, and dynamic assessment (De Lamo White & Jin, 2011). Ethnographic interviews and observations have long been utilized in social and anthropological research because they help build rapport among relevant parties by shifting the focus away from the interviewer's perspective and limiting the influence of external factors (Roseberry-McKibbin, 2008). In turn, the process is more authentic, naturalistic, holistic, and family-centered. A socio-cultural approach is intensive and unlikely to solve every challenge faced by the assessment team (De Lamo White & Jin, 2011). However, it affords the CLD individual with CCN the greatest opportunity to demonstrate their current level of communicative competence, a benefit that greatly outweighs any logistical disadvantages.

To support a socio-cultural approach, tools are available for SLPs and other professionals to facilitate the assessment process and to encourage skill development related to AAC evaluations with people from CLD backgrounds. Robinson and Solomon-Rice (2009) compiled an adapted list of AAC self-efficacy assessment questions (Parette & Dempsey Marr, 1997; Wilcox, Weintraub, & Aier, 2003) to assist professionals less familiar with the complexities of an AAC evaluation. Huer (1997) designed the Protocol for Culturally Inclusive Assessment of AAC that includes a section for assessment of communication needs, capability, and technology. Many of the tools that strengthen the evidence-based assessment process for people with CCN can be utilized with CLD clients and families. Some may require adaptations or enhancements to meet the specific cultural and linguistic needs of the client. Translations of informal assessment tools (e.g., case history forms, caregiver questionnaires) reduce cognitive load on the interpreter and ensure questions are asked and answered as intended. Other assessment tools to consider include the AAC Profile: A Continuum of Learning (Kovach, 2009), Checklist of Communication Competencies, revised (Bloomberg, West, Johnson, & Iacono, 2009), Functional Communication Profile, revised (Kleiman, 2003), AAC Assessment Checklist (Karnezos, 2018), Augmentative Communication Assessment Protocol for Symbolic Augmentative Systems (Gamel-McCormick & Dymond, 1994), and Test of Aided-Communication Symbol Performance (TASP; Bruno, 2010). Multilingual assessment tools specifically developed for use with CLD individuals with disabilities include the Ventura County Comprehensive Alternate Language Proficiency Survey for Students with Moderate-Severe Disabilities (VCCALPS, 2017), Communication Matrix (Rowland, 2004), Dynamic AAC Goals Grid-2 (DAGG-2; Dynamic Therapy Associates & Tobii-Dynavox, 2014), and Social Networks: A Communication Inventory for Individuals with Complex Communi-

cation Needs and Their Partners, revised (Blackstone & Hunt Berg, 2012).

Intervention-Specific Solutions

Closely examining the choice of language in intervention is a solution for improving service across different communication disorders and disability groups (Gutierrez-Clellen, 1999). Few true choices in language have been offered historically to families of children with CCN (Marinova Todd et al., 2016; Yu, 2013). Recognition of the disadvantages experienced by bilingual children if one of their languages is suppressed in intervention is an initial step. The sacrifice of home language in intervention may result in a loss of home language-specific knowledge alongside the invaluable home language interactions that promote socioemotional development (Kremer-Sadlik, 2005; Wong Fillmore, 2000). Conversely, monolingual caregivers grow concerned about their child's ability to perform in a majority-language educational environment when the language of instruction is limited to the home language (Peña, 2016). Caregivers are not at fault in thinking that there is a need to simplify learning as they likely recognize that typical home language input cannot support all of their bilingual child's language needs. Health care and educational professionals along with caregivers must demonstrate adding diverse supports for language, rather than urging caregivers to sacrifice the home language. Bilingual children's knowledge is distributed across two languages (Core, Hoff, Rumiche, & Señor, 2013; Oller, 2005). CLD children with CCN possess language-specific knowledge that warrants maintenance.

A main solution is taking a bilingual approach to intervention. This is consistent with converging evidence that bilingual children who have a developmental disability can learn two languages, and are best supported by a bilingual approach to intervention (Kohnert & Medina, 2009; Kay-Raining Bird et al., 2016). Although there is a push for children with CCN to be included in general education classrooms (Office of Administration for Children and Families, 2016; Office of Civil Rights, 2015), they often do not have the opportunity to learn their two languages based on policies implemented and resources available at their school (Pesco et al., 2016). The perceived barriers to accessing second-language education are more considerable for children who have more severe developmental disabilities. This was evident in an international sample of SLPs and educators that reported more neutral perspectives about second language learning toward children with severe disabilities than those with milder degrees of disability (Marinova-Todd et al., 2016). All bilingual or multilingual children with CCN should have the option of a bilingual approach to intervention.

SLPs and other professionals must respond with a paradigm shift to follow empirical evidence supporting a bilingual approach. This shift should move away from the notion that a bilingual approach is maintained only when a teacher or SLP has an interest in other languages (Pickl, 2011). Rather, the starting place for intervening with CLD children who have CCN should be finding solutions that provide a bilingual approach.

Solutions are needed that broadly educate caregivers, educators of all types, and health care professionals about the importance of promoting both or all languages in development. Additionally, intervention materials in a variety of languages providing customizable access for multiple languages are needed. Using culturally-appropriate, language-specific symbols

in a format that alternated languages was found to be viable and effective in a case study of a young girl with ASD (Johnston, O'Neill, & Schumann, 2018). Alternating treatments mimicked the language environment as the child moved from school to home each day and resulted in meeting criterion in both languages through functional communication training. Important issues arose in this case study that require more evidence. First, the research team made the decision to use two distinct symbols to represent two languages, which is responsive to the typological differences and cultural depictions of words between the two languages. There is still a paucity of research in the use of distinct representations of two linguistic systems within one device. Second, this child benefitted from a carryover effect across languages, a natural and positive aspect of dual-language development. If the child did not reach criterion in both languages, the SLP would hopefully still advocate that the less-proficient language would not be dropped from intervention so long as both languages are present in the linguistic environment.

Another solution pertains to adjustments to existing interventions that will enhance communication for a CLD individual with CCN and his or her family. Interventions and adaptations of interventions should respectfully use materials that reflect that family's culture (Castro, Barrera, & Martinez, 2004; Droop & Verhoeven, 1998; Mendez, Crais, Castro, & Kainz, 2015). Notably, Soto (2012) stated that "AAC devices should include symbols that incorporate glosses, designs, colors, and referents that are compatible with the home culture as well as vocabulary that is functional and culturally valued" (p. 148). Using culturally relevant content, such as pictures that are relevant to an individual's ethnic background (Pickl,

2011), increases buy-in from the family and stands to increase the amount of communication occurring in the home language. This in turn gives added importance and impetus to integrate the device at home (Pickl, 2011). In the process of goal-setting the SLP should take into consideration the potential for both the target and the intervention materials to be culturally meaningful.

Families and clinicians alike have expressed a need for increased flexibility of devices to switch between languages (Soto & Yu, 2014, Wagner, 2018). In a review of symbol-based apps (Wagner, 2018), several were reported to have bilingual design elements with varying degrees of accessibility. User experiences ranged from the expressive output being completely bilingual to being limited by simple restrictions (e.g., having to clear the message bar before switching languages) to more overt barriers (e.g., requiring additional fees to access bilingual voices). However, a solution may not be as simple as switching a setting. Incorporating typological differences between languages is a step to promoting a bilingual user's experience with a device. Code-switching is merely one facet of a bilingual individual's language development. Considering other typical processes in language development (e.g., interlanguage use, positive and negative transfer, borrowing) will give CLD users with CCN a way to experiment with language on their AAC device that mimics dual language development (Wagner, 2018).

Consider the following case study of a Chinese-American family. Imagine yourself as the SLP tasked with working with the family.

Min. Min was a twenty-year-old high school student with Autism Spectrum Dis-

order. He lived at home with his mother, father, grandmother, and his younger sister. His mother, Chen, was concerned about his transition from being in a self-contained classroom to the home environment as reported to the SLP in an interview. Min's plans after high school included participation in community activities through a local center for individuals with disabilities. His family felt he did not have sufficient communication to seek employment. Min used some speech that was moderately intelligible to his teachers and classmates, though Chen had concerns about his ability to interact with unfamiliar communication partners. His spontaneous communication typically used a combination of communication boards and a tablet-based application.

Min had a history of challenging behaviors in the classroom in his early school years and Chen reported that she had often experienced judgment around remediation of his behaviors. She reported that in his adolescence his behaviors had changed to be more "in harmony," meaning fewer challenging behaviors observed. She expressed gratitude that she could always count on family support for caregiving. However, Min's grandmother did not seem to accept Min's diagnosis and believed Min would eventually get better, according to Chen's report. Chen and her husband, both bilingual in English and Mandarin, primarily spoke to Min in English, but Min's grandmother exclusively spoke to him in Mandarin. Chen expressed concerns about Min's future, saying "What will happen to him when we are gone?"

The SLP gained valuable knowledge about the circumstances surrounding Min's family by adopting a sociocultural approach. How might the SLP collaborate with Chen in assessment to inform dual-language intervention that is consistent with Min's home environment?

Work Collaboratively

Collaboration is a vital solution in AAC implementation, whether specific skills or cultural, and linguistic knowledge are readily available or not. Incorporating different professionals' and stakeholders' perspectives through a team approach is well-documented in the provision of AAC services (Binger et al., 2012; Blackstone, Williams, & Wilkins, 2007; McNaughton et al., 2019). When serving people with CCN who come from CLD backgrounds, "culturally responsive teaming" is critical and must extend beyond the initial assessment into intervention services.

Although a team approach may not always be the easiest solution for professionals, it will bring the best outcomes for clients and their families. Beukelman and Mirenda (2013) outline the four most important processes to promote positive interdependence and support efficient team functioning including (a) discussing individual philosophies, goals, roles, and needs, (b) identifying learning and work-style needs, (c) agreeing on mutual team goals, and (d) creating positive resource, role, task, and reward interdependence. As with any aspect of service provision, unanticipated changes and challenges are likely to arise within a group dynamic, so regular opportunities to meet and openly reflect with team members without judgment is necessary for adequate problem-solving and prevention.

For monolingual SLPs serving people with CCN from CLD backgrounds, it is best to use an interpreter who can serve as both a cultural and linguistic broker (ASHA, n.d.; Hyter & Salas-Provance,

2019). A cultural broker identifies cultural practices and community characteristics (e.g., caregiving routines, beliefs about the origins of disabilities, expectations about the health care or education systems, cultural norms for interpersonal communication). Community advocates who are not trained in interpreting may also aid in the identification of these aspects of communication. As an example, a community broker may offer advice to an SLP about consistency of AAC use at school when families do not wish to protest out of deference to a professional. A linguistic broker identifies sociolinguistic norms in the client's speech (e.g., grammaticality, phonetic productions, semantics, pragmatics, common dialectal variations). Use of interpreters in assessment and intervention requires consistency. The SLP and interpreter continuously communicate about changes to the AAC system and may often spend time talking outside the session. The benefits of using an interpreter, including generalization, patient satisfaction, and expedited problem-solving, far outweigh the inconveniences.

Assessment-Specific Solutions

> "The vocabulary is sometimes so specific and the concept is so challenging to introduce, that the addition of the language barrier can make the process feel three times longer."
>
> —SLP

A team approach is critical to ensuring success across models of AAC assessment. Effective collaboration between professionals, clients, and families during the assessment process is central to this goal.

Before starting the assessment, the team should predetermine who will be involved at each step and describe each team member's role in accomplishing those steps. Due to the SLP's unique background and training, they may be the most likely candidate to serve as the team leader for an AAC assessment, making them responsible for facilitating participation and effective communication between team members. This is particularly important when working with CLD clients and families due to the critical need for extra preparation such as scheduling interpreters and translation services. Without the appropriate use of interpreters and inclusion of cultural/linguistic advocates, the team will not be able to effectively build trust and communication with the client and family. For instance, making assumptions about family members' cultural beliefs and levels of proficiency in speaking/listening and reading/writing can contribute to miscommunication and misunderstanding among team members resulting in poor planning, an absence of cultural responsivity, and less comprehensive results. Instead, team members should involve interpreters and cultural/linguistic brokers to some degree throughout planning and implementation of the evaluation, taking care to inquire with family members in advance regarding practical issues and constraints (e.g., schedule availability, transportation, language preference, comfort level with communication modalities). SLPs should approach the assessment process with humility by honoring differences, explicitly stating the limitations of their own lens, and reducing assumptions and expectations.

The steps of an AAC assessment are similar to that of any speech-language evaluation, although specific procedures to address the assessment goals may differ somewhat. General steps include referral, collecting case history, developing diagnostic questions, implementing evaluation procedures, identifying and recommending AAC interventions, securing funding, and monitoring progress through ongoing assessment (Binger et al., 2012).

Several important assessment components with corresponding goals and procedures must be carefully planned by the team evaluating the individual with CCN. Components of an AAC evaluation include the identification of communication needs, determination of goals and priorities, assessment of language and skills, identification of supports and barriers, intervention planning to enhance communicative competence, intervention planning for facilitators, and evaluation of intervention efficacy (Light, Roberts, Dimarco, & Greiner, 1998). The team must prepare specific procedures to ensure each component and goal is comprehensively addressed, such as trialing various devices, assessing the individual's ability to identify and use an assortment of symbols, evaluating potential access methods and modalities, teaching the individual and caregivers how to use the AAC system, and personalizing the system to meet the individual's needs (Dietz, Quach, Lund, & McKelvey, 2012).

With an AAC assessment, there may also be additional team members than those who would typically be involved in an assessment for a person without CCN. For example, there may be specialty personnel involved at various stages of the assessment process, which may include but is not limited to an an AAC finder, AAC clinical specialist, AAC research/policy specialist, AAC manufacturer/vendor, AAC funding agency, and AAC technology trainer (Binger et al., 2012). Having additional team members creates more lines of communication, thus the SLP's role as gatekeeper becomes increasingly important so that family members are not left out of the loop due to a language barrier. Additionally, multilingual people with CCN need to have consistent access to all of their languages for effective communication, and AAC specialists are team assets whose roles can alleviate some burden, because they will have the most up-to-date information regarding language availability across systems and devices.

Intervention-Specific Solutions

Facilitating a team approach when working in intervention services is a solution to many implementation problems, particularly generalization. CLD family members should have opportunities to offer insight and perspectives throughout treatment to ensure that solutions are generalized in the home and in other environments (e.g., schools, clinics, hospitals, and private practices). Notably, finding professional interpreting options that are consistently available for intervention can be a challenge with limited numbers of interpreters available and growing caseload sizes. Although interpreters cannot be replaced, working with minority-language speaking school professionals, bilingual family members, cultural and linguistic brokers, or remote bilingual therapists can inform intervention if limited options are available.

Intervention with the device should begin with a comprehensive understanding of language use in the household. First, and critically, all languages used in the household should be represented on the device. This will promote the integration of all communication partners in the household, which will lead to greater input delivered to the individual with CCN. The SLP ideally should provide direct instruc-

tion to all family members who communicate with the individual with CCN, including siblings, extended family who may be living in the home, and other individuals responsible for caregiving. Finally, the SLP should continuously work with the family to understand the dynamics of language use in the home. Language dominance may change over time and may depend on context. All people with CCN will enter and leave different social contexts over time, and the SLP should anticipate language growth, shifting dominance, and capacity for dynamic communication over time in order to reduce the risk of abandonment.

Consider the following case study, which profiles a Spanish-English-speaking child with Down syndrome and the solutions developed by the AAC team in collaboration with the family.

Carmen. Carmen was a 4-year-old girl with Down syndrome who lived at home with her mother, father, and maternal grandparents. Carmen's mother Lidia spoke Spanish and English and worked in the front office at the dual language school where her daughter attended preschool. Lidia used both languages to communicate with her daughter at home, although Carmen's father and grandparents spoke limited English, and so Spanish was the primary home language. Carmen's preschool teachers, special education teacher, SLP, and related-service providers worked together with Carmen's family to ensure she was receiving inclusive early services that would prepare her for a successful future. The SLP provided two sessions a week in the classroom, and one session a week outside of the classroom for one-on-one treatment. When possible, Lidia took breaks at work during scheduled speech-language therapy sessions to learn by observing or through informal coaching. Lidia made a point to check-in with team members to discuss her daughter's progress, ask what she could be doing at home, and bring up any new issues or questions regarding her daughter's treatment goals. The SLP and teachers debriefed weekly to support shared goals, encourage generalization of newly taught skills across contexts and settings, and send home progress summaries or ideas for carryover at home. Additionally, Lidia became more involved in advocacy efforts and began to attend events and workshops regularly hosted by the local chapter of the Down Syndrome Guild. Carmen continued to learn and use both Spanish and English and successfully expressed herself using a combination of single words, verbal approximations, gestures, signs, and visuals at home and in the classroom. Carmen thrived socially and especially enjoyed playing with her peers during centers. At the end of Carmen's preschool year, her IEP and kindergarten transition meeting was scheduled to address her progress and the plan for her service in kindergarten.

The team working with Lidia and Carmen maximized generalization of intervention into different settings and collaborated to promote intervention efforts in both languages. How might the team approach benefit Carmen as she transitions into kindergarten?

Prioritize the Family and Their Values

> "One thing that helps is to start the therapeutic relationship by building trust and rapport with the family, not just the child"
>
> —SLP

It is imperative that client and family member perspectives are explicitly sought and valued by the team. For many families, the opportunity for their child with disabilities to maintain their linguistic and cultural heritage is highly valued and can be more easily achieved through supportive relationships built with the child's educators and the SLP (Soto & Yu, 2014). It is the role of professionals to involve families equally in the process and take care not to treat them as afterthoughts or fringe team members (Beukelman & Mirenda, 2013). Clients and their families are primary team members, and should be considered as such from the onset of evaluation. This is especially important when the professional team members speak the majority language and when clients and their families speak a minority language. Participation may be wholly dependent on access to the minority language. As SLPs and families make decisions about AAC services for CLD individuals, a primary solution should be to integrate family input both initially and in ongoing consultation. Using a family-centered model for *all* patients and clients, regardless of cultural or linguistic background is a solution (Mandak, O'Neill, Light, & Fosco, 2017).

Considering the composition of the family unit is critical in AAC services. Diverse communicative family partners may be wishing to join the conversation about services for their family member with CCN. Families may be multigenerational or may include "nonbiologic kin" (Battle, 2012, p. 250). Additional family caregivers can ease caregiver burden when more agents are involved; however, it may also mean that primary caregivers have multiple family members for whom they are providing care or that there is not a true *primary* caregiver. More caregivers may also lead to diversity of languages, a range of proficiency in languages spoken in the home environment, and distinct beliefs about disabilities across generations. SLPs need to view family caregivers as additional communication partners to train and integrate into treatment. Understanding each family member's role in the home can provide valuable information for assessment and intervention.

Families may have opinions related to culturally loaded content that is present on devices. For emergent and competent communicators, culturally-loaded icons should depict an individual who is of the same racial or ethnic background as the family. For people with CCN, who possess literacy skills in any or multiple languages, cross-linguistic comparison of orthographic systems and re-examination of the organization of icons are necessary steps for the SLP to address alongside the family. When structures are shared across languages, the system might represent translation equivalents in both languages with a shared icon or with distinct icons. SLPs should consider implications of both scenarios for facilitating communication and which system best represents the family's communication. When divergent forms are present across languages, SLPs should ensure that AAC systems include both forms and that icons accurately indicate and differentiate targets. Additionally, families will make contributions about voices used in speech-generating devices that most accurately represent their family members with CCN. SLPs should work to value that input and provide options for CLD families.

Assessment-Specific Solutions

The roles of family members are particularly important in AAC assessment, as they are often primary communication partners who will serve as AAC facilitators. By consistently involving the family in the assessment process, the SLP can foster a system of trust and two-way communication, ensuring the opportunity to be heard and to share specialized knowledge. Ultimately this promotes collaborative decision-making and initial rapport building.

For a multilingual individual, it is imperative to assess skills in both or all languages. This includes evaluating all linguistic domains (semantics, phonology, morphology, syntax, and pragmatics) across all languages to determine areas of strength and need. In turn, the evaluation process tends to be more time-consuming with CLD populations. Furthermore, certain aspects of the evaluation may require more direct input from the client and family if the SLP has limited familiarity with the language or culture. For example, device features vary substantially, and how well they match with the client's cultural and linguistic background must be carefully considered to ensure appropriate selection of vocabulary, symbols, icons, and voice settings.

When assessing a CLD client with CCN, collecting information regarding their communication partners' language skills is also important because different partners may speak different languages and interactions with certain partners may occur more frequently within specific settings or contexts. For example, it is not uncommon for a child with CCN to attend school where the majority of communication partners speak English but reside in a home where English is not spoken by the primary caregivers. However, it is also likely that the child with CCN has friends at school or in the community who speak the home language and siblings who speak both English and the home language, thus complicating their ability to communicate functionally. Having access to an AAC system that easily allows a person to switch between languages is a priority. Ideally, a system that allows both languages to be used within a single utterance is preferred. For these reasons, the importance of language access may override other best matched features for multilingual people with CCN with respect to selecting an AAC platform and software application.

Intervention-Specific Solutions

> "I've come to learn that if you have the right AAC system, AAC therapy looks exactly the same as any other language therapy, with the same skilled interventions, just a different modality."
>
> —SLP

Extant literature on AAC interventions and on bilingual approaches to intervention provides some guidance on targets for CLD people with CCN. The AAC team must talk in an ongoing fashion with the family to identify *culturally congruent* practices (Guiberson & Ferris, 2018; Wing et al., 2007). Culturally congruent practices are those that capitalize upon existing cultural practices or routines for use in intervention. The result is that goals are both culturally appropriate and mutually motivating (Verdon, McLeod, & Wong, 2015). Leveraging existing routines also increases buy-in and likelihood of carryover with home-based interventions (Kummerer, 2012; Kummerer & Lopez-Reyna, 2009; Nunes & Hanline, 2007). These considerations require seeking input on initial goal-setting and engag-

ing in continued dialogue with family partners for progress monitoring on goals (Soto, 2012). Furthermore, intervention should support a family's learning of school culture and expectations, which is inclusive of conversational topics and typical interactions in the classroom (Soto, Solomon-Rice, & Caputo, 2009). Soto (2012) provided a list of open-ended relevant questions for gathering information from caregivers to identify intervention targets, including information such as languages that the individual needs to use at home, information the individual might wish to communicate, communication style of that individual, appropriate times to use AAC, and the effectiveness of intervention strategies performed in daily routines. A focus on the family's routines is a solution-oriented lens for SLPs and CLD families.

A primary goal of intervention is to teach all caregivers whose family members use AAC about aided language input (Wagner, 2018). First, the SLP must consider the family's home language environment, including which is the primary home language, which is the language being learned, and which is the preferred language for everyday activities. A child may be learning two languages simultaneously; that is, they are exposed to two languages in some proportion in the home environment. A child may also be sequentially learning two languages when he or she acquires at least in part one language before adding another language. Wagner suggested that an AAC system itself constitutes a third language to learn, and that CLD children with CCN who hear two languages may in fact be gaining a third language when they add an AAC system (Wagner, 2018). This notion gives importance to the provision of the native language, the second language, and/or bilingual input using the AAC system. Appropriate language input must be available in the AAC system.

Critically, caregivers should be directly instructed how to model input using AAC. For young children with CCN, this early language input is necessary to promote early interaction and achieve language milestones (e.g., AAC babbling, word combinations). When input is provided in multiple languages, children and caregivers need opportunities to practice in both languages (Wagner, 2018). Caregiver modeling using aided input is a key to giving a child communicative power. SLPs should request that a family give examples of functional phrases in the home language to determine appropriate input and maximize authenticity (Wagner, 2018). Furthermore, without seeing AAC used at home and without seeing it used bilingually with a variety of caregivers of varying language proficiencies, caregivers may not observe added benefits of having the system or device in the home (Soto, 2012; Stuart & Parette, 2002).

■ Special Considerations Across the Lifespan for People Who Use AAC

> "Our lives depend on this job. He was already fighting to keep the job with a language barrier. What's to stop them from firing him now that he uses a device to communicate?"
>
> —Caregiver

As stated earlier, ethnicity-based disparity in access is a challenge in providing AAC devices (Eneriz-Wiemer, Sanders, Barr, & Mendoza, 2014; Kay, Yeager, & Reed, 2008; Lindsay & Tsybina, 2011). This is apparent across the lifespan for people who rely on AAC. As the U.S. population ages and diversifies, SLPs are much more likely to play a role in service to CLD people with CCN who are experiencing acute and chronic health scenarios or end-of-life issues that lead them to AAC system use. When people with CCN are receiving medical care and come from CLD backgrounds, communication between providers is essential for patient safety, for transmission of health information to patient and caregiver, and for ethical care provision that takes into consideration health literacy, and is inclusive of vulnerable populations (Blackstone, Ruschke, Wilson-Stronks, & Lee, 2011). Thanks to technology, a burgeoning solution is the use of AAC options in acute health scenarios (e.g., ICU visits). They are suggested ways to improve the patient experience, facilitate communication between nonspeakers of English and English-only providers, and reduce the number of health care-related accidents (Hurtig, Czerniejewski, Bohnenkamp, & Na, 2013; Rodriguez et al., 2016).

High-tech options in AAC have proliferated in the last decade, which has advantages for patients, including increased customization of languages for CLD families and web-based searches for language-specific resources. Current technology also allows for easy creation of videos and recordings that are useful in intervention. However, older or nontechnology-oriented patients may also prefer low-tech AAC options for learning a new technology. It becomes critical to dialogue with CLD families about what is important for their family member with CCN for daily functional communication (World

Health Organization, 2001), and for end-of-life scenarios where appropriate (Kane, 2013). Still, culturally appropriate iconography for end-of-life rituals and routines is lacking. Additional efforts are needed to deliver better service to CLD families and individuals affected later in life.

Consider the following case study of a bilingual individual who has an acute need for AAC and the responsiveness to family engagement and values shown by the monolingual SLP.

Sergio. Sergio was a 65-year-old man who suffered a stroke while on an out-of-state visit to see his children and grandchildren. Sergio and his wife were traveling from a majority Spanish-speaking region, and neither spoke English. Sergio's son and granddaughter spoke English and were present at the time of the CVA to assist with interpreting and hospital intake. Sergio's communicative abilities were initially evaluated by a Spanish-speaking SLP, and, as he transitioned into outpatient care, he was assigned to an English-speaking therapist. His chief symptoms were characterized by general muscle weakness, severe apraxia of speech, and mild-to-moderate receptive aphasia. Prestroke, Sergio had some Spanish reading and writing abilities, having completed formal education through 4th grade. Sergio's wife's Spanish literacy skills were more limited as she did not complete school, and Spanish was her second language.

At baseline, Sergio was heavily reliant on gestures. He used some speech when answering yes/no questions, but his responses did not consistently correspond to the accompanying head gesture. With visual and verbal cues, he was able to imitate a limited repertoire of sounds and complete two-step directions with

minimal cues about half the time. The main challenges expressed by the family centered around Sergio communicating with staff. Therapy sessions and scheduling appointments required a bilingual family member's presence. Sergio's wife reported that his work as a mechanic and coach required both physical and communication capabilities that he was unable to perform post-stroke. The outpatient SLP worked to create materials for family training. "Homework" was key in the therapeutic approach, and all instructions were provided in written form, in-person, and with video demos in both languages for family members. The SLP worked extensively with members of the family to support material creation that matched Sergio's needs as he prepared to return to his home state.

The SLP worked with Sergio and his wife to incorporate the family's perspectives in creating materials appropriate for his unique circumstances. What other strategies might the SLP consider to help Sergio and his family transition back home?

■ Overcoming Abandonment of AAC

"I might know that eventually we are going to have to try a core board, or a speech generating device, but if I rush into that decision, the system will inevitably get abandoned."
—SLP

Not every implementation of an AAC system will end in success. Device abandonment occurs when a family no longer uses an AAC option for communication, and this may result in a lost investment of time and energy that a family and an AAC team exerted to obtain a device, or to develop an appropriate AAC system. On average, within the first three months of us, a third of devices are abandoned, with reports of nonuse as high as 75% (Phillips & Zhao, 1993; Scherer & Galvin, 1994). Several reasons may contribute to abandonment or inefficiency of an AAC system. Unnatural synthetic speech quality, unappealing cosmetic features, and inadequate portability or mounting of AAC systems have all been cited as contributing factors to device abandonment (Jinks & Sinteff, 1994; Riemer-Reiss & Wacker, 2000). Research has shown that the disadvantages related to the use of digitized speech can be especially problematic for CLD families whose negative experiences tend to be disproportionately higher than those of English-speaking individuals who use AAC (Alamsaputra, Kohnert, Munson, & Reichle, 2006; Axmear et al., 2005). Furthermore, inadequate communication partner training, environmental access restrictions, inappropriate vocabulary selection, and limited understanding of the multimodal nature of communication can also reduce the likelihood of an AAC system being maintained by the user and family (Murphy, Marková, Moodie, Scott, & Boa, 1996). Not surprisingly, making important AAC decisions via a professional-centered approach instead of a family-centered approach frequently leads to abandonment of an AAC system (Riemer-Reiss & Wacker, 2000), and CLD families are at a particularly high risk due to bias among team members and linguistic/cultural barriers. Unfortunately, abandonment can stem from a fractured or misguided effort on the part of the AAC team and other professionals. In semi-structured interviews with caregivers who had abandoned AAC devices, rejection of AAC devices occurred: when parents were influenced by the attitudes or lack of support from professionals, including SLPs; when ineffective communication occurred between professional stakeholders; and when AAC was being implemented in a community that did not support its use (Moorcroft, Scarinci, & Meyer, 2019). Along with the above-mentioned factors, CLD families face additional challenges that contribute to device abandonment.

Several suggestions may reduce device abandonment among CLDs families. First, the home communication may be more expedient than the AAC system. If that inefficiency is also compounded by a mismatch in cultural communication styles, the likelihood of continued use in the home environment is low. One possible solution can come from continued communication about goals with CLD families. SLPs can increase expediency of communication by selecting intervention targets that reflect established sources of communicative difficulty in the home.

Second, current AAC systems may lack the diversity of voices or languages for a family to develop familiarity. In work pertaining to training CLD partners for AAC, Soto states that "As long as the AAC device is not able to produce voice output in the home language, it will continue to be a less useful tool for the family" (Soto, 2012, p. 148). Ultimately a mismatch in language or voice output fails to be responsive to a family's home environment and communication style. Families may choose not to use AAC systems when they wish to build intimacy or to use humor with their family member with CCN. Building intimacy across cultural groups may require nuanced understanding of communication styles. SLPs should advocate for family-specific expressions of intimacy and humor to be included in communication devices.

When abandonment of an AAC system seems inevitable or has already occurred, it is critical to revisit the family's initial questions about the AAC system. Does it coincide with ongoing treatment targets? Was the family's message misconstrued along the way? Has communication in the home changed? Revisiting initial questions and engaging in ongoing dialogue about the AAC system, its implementation, and its potential for generalization can aid in continued use and in improvements to solutions on subsequent attempts. With the rapid evolution of technology, teams must revisit options as they become available to the public.

■ Concluding Remarks

Variety in the cultural and linguistic landscapes of schools, clinics, and hospitals is a reality and a gift. The recommendations contained in this chapter are not exhaustive. They are a starting place. Through self-examination, collaboration, and cultural humility, SLPs and other providers have the opportunity to improve service delivery for an underserved population.

■ References

Alamsaputra, D. M., Kohnert, K. J., Munson, B., & Reichle, J. (2006). Synthesized speech intelligibility among native speakers and non-native speakers of English. *Augmentative and Alternative Communication*, 22(4), 258–268. https://doi.org/10.1080/00498250600718555

American Speech-Language-Hearing Association. (n.d.). *Bilingual service delivery* [Practice portal]. Retrieved from http://www.asha.org/Practice-Portal/Professional-Issues/Bilingual-Service-Delivery

American Speech-Language-Hearing Association. (2016). *Code of ethics* [Ethics]. Retrieved from http://www.asha.org/policy/

American Speech-Language-Hearing Association. (2016). *Scope of practice in speech-language pathology* [Scope of practice]. Retrieved from http://www.asha.org/policy/

American Speech-Language-Hearing Association. (2018). *Demographic profile of ASHA members providing bilingual services, year-end 2018*. Retrieved from https://www.asha.org/uploadedFiles/Demographic-Profile-Bilingual-Spanish-Service-Members.pdf

Arias, G., & Friberg, J. (2017). Bilingual language assessment: Contemporary versus recommended practice in American schools. *Language, Speech, and Hearing Services in Schools, 48*, 1–15.

Axmear, E., Reichle, J., Alamsaputra, M., Kohnert, K., Drager, K., & Sellnow, K. (2005). Synthesized speech intelligibility in sentences. *Language, Speech, and Hearing Services in Schools, 36*(3), 244–250. https://doi.org/10.1044/0161-1461

Battle, D. E. (2012). *Communication disorders in multicultural and international populations*. Elsevier/Mosby.

Beukelman, D., & Mirenda, P. (2013). *Augmentative and alternative communication: Supporting children and adults with complex communication needs* (4th ed.). Brookes.

Binger, C., Ball, L, Dietz, A., Kent-Walsh, J., Lasker, J., Lund, S., . . . Quach, W. (2012). Personnel roles in the AAC assessment process, *Augmentative and Alternative Communication, 28*,4, 278–288. https://doi.org/10.3109/07434618.2012.716079

Blackstone, S. W., & Hunt-Berg, M. (2012). *Social networks: A communication inventory for individuals with complex communication needs and their communication partners*. Attainment Company.

Blackstone, S. W., Ruschke, K., Wilson-Stronks, A., & Lee, C. (2011). Converging communication vulnerabilities in health care: An emerging role for speech-language pathologists and audiologists. *SIG 14 Perspectives on Communication Disorders and Sciences in Culturally and Linguistically Diverse (CLD) Populations, 18*(1), 3–11.

Blackstone, S. W., Williams, M. B., & Wilkins, D. P. (2007) Key principles underlying research and practice in AAC. *Augmentative and Alternative Communication, 23*(3), 191–20. https://doi.org/10.1080/074346107 01553684

Bloomberg, K., West, D., Johnson, H., & Iacono, T. (2009). *Triple C: Checklist of communication competencies*. SCOPE: Victoria.

Bruno, J. (2010). *Test of aided-communication symbol performance*. Dynavox Mayer Johnson.

Caesar, L. G., & Kohler, P. D. (2007). The state of school-based bilingual assessment: Actual practice versus recommended guidelines. *Language, Speech, and Hearing Services in Schools, 38*, 190–200. https://doi.org/10.1044/0161-1461(2007/020)

Castaño, M. T., Biever, J. L., González, C. G., & Anderson, K. B. (2007). Challenges of providing mental health services in Spanish. *Professional Psychology: Research and Practice, 38*, 667–673. https://doi.org/1037/0735-7028.38.6.667

Castro, F. G., Barrera, M., & Martinez, C. R. (2004). The cultural adaptation of prevention interventions: Resolving tensions between fidelity and fit. *Society for Prevention Research, 5*, 41–45.

Core, C., Hoff, E., Rumiche, R., & Señor, M. (2013). Total and conceptual vocabulary in Spanish–English bilinguals from 22 to 30 months: Implications for assessment. *Journal of Language, Speech, and Hearing Research, 56*, 1637–1649. https://doi.org/10.1044/1092-4388(2013/11-0044)

De Lamo White, C., & Jin, L. (2011). Evaluation of speech and language assessment approaches with bilingual children. *International Journal of Language & Communication Disorders, 46*(6), 613–627.

Dietz, A., Quach, W., Lund, S. K., & McKelvey, M. (2012). AAC assessment and clinical decision making: The impact of experience. *Augmentative and Alternative Communication, 28*(3), 148–159.

Droop, M., & Verhoeven, L. (1998). Background knowledge, linguistic complexity, and second-language reading comprehension. *Journal of Literacy Research, 30*, 253–271. https://doi.org/10.1080/1086296 9809547998

Dynamic Therapy Associates & Tobii-Dynavox. (2014). *Dynamic AAC Goals Grid* (2nd ed.).

Ereniz-Wiemer, M., Sanders, L. M., Barr, D. A., & Mendoza, F. S. (2014). Parental limited English proficiency and health outcomes for children with special health care needs: A systematic review. *Academy of Pediatrics, 14*, 128–136. https://doi.org/10.1016/j.acap .2013.10.003.

Esping-Andersen, G., Garfinkel, I., Han, W., Magnuson, K., Wagner, S., & Waldfogel, J. (2012). Child care and school performance in Denmark and the United States. *Children and Youth Services Review, 34*, 576–589. https://doi.org/10.1016/j.childyouth .2011.10.010

Flores, G. (2005). The impact of medical interpreter services on the quality of health care: A systematic review. *Medical care research and review, 62*(3), 255–299.

Gamel-McCormick, M., & Dymond, S. (1994). *Augmentative communication assessment protocol for symbolic augmentative systems*. Virginia Commonwealth University.

Guiberson, M. & Ferris, K. P. (2018). Early language interventions for young dual language learners: A scoping review. *American Journal of Speech-Language Pathology, 28*, 945–963. https://doi.org/10.1044/2019 _AJSLP-IDLL-18-0251

Gutierrez-Clellen, V. F. (1999). Language choice in intervention with bilingual children. *American Journal of Speech-Language Pathology, 8*, 291–302. https://doi.org/10 .1044/2019_AJSLP-IDLL-18-0251

Hoff, E., & Core, C. (2015). What clinicians need to know about bilingual development. *Seminars in Speech and Language, 36*, 89–99.

Huer, M. B. (1997). Culturally inclusive assessments for children using augmentative and alternative communication (AAC). *Journal of Children's Communication Development, 19*(1), 23–34. https://doi.org/10.1177/152574019701900104

Huer, M. B., Parette, H. P., & Saenz, T. I. (2001). Conversations with Mexican Americans regarding children with disabilities and augmentative and alternative communication. *Communication Disorders Quarterly, 22*(4), 197–206.

Hurtig, R., Czerniejewski, E., Bohnenkamp, L., & Na, J. (2013). Meeting the needs of limited English proficiency patients. *Perspectives on Augmentative and Alternative Communication, 22*, 91–101. https://doi.org/10.1044/aac22.2.91

Hyter, Y. (2014). A conceptual framework for responsive global engagement in communication sciences and disorders. *Topics in Language Disorders, 34*, 103–120.

Hyter, Y. D., & Salas-Provance, M. B. (2019). *Culturally responsive practices in speech, language, and hearing sciences*. Plural Publishing.

Individuals with Disabilities Education Act, 20 U.S.C. § 1400 et seq. (2004).

Jinks, A., & Sinteff, B. (1994). Consumer response to AAC devices: Acquisition, training, use, and satisfaction. *AAC: Augmentative and Alternative Communication, 10*(3), 184–190. https://doi.org/10.1080/07434619412331276890

Johnston, S. S., O'Neill, R. E., & Schumann, J. (2018). Assessing symbol acquisition and preference during functional communication training with English language learners who use augmentative and alternative communication. *Perspectives of the ASHA Special Interest Groups, 3*(4). Retrieved from https://pubs.asha.org/doi/10.1044/persp3.SIG12.164

Kane, C. (2013). Supporting adults with intellectual and developmental disabilities and communication disorders to express end-of-life wishes. *Perspectives on Gerontology, 18*(3), 80. https://doi.org/10.1044/gero18.3.80

Karnezos, J. L. B. (2018). *The effect of a checklist on school teams' plans for augmentative and alternative communication assessment* (Doctoral dissertation). Pennsylvania State University, University Park, PA.

Kay-Raining Bird, E., Genesee, F., & Verhoeven, L. (2016). Bilingualism in children with developmental disorders: A narrative review. *Journal of Communication Disorders, 16*, 1–13. https://doi.org/10.1016/j.jcomdis.2016.07.003

Kaye, H. S., Yeager, P., & Reed, M. (2008). Disparities in usage of assistive technology among people with disabilities. *Assistive Technology, 20*, 194–203. https://doi.org/10.1080/10400435.2008.10131946

Kleiman, L. (2003). *Functional Communication Profile, Revised*. LinguiSystems.

Koball, H. & Jiang, Y., (2018). *Basic facts about low-income children: Children under 18 years, 2016*. National Center for Children in Poverty, Mailman School of Public Health, Columbia University.

Kohnert, K., & Medina, A. (2009). Bilingual children and communication disorders: A 30-year research retrospective. *Seminars in Speech and Language, 30*, 219–233. https://doi.org/10.1055/s0029-1241721.

Kovach, T. M. (2009). *AAC Profile: A continuum of learning*. LinguiSystems.

Kremer-Sadlik, T. (2005). To be or not to be bilingual: Autistic children from multilingual families. *Proceedings of the 4th International Symposium on Bilingualism, 5*, 1225–1234. Retrieved from http://www.cascadilla.com/isb4.html

Kummerer, S. E. (2012). Promising strategies for collaborating with Hispanic parents during family-centered speech-language intervention. *Communication Disorders Quarterly, 33*, 84–95. https://doi.org/10.1177/1525740109358453

Kummerer, S. E., & Lopez-Reyna, N. A. (2009). Engaging Mexican immigrant families in language and literacy interventions: Three case studies. *Remedial and Special Education, 30*(6), 330–343. https://doi.org/10.1177/0741932508321014

Light, J. C., Roberts, B., Dimarco, R., & Greiner, N. (1998). Augmentative and alternative communication to support receptive and expressive communication for people with autism. *Journal of Communication Disorders, 31*, 153–180.

Lindsay, S. & Tsybina, I. (2011). Predictors of unmet needs for communication and mobility assistive devices among youth with a disability: The role of socio-cultural factors. *Disability and Rehabilitation: Assistive Technology, 6*, 10–21. https://doi.org/10.3109/17483107.2010.514972

Mandak, K., O'Neill, T., Light, J., & Fosco, G. M. (2017). Bridging the gap from values to actions: A family systems framework for family-centered AAC services. *Augmentative and Alternative Communication, 33*(1), 32–41. https://doi.org/10.1080/07434618.2016.1271453

Marinova-Todd, S. H., Colozzo, P., Mirenda, P., Stahl, H., Kay-Raining Bird, E., Parkington, K., . . . Genesee, F. (2016). Professional practices and opinions about services available to bilingual children with developmental disabilities: An international study. *Journal of Communication Disorders, 63*, 47–62. Retrieved from https://doi.org/10.1016/j.jcomdis.2016.05.004

Mazor, S. S., Hampers, L. C., Chande, V. T. & Krug, S. E. (2002). Teaching Spanish to pediatric emergency physicians: Effects on patient satisfaction. *Archives of Pediatric and Adolescent Medicine, 156*, 693–695.

McCord, M. S., & Soto, G. (2004). Perceptions of AAC: An ethnographic investigation of Mexican-American families. *Augmentative and Alternative Communication, 20*(4), 209–227. https://doi.org/10.1080/07434610400005648

McNamara, E. (2018). Bilingualism, augmentative and alternative communication, and equity: Making a case for people with complex communication needs. *Perspectives of the ASHA Special Interest Groups, 3*(4), 138–145.

McNaughton, D., Light, J., Beukelman, D. R., Klein, C., Nieder, D. & Nazareth, G.

(2019). Building capacity in AAC: A person-centered approach to supporting participation by people with complex communication needs. *Augmentative and Alternative Communication, 35*, 56–68, https://doi.org/10.1080/07434618.2018.1556731

Méndez, L. I., Crais, E. R., Castro, D. C., & Kainz, K. (2015). A culturally and linguistically responsive vocabulary approach for young Latino dual language learners. *Journal of Speech, Language, and Hearing Research, 58*(1), 93–106. https://doi.org/10.1044/2014_JSLHR-L-12-0221

Mills-Koonce, W., Willoughby, M., Garrett-Peters, P., Wagner, N., & Vernon-Feagans, L. (2016). The interplay among socioeconomic status, household chaos, and parenting in the prediction of child conduct problems and callous–unemotional behaviors. *Development and Psychopathology, 28*, 757–771. https://doi.org/10.1017/S0954579416000298

Mindel, M., & John, J. (2018). Bridging the school and home divide for culturally and linguistically diverse families using augmentative and alternative communication systems. *Perspectives of the ASHA Special Interest Group, 3*(4), 154–163. Retrieved from https://pubs.asha.org/doi/10.1044/persp3.SIG12.154

Moorcroft, A., Scarinci, N., & Meyer, C. (2019). A systematic review of the barriers and facilitators to the provision and use of low-tech and unaided AAC systems for people with complex communication needs and their families. *Disability and Rehabilitation: Assistive Technology, 14*, 710–731. https://doi.org/10.1080/17483107.2018.1499135

Morgan, P. L., Farkas, G., Hillemeier, M. M., Li, H., Pun, W. H., & Cook, M. (2017). Cross-cohort evidence of disparities in service receipt for speech or language impairments. *Exceptional Children, 84*(1), 27–41. https://doi.org/10.1177/0014402917718341

Mueller, T. G., Singer, G. H. S., & Carranza, F. D. (2006). A national survey of the educational planning and language instruction practices for students with moderate to severe disabilities who are English language learners. *Research and Practice for Persons with Severe Disabilities*, 31(3), 242–254. https://doi.org/10.1177/154079690603100304

Murphy, J., Marková, I., Moodie, E., Scott, J., & Boa, S. (1996). AAC systems: Obstacles to effective use. *European Journal of Disorders of Communication*, *31*, 31–44.

National Center for Education Statistics. (2018). *The condition of education 2018.* Retrieved from https://files.eric.ed.gov/full text/ED583502.pdf

Nunes, D., & Hanline, M. F. (2007). Enhancing the alternative and augmentative communication use of a child with autism through a parent-implemented naturalistic intervention. *International Journal of Disability, Development and Education*, *54*, 177–197. https://doi.org/10.1080/1034 9120701330495

Office of Administration for Children and Families. (2016). *Policy statement on supporting the development of children who are dual language learners in early childhood programs.* Retrieved from https://sites.ed.gov/underservedyouth/files/2017/01/Policy-Statement-on-Supporting-the-Develop ment-of-Children-who-are-Dual-Language-Learners-in-Early-Childhood-Programs.pdf

Office of Civil Rights. (2015). *Dear colleague letter: English learner students and limited English proficient parents.* Retrieved from https://www2.ed.gov/about/offices/list/ocr/letters/colleague-el-201501.pdf

Oller, D. K. (2005). The distributed characteristic in bilingual learning. In J. Cohen, K. T. McAlister, K. Rolstad, & J. MacSwan (Eds.), *Proceedings of the 4th International Symposium on Bilingualism.* (pp. 1744–1749). Cascadilla Press.

Parette Jr, H. P., & Dempsey Marr, D. (1997). Assisting children and families who use augmentative and alternative communication (AAC) devices: Best practices for school psychologists. *Psychology in the Schools*, *34*(4), 337–346.

Peña, E. D. (2016). Supporting the home language of bilingual children with develop-

mental disabilities: From knowing to doing. *Journal of Communication Disorders*, *63*, 85–92.

Pesco, D., MacLeod, A. A. N., Kay-Raining Bird, E., Cleave, P., Trudeau, N., . . . Verhoeven, L. (2016). A multi-site review of policies affecting opportunities for children with developmental disabilities to become bilingual. *Journal of Communication Disorders*, *63*, 15–31.

Pham, G., Kohnert, K., & Mann, D. (2011). Addressing clinician-client mismatch: A preliminary intervention study with a bilingual Vietnamese-English preschooler. *Language, Speech, and Hearing Services in the Schools*, *42*, 408–422. https://doi.org/10.10 44/0161-1461(2011/10-0073)

Phillips, B., & Zhao, H. (1993). Predictors of assistive technology abandonment. *Assistive Technology*, *5*, 36–45.

Pickl, G. (2011). Communication intervention in children with severe disabilities and multilingual backgrounds: Perceptions of pedagogues and parents. *Augmentative and Alternative Communication*, *27*(4), 229–244. https://doi.org/10.3109/0743461 8.2011.630021

Riemer-Reiss, M. L., & Wacker, R. R. (2000). Factors associated with assistive technology discontinuance among individuals with disabilities. *Journal of Rehabilitation*, *66*, 44–50.

Ripat, J. & Woodgate, R. (2011). The intersection of culture, disability and assistive technology. *Disability and Rehabilitation: Assistive Technology*, *6*, 87–96. https://doi.org/10.3109/17483107.2010.507859

Robinson, N. R., & Solomon-Rice, P. L. (2009). Supporting collaborative teams and families in AAC. In G. Soto & C. Zangari (Eds.), *Practically speaking: Language, literacy, and academic development for students with AAC needs* (pp. 289–312). Brookes.

Rodriguez, C. S., Rowe, M., Thomas, L., Shuster, J., Koeppel, B., & Cairns, P. (2016). Enhancing the communication of suddenly speechless critical care patients. *American Journal of Critical Care*, *25*(3), e40–e47. https://doi.org/10.4037/ajcc2016217

Roseberry-McKibbin, C. (2008). *Multicultural students with special language needs* (3rd ed.). Academic Communication Associates.

Rowland, C. (2004). *Communication matrix* (Rev. ed.). Oregon Health & Science University, Design to Learn Projects.

Scherer, M. J., & Galvin, J. C. (1994). Matching people with technology. *Rehabilitation Management, 7*(2), 128–130.

Solomon-Rice, P. L., Soto, G., & Robinson, N. B. (2018). Project building bridges: Training speech-language pathologists to provide culturally and linguistically responsive augmentative and alternative communication services to school-age children with diverse backgrounds. *Perspectives of the ASHA Special Interest Groups, 3*(4), 186–204.

Soto, G. (2012). Training partners in AAC in culturally diverse families. *Perspectives of the ASHA Special Interest Groups,* 144–150.

Soto, G., Solomon-Rice, P., & Caputo, M. (2009). Enhancing the personal narrative skills of elementary school-aged students who use AAC: The effectiveness of personal narrative intervention. *Journal of Communication Disorders, 42,* 43–57.

Soto, G., & Yu, B. (2014). Considerations for the provision of services to bilingual children who use augmentative and alternative communication. *Augmentative and Alternative Communication, 30*(1), 83–92. https://doi.org/10.3109/07434618.2013.878751

Stuart, S., & Parette, H. P. (2002). Native Americans and augmentative and alternative communication issues. *Multiple Voices, 5*(1), 38–53.

Suphanchaimat, R., Kantamaturapoj, K., Putthasri, W. & Prakongsai, P. (2015). Challenges in the provision of healthcare services for migrants: A systematic review through providers' lens. *BMC Health Services Research 15,* 390. https://doi.org/10.1186/s12913-015-1065-z

U.S. Census Bureau. (2017). *New Census Bureau report analyzes U.S. population projections.* Retrieved from https://www.cen sus.gov/newsroom/press-releases/2015/cb15-tps16.html

Ventura County Special Education Local Plan Area. (2017). *Ventura County comprehensive alternate language proficiency survey for students with moderate-severe disabilities.* Retrieved from https://www.vc selpa.org/LinkClick.aspx?fileticket=QUL LcSs2dY%3D&portalid=0

Verdon, S., McLeod, S., & Wong, S. (2015). Supporting culturally and linguistically diverse children with speech, language and communication needs: Overarching principles, individual approaches. *Journal of Communication Disorders, 58,* 74–90. https://doi .org/10.1016/j.jcomdis.2015.10.002

Wagner, D. K. (2018). Building augmentative communication skills in homes where English and Spanish are spoken: Perspectives of an evaluator/interventionist. *Perspectives on Augmentative and Alternative Communication, 3,* 172–185. https://doi.org/10.1044/persp3.SIG12.172

Wilcox, M. J., Weintraub, H .L., & Aier, D. (2003). *Confidence in use of assistive technology by early interventionists.* Paper presented to the annual meeting of Center for Exceptional Children, Division for Early Childhood, Washington, DC.

Wing, C., Kohnert, K., Pham, G., Cordero, K. N., Ebert, K. D., Kan, P. F., & Blaiser, K. (2007). Culturally consistent treatment for late talkers. *Communication Disorders Quarterly, 29,* 20–27.

Wong Fillmore, L. (2000). Loss of family languages: Should educators be concerned? *Theory Into Practice, 39*(4), 203–210.

World Health Organization. (2001). *International classification of functioning, disability and health: ICF.* Author.

Yu, B. (2013). Issues in bilingualism and heritage language maintenance: Perspectives of minority-language mothers of children with autism spectrum disorders. *American Journal of Speech-Language Pathology, 22,* 10–24.

PART V
Final Thoughts

14

Becoming a Solution-Oriented AAC Provider

Billy T. Ogletree and Kelsey Williams

This book features both challenges and solutions central to AAC service provision. Authors generated their chapters to address two simple questions: (1) What challenges have you encountered in AAC-related practice? and (2) What evidence-based solutions or well-reasoned speculations about possible solutions are worthy of consideration by stakeholders and service providers? At the start of the book, we acknowledged that not all challenges are examined here. The ones that are, however, span a range of populations, disabilities, and service settings. Furthermore, chapter authors offer unique insights into how researchers and master clinicians approach challenges in their practices.

Our final chapter pulls from the chapters that precede it to examine the idea of solution-oriented AAC practice. Chapter 1 suggests that many professionals who serve individuals relying on AAC systems and devices are likely to be solution-oriented. It also suggests that AAC stakeholders often exhibit "grit and resilience" in their pursuit of solutions and that these qualities may be central to effective AAC outcomes. "Grit" is described by terms like "perseverance," "passion," and "sustained commitment," whereas "resilience" is portrayed as an ability to "bounce back" after hardship (Duckworth, Peterson, Matthews, & Kelly, 2006; Tempski et al., 2015; Shi, Wang, YuGe, & Wang, 2015). Resilience is suggested to be an essential feature of grit (Stoffel & Cain, 2018). For anyone who has had the good fortune to observe ideal AAC services, the notion of grit and resilience as characteristics of providers should feel familiar.

If grit and resilience are critical to ideal solution-oriented AAC service provision, how are these attributes fostered? Chapter 1 suggests that past AAC success, empathy, spirituality, and encouragement may fuel provider grit and resilience. This chapter takes these speculations further by offering a model to guide AAC stakeholders as they pursue solution-oriented practices. Components of this model are illustrated with examples drawn from the chapters of this book. Finally, readers are charged with a call to be solution-oriented.

Human Problem-Solving

Before considering human problem-solving as a process, it is interesting to note that problem-solving abilities do not always lead to solutions. That is, human problem-solving is impacted by a host of variables. Among other things, these include extrinsic and intrinsic motivational factors. For example, assuming some problem-solving capacity, extrinsic motivators such as financial gain or professional notoriety may encourage an individual to work hard to achieve a desirable solution. Similarly, intrinsic motivators like grit and resilience may drive the capable problem-solver to elegant and innovative solutions. We'll return to the key concepts of grit and resilience in our model for solution-oriented providers later in this chapter. What follows is a brief review of human problem-solving in general.

In a broad sense, arriving at solutions to problems, even commonplace ones, is an innate human ability. That is, humans face and address problems daily and have done so for millennia. Some clearly do this better than others, making the process of human problem-solving both interesting and worthy of examination, especially as it applies to AAC decision-making.

Current Thought About Human Problem-Solving

Our present knowledge of problem-solving is rich, but incomplete. What is known suggests that humans approach this process with some commonalities. It has been proposed that we reduce problems to three factors: *givens, goals,* and *operations* (Wang & Chiew, 2010). *Giv-*

ens are pieces of information available as part of the problem, *goals* are the desired termination states of a solution to the problem, and *operations* are potential actions executed to achieve the goal of the problem, a termination state. For every problem to be solved, there is a corresponding *problem space* containing all known possible goals and paths related to the problem.

Humans have been observed to employ various strategic approaches to problem-solving. Wang and Chiew (2010) described these as *direct facts, heuristic, analogy, hill climbing, algorithmic deduction, exhaustive search, divide-and-conquer,* and *analysis and synthesis.* Labels for these approaches reflect processes employed during each. *Direct facts, algorithm deduction, analysis and synthesis,* and *analogy* problem-solving involve solutions to new problems based on known solutions to similar problems. In contrast, a *heuristic* approach requires adopting the most probable solutions as a rule of thumb as problems are addressed. *Hill climbing* and *divide and conquer* both involve reductionist methods to problems that utilizes small solutions to move slowly toward broad resolutions. Finally, an *exhaustive search* approach includes systematically examining all possible solutions.

Although strategies are helpful when solving problems, they do not guarantee solutions. In fact, the process of problem-solving is recursive in that as one portion of a problem is solved, many others may be revealed. As problems arise and expand, individual differences among problem-solvers may impact the likelihood of eventual solutions (Delaney, Ericsson, & Knowles, 2004). For example, one's knowledge of the complexities of a problem at hand or their past positive and negative experiences with comparable situations may make solutions more or less probable (Duris, 2018; Lovett & Anderson, 1996; Ross, 1987; Wang & Chiew, 2010). Furthermore, some problem solvers may be particularly efficient with approaches or strategies, making their efforts more productive (Bassok et al., 2004). It appears, then, that myriad variables contribute to effective problem-solving.

Mechanisms of Effective Problem Solvers

Thus far, we have suggested that there are common strategic approaches utilized by humans as they solve problems. We've also noted that as problems are solved, unexpected new problems may arise. Finally, we have suggested that some individuals perform well as problem-solvers due to their knowledge and experiences. What follows is the presentation of several mechanisms used by effective problem-solvers. Mechanisms can be thought of as larger theoretical orientations. The likely strategies associated with each mechanism are mentioned within the context of AAC problem-solving.

Mechanism 1: Similarity Discovery

Similar problems often have similar solutions. Duris (2018) refers to the process of comparing current and past problems as case-based reasoning. To use this mechanism, a problem-solver identifies a set of problem concepts that relate to previously solved problems. By doing this, the solver can apply historically effective solutions, expediting the problem-solving process.

This mechanism is intuitive and familiar to most of us. For example, in the world of AAC, we have all encountered problems that are familiar. Positioning, access, technological competence, and funding all come to mind. The similarity discovery mechanism simply suggests that our previous problems inform our approach to new problems (Bassok, 2003; Lovett & Anderson, 1996; Ross, 1987). Similarity discovery as a mechanism seems to invoke the *algorithm deduction, analysis and synthesis*, and *analogy* problem-solving strategies described above (Wang & Chiew, 2010).

Mechanism 2: Relation and Association Discovery

Effective problem-solvers identify facts, problems, and/or situations related to the problem to be solved, subsequently creating relationships and associations useful in their problem-solving journey. They use this mechanism to process possible solutions, while filtering out unimportant information. Duris (2018) notes that effective problem solvers' ability to both link important data and filter out that which is unimportant, contributes to effective and efficient solutions.

Once again, drawing from relationships and associations appears to be a relevant mechanism applied by AAC providers. For example, prioritizing the desires and preferences of the individual using AAC and their stakeholders may well lead to the creation of relationships and associations as solutions are generated that embrace multiple, meaningful perspectives. This mechanism pairs nicely with *hill climbing* and *divide and conquer* strategic problem-solving (Wang & Chiew, 2010).

Mechanism 3: General Solutions

As processors, humans are most likely to remember general yet crucial aspects of information or experiences useful in problem-solving. These easily recalled memories are often vital when searching for solutions. Duris (2018) notes effective problem-solvers are known to look first at promising, big picture (general) solutions, then narrow down the details later (Bassok, 2003; Duris, 2018; Lovett & Anderson, 1996; Ross, 1987). Given that a solution to one problem may, in fact, uncover associated problems, use of a general solution-oriented approach to problem-solving can provide a broad-based solution orientation helpful with addressing unexpected problems along the way.

The use of a general, big-picture solution mechanism should certainly be familiar to those in the world of AAC. In fact, the undergirding emphasis upon grit and resilience in this chapter's AAC problem-solving model (see Figure 14–1, ahead) likely reflects a general solution perspective. That is, effective AAC providers and teams see the ultimate "big picture" prize and persevere until it becomes a reality. All of Wang and Chiew's (2010) problem-solving strategies appear to be involved in a general solution mechanism.

Mechanism 4: Abstraction

As with previous mechanisms, abstraction allows problem-solvers to break down problems into a representation of those features that are related to the problem's general pattern (Anderson, 1983; Bassok, 2003; Duris, 2018). This concept, although related more closely to mathematical problems, can also inform human problem solving. By breaking down a problem into its most essential parts, an effec-

tive problem-solver can clearly see the most important parts of the problem to address.

Most AAC teams use abstraction. In fact, teams may divide and conquer problems as an efficient way to arrive at solutions. If, for example, device procurement is the big problem for a team, some team members may explore funding options while others seek devices for a trial run to support funding. Here, all team members are working toward solving a large problem by utilizing their varied experiences, contacts, and resources. Abstraction aligns closely with Wang and Chiew's (2010) exhaustive search solution strategy.

Mechanism 5: Intuition

Intuition enables problem-solvers to pursue solutions even though the solver cannot articulate the reasons why she should do so (Duris, 2018; Style, 1979). Effective problem-solvers often rely on intuition as much as data. Intuitive thinking may expedite solutions by providing possible directions to pursue (Duris, 2018; Style, 1979).

Although there is little to support a contention that effective AAC providers are intuitive, the idea is appealing. Furthermore, an intuitive mind may well be key to developing grit and resilience, with the solution seeker driven by informed hunches about probable success. Again, an intuitive solution-oriented perspective would seem to be aided by all of Wang and Chiew's (2010) strategies.

Mechanism 6: Context Sensitivity

Context sensitivity, as a problem-solving mechanism, is centered in the observation that things or situations can behave, respond, or be interpreted differently depending on context. In the process of problem-solving, context is vitally important (Duris, 2018). This mechanism mostly involves ruling out solution options that do not fall within the context of the problem to be solved.

In the AAC world, there are solutions that might work in one context but not in another. Effective providers utilize all of Wang and Chiew's (2010) solution strategies to resolve problems in ways sensitive to contextual variance.

Clearly, with appropriate strategies and mechanisms, we all solve problems every day. For the AAC provider or team, problem-solving is central to the generation of effective solutions for individuals with complex communication needs across myriad life settings. What follows is a model describing a process leading to solution-oriented practice. Although our model may not apply to all who pursue it as a guide, we believe it provides one path to effective AAC solutions.

■ A Model to Guide Solution-Oriented AAC Practice

The reality of AAC challenges and the need for effective AAC solutions is not new. Since the very early days of the discipline, providers have faced challenges related to decision-making and practice. As the field evolved, the experiences (successes and failures) of early providers informed those who followed. Over time, practice patterns became established and subsequently modified by research findings and technological innovations. To guide AAC practice, researchers utilize illustrative models to describe commu-

nication processes as well as assist with assessment and intervention practices (Lloyd, Quist, & Windser, 2009; Loncke, 2014). This chapter offers such a model for solution-oriented AAC practice. The model, illustrated in Figure 14–1, features several key components. Model elements are presented within a framework of two concentric circular patterns. The inner circle moves left to right and includes variables that contribute to the solution-oriented practice of AAC. The outer circle represents the importance of grit and resilience as overarching attributes of a solution-oriented perspective. A discussion of the model follows.

Solution-Oriented AAC

Our model is not intended to describe "the path" to becoming a solution-oriented AAC provider, but to guide that process by identifying and describing central and critical points to ponder. With that in mind, we'll consider each component of the model before examining it as a whole, and eventually tying the model to notable examples of problem-solving presented in the chapters of this book.

Becoming a Critical Observer

Experienced AAC providers know the value of critical observation. Critical observers observe both people and processes (Eudy, 2019). The solution-oriented AAC provider must critically observe people who use AAC, their partners, and their environments to know that challenges exist. They must also observe nuanced aspects of individual lives and where communication failures arise. Sometimes challenges are subtle. These may include, among other things, covert yet negative

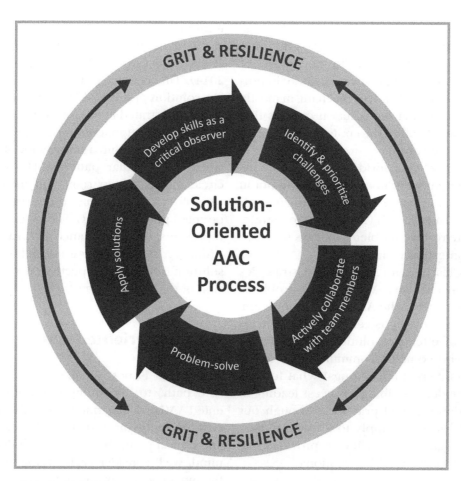

Figure 14–1. A model of solution-oriented AAC practice.

attitudes of communicative partners, discomfort with altered communicative roles caused by acquired impairments, or reduced communicative opportunities due to faulty assumptions about abilities or interests. Of course, challenges can be obvious as well, such as physical barriers limiting access to communication and denials of services or technology based upon inadequate resources or arbitrary eligibility requirements.

This notion of observing is not new to AAC. Beukelman and Light (2020) charged providers to observe and address several barriers that impact individuals with com-

plex communication needs (CCN). In our model, we encourage AAC professionals to critically observe the everyday lives of those they serve. We take this a step further and suggest that the best critical observers will establish authentic and meaningful relationships with those using AAC and their stakeholders, which leads to honest discussions of challenges. As providers, observations we make in isolation are ours alone. Our observations, even if obtained through critical and comprehensive efforts, must be validated through dialogue with those we serve and their communicative partners.

Identifying and Prioritizing Challenges

The second step of our model includes the identification and prioritization of AAC challenges. Critical observations will undoubtedly lead to lists of potential challenges. These can be confirmed or refuted by the individual who uses AAC and their stakeholders. Again, it simply cannot be overstated that provider observations need to be validated by others, especially individuals with CCN seeking AAC solutions.

After a list of challenges is compiled, providers are tasked with prioritizing the needs requiring immediate attention. A logical first step is to ask the person who uses AAC. Obviously, the individual with CCN has the most important voice in the selection of priority challenges. Prioritization could also be based upon the perceived urgency of stakeholders, the effects on participation and inclusion for the person with CCN, and the likelihood of impact beyond the challenge selected. For example, other stakeholders may have critical insights specific to the relative importance of challenges due to their multiple and varied perspectives. Furthermore, challenges that prevent individuals with CCN from participating with ACC and included as members of their communities are certainly deserving of attention. Finally, addressing some challenges may have positive cascading effects on others. That is, a solution for one challenge may alleviate other problems yet to be addressed. Addressing the need for an effective communication system across settings, for example, may open doors to employment and social opportunities that previously seemed closed.

It is fair to say that the identification and prioritization of challenges is a task worthy of careful consideration and multiple perspectives, one that likely motivates our next model component, utilizing a collaborative team perspective.

Collaborating as a Team

Ogletree (1999) defined a team as two or more people working together to solve a problem. Clearly, a team orientation helps with most challenges, and is an important part of all aspects of this model; teams of observers can assist with assuring the validity of observations, and teams of stakeholders, including the person using AAC, can provide invaluable insights into challenge identification and prioritization.

As providers move to the problem-solving step of our model, it will be useful to have a team in place. This may require the more formal creation of a team structure involving the solicitation of team members and some discussion about team functioning. With respect to membership, teams must involve those closest to prioritized challenges. This will involve both the individual with CCN using AAC, as well as their communicative partners in settings where selected challenges are prevalent. It may also be helpful to have individuals involved with the authority to alter policies or practices central to many AAC challenges. For example, if a team identifies and prioritizes a challenge specific to device access in multiple school settings, a team member with administrative authority in the school may be critical to enacting needed change.

Ogletree (1999) points to several characteristics of effective teams that should inform team functioning. These include, among other things, commitment to open communication and respect for every team member's opinions and contributions. With an efficient and committed team in place, solutions to AAC challenges become more likely.

This model component is based upon collaboration, emphasizing that teams are not as effective unless they work together. Ogletree (1999) mentions three common team models in his description of teaming (i.e., multidisciplinary, interdisciplinary, and transdisciplinary) and identified that all models create the possibility for collaboration as problems arise. This said, he notes that interdisciplinary and transdisciplinary teams identify collaboration as a key to their success making them well-suited for AAC assessment and intervention.

Problem-Solving

This chapter has provided some limited insights into the strategies and mechanisms used by effective problem-solvers. In sum, teams and the individuals who comprise them will potentially apply a host of problem-solving strategies in their efforts to generate AAC solutions. No doubt, team members may approach challenges from differing perspectives and with different ideas for solutions. We see this as a positive attribute of teaming, one that will improve eventual solution choices, assuming teams work collaboratively.

Whether providers and teams utilize one or more of Duris' (2018) mechanisms of effective problem-solving and/or apply any of the many strategic approaches to solving problems described by Wang and Chiew (2010) (all reviewed earlier), there is little doubt that there will be the need for problem-solving during AAC service delivery. In all stages of AAC assessment, challenges arise. These may relate to determining team composition and func-

tioning, access and positioning, obtaining representative and reliable results across assessment domains, sharing findings, trialing and procuring devices, and securing funding, among other things. Likewise, in AAC intervention problems are common. Problems persist at every turn. Challenges surface as providers transition assessment findings into effective everyday solutions across life settings, create socially valid objectives for treatment, acquire participation of all stakeholders, monitor progress, and alter treatment plans.

It seems almost too obvious to include problem-solving as one of our model components, yet by doing so we hope to heighten awareness to the simple fact that effective AAC services seldom come easily. The process of AAC assessment and intervention is complex, not only involving the individual with CCN, but everyone in their world, and every environment encountered. Challenges are inevitable and will require a commitment to effective problem-solving by all involved.

Applying Solutions

The final component to the inner circle of our model is the application of AAC solutions. One might think that once generated, AAC solution application should be simple. Although this can be the case, applying solutions may well generate new problems, sending providers and teams back into the spiral of our model. For example, assume a device is selected for an individual with CCN and several associated problems are addressed in this process via observation, prioritization, team collaboration, and problem-solving. Although generally successful when the device is used in a specific, yet critical work setting, communication failures occur at an unexpectedly high rate. Here, the team may need to apply the effective problem-solving features of our model again, relative to this one setting of concern.

The Role of Grit and Resilience

As noted, when first describing our model, grit and resilience fill the outer of the two concentric circles illustrated in Figure 14–1, emphasizing the foundational role of these concepts in solution-oriented AAC processes. At each stage of the model, whether observing, prioritizing, team building, problem-solving, or applying solutions, we are confident that grit and resilience underlie success. Earlier, descriptive characteristics tied to grit and resilience such as "perseverance," "passion," and "sustained commitment," were suggested to be evident in many AAC providers. Let's face it, if grit and resilience are absent, failures will abound in life as well as in AAC service delivery.

We propose that success at each stage of the AAC assessment and intervention process is dependent upon grit and resilience—an undeterred spirit that pushes through challenges to achieve optimal outcomes. Our guess is that these qualities are evident in many individuals who choose the health and educational professions involved in AAC services. They are also likely present in individuals with CCN, family members, and other stakeholders. If someone enters the field of AAC without grit and resilience, it is our experience that they can learn to embrace these characteristics as they encounter them in others. That is, as they see others persevere to break barriers, obtain needed technologies, and build necessary

coalitions to achieve success, they too will likely be motivated to persevere.

Finally, as chapter authors, we call upon researchers to examine the concepts of grit and resilience empirically, to both define these ideas in ways that can be measured, and to determine their potential role in successful AAC service delivery. Too often, preprofessional preparation in allied health and educational fields has avoided potentially meaningful instruction in areas perceived as "soft" or less data-driven. The likely value of spirituality in professionals, and those they serve, is a prime example (Zollfrank et al., 2015). If, indeed, grit and resilience are potentially fundamental to provider and team success, they deserve empirical validation and attention in the preservice curricula of the AAC providers of the future.

Considered collectively, our model is simply a guide to solution-oriented AAC practice. It is our hope that readers will use it to reflect on their actions as AAC providers and team members. The individual components of the inner circle of the model, when applied with grit and resilience, (represented by the outer circle), can help providers find their way to small and large solutions to challenges encountered throughout AAC services.

If our model has validity, we should be able to identify examples of its components in a book dedicated to AAC challenges and solutions. What follows are examples from earlier chapters that illustrate our solution-oriented model.

Solution-Oriented AAC: Illustration of a Model

This book has highlighted AAC challenges and solutions across both the lifespan and across disabilities. Although aspects of our solution-oriented model are evident in all chapters, here we simply highlight illustrative instances of inner-circle components of the model to demonstrate its validity and usefulness. We begin by considering critical observation, challenge identification, and challenge prioritization collectively. Thereafter, we provide key examples of other model components individually.

Supporting grit and resilience (the model's outer circle) through specific examples is more difficult. This is due to the more nebulous nature of these concepts. Accordingly, we offer the outer circle of our model as more speculative and, as is mentioned earlier, deserving of empirical study.

Critical Observation, Challenge Identification, and Challenge Prioritization

Obviously, observation is a vital tool in AAC services. It aids providers and stakeholders at every step of decision-making. Although many examples of critical observation are present throughout this book, we focus on three chapters stressing observation, challenge identification, and prioritization. First, Sigafoos, Roche, and Tate (Chapter 9) provide readers with solid examples of observation in their descriptions of challenges associated with Sarah and Robert, two people with CCN who present profound intellectual and multiple disabilities. Critical observations of these individuals and their communicative partners and environments lead to the identification of three specific challenges often problematic in service provision with this population: the identification of reinforcers and viable response topographies, fostering biobehavioral states con-

ducive to learning, and accommodating developmental reflexes. One can certainly extrapolate how, once identified, these challenges could be prioritized based upon individual or situational needs.

Fager, Gormley, and Sorenson (Chapter 8) illustrate the value of critical observation in the identification and prioritization of AAC as they consider access issues in early recovery for adults with acquired communication and language impairments. These authors structure their chapter by describing several key problems observed during their extensive clinical experiences with patients regarding access issues, including where to introduce access to AAC systems within health care settings; and addressing tracheostomy or ventilator dependence, co-occurring cognitive deficits, limited treatment opportunities, and communicative partners naïve to access solutions. As in the example from Sigafoos et al. above, once identified, the prioritization of these challenges can occur more easily, based upon the needs of individuals who rely on AAC as well as their partners and environments.

Finally, in the chapter addressing AAC challenges and solutions in the first years of life, Sevcik, Romski, Walters, and Kaldes (Chapter 2) provide several examples illustrating the value of critical observation. The authors stress the importance of confronting frequently held assumptions limiting access to AAC at very early ages, such as a child who is thought to be too young or too impaired to benefit from AAC services. Sevcik et al. masterfully offered research findings based upon critical observations of children and their communicative partners to support AAC access for all, including those who are chronologically and developmentally young.

Active Collaboration With Team Members

Many of this book's chapters emphasize the value of teams. Wofford and Hodge (Chapter 13) discuss team collaboration as a key component in solution-oriented practice, stating, "The SLP and teachers debriefed weekly to support shared goals, encourage generalization of newly taught skills across contexts and settings, and send home progress summaries or ideas for carryover at home" (p. 354 in this text). These authors go on to support team collaboration when discussing challenges associated with the rapid evolution of technology, reporting that teams are central vehicles for acquiring and sharing knowledge about innovative systems and devices. Likewise, Robinson and Soto (Chapter 4) repeatedly describe teaming as critical to the success of inclusive AAC services in today's schools. These authors extend the simple idea of teaming in their advocacy for broad-based practice changes driven by interprofessional education and services for AAC providers. In a final example, Fager, Gormley, and Sorenson (Chapter 8), speak directly to the value of collaborative teams in reducing demands on patients while facilitating effective treatments. Fager and colleagues report, "Coordination across the interdisciplinary team members to cluster patient cares, offer co-treatments, establish a schedule, and minimize cognitive demands to support patient alertness and engagement is key to supporting these patients" (p. 204 in this text).

Problem-Solving

Each chapter offers insights relative to problem-solving AAC challenges. In fact, problem-solving is so ubiquitous throughout the book, it is difficult to isolate and feature examples. In our review of contributions, we noted applications of several of the previously discussed problem solving mechanisms and their associated strategies.

Examples of similarity discovery and general solutions as applied mechanisms were obvious in the chapters offered by Chavers, Cheng, and Koul (Chapter 6) and McLaughlin and colleagues (Chapter 7). Possibly, some of the more unique problem-solving occurred in chapters devoted to special populations and issues. Erickson, Geist, Hatch, and Quick (Chapter 10), Schlosser and colleagues (Chapter 11) and Wilkinson, Na, Rangel-Rodriguez, and Sowers (Chapter 12) all utilized general solutions, abstraction, and intuition as they negotiated complex issues, such as extending vocabulary choice for individuals with more significant disabilities, using visuals for individuals with autism, and promoting emotional expression in young children. Likewise, McNaughton and Babb (Chapter 5) used similarity discovery, abstraction, and intuition in their pursuit of aids to support participation and communication in prevocational activities for adolescents with intellectual disabilities.

Applying Solutions

When invited to contribute to this text, all authors were asked to pose both AAC challenges and solutions from their experiences as researchers and practitioners in the field. Accordingly, each chapter applies AAC solutions based on either empirical data or well-reasoned ideas.

The idea of generating solutions needs little support. That is, our experiences tell us that the AAC processes culminate, at least temporarily, in solutions. The arrows of the inner circle of our model in Figure 14–1 suggest that applying a solution will likely only address a challenge in the moment and that other challenges will inevitably arise, causing individuals with CCN, providers, and other stakeholders to begin a process of problem-solving once again.

Becoming a Solution-Oriented AAC Provider: A Final Charge

During this book project, I (the first author of this chapter and book editor) was confronted with a question by a chapter contributor whom I've known for some time. She said, "Bill, aren't all AAC providers supposed to be solution-oriented?" I quickly responded with, "Absolutely," then added the following question of my own—"But are they?" Do we, as a collective group, do everything within our power to assure optimal outcomes for individuals with CCN?

I think many of us became involved with AAC because we were attracted to the idea of finding solutions for individuals with limited to no speech. As that idea became our daily job, we saw just how difficult solutions could be. A few of us likely became discouraged to the point of frustration—maybe some pursued professional redirection. Many, however, had one or more experiences that drove us to persevere. Possibly, we saw individuals communicate their preferences for the first time, be included with typical peers, express personal feelings with loved ones, re-enter the work force—all because they gained or regained communicative abilities. These moments must energize us during the more difficult, and often more prevalent, challenges of ongoing AAC practice. They can be a source of the grit and resilience referred to in this chapter.

The moment that motivates my perseverance occurred 30 years ago. I evaluated a 12-year-old girl who had no conventional communication. She presented with profound intellectual disabilities and concomitant physical and health limitations. Prior to the evaluation, her parents shared that they had very limited expectations of my time with their daughter. Frankly, I also had doubts that I could be helpful. During the assessment, I took the opportunity to move back and forth with the child while holding her in a playful manner. After a few turns, she oriented toward me, smiled, and kicked to reinitiate the movements. Both parents, who were watching, immediately burst into tears, sharing that they had never seen their daughter initiate communication. This epiphany was the beginning of several new opportunities for their child and provided me with motivation on those days when solutions are hard to find.

As a reader of this book, the choice is yours. You can find sources of grit and resilience that motivate you when challenges mount. You can even use the solution-oriented model provided here, or create your own similar practice guide. Either way, it is my hope that you choose a solution-oriented AAC path and that the ideas provided in this book assist you in your journey.

■ References

Anderson, J. R. (1983). A spreading activation theory of memory. *Journal of Verbal Learning and Verbal Behavior, 22*(3), 261–295.

Bassok, M. (2003). Analogical transfer in problem solving. In J. Davidson & R. Sternberg

(Eds.), *The psychology of problem solving* (pp. 343–370). Cambridge University Press. https://doi.org/10.1017/CBO978051161 5771.012

Beukelman, D. R., & Light, J. C. (2020). *Augmentative & alternative communication: Supporting children & adults with complex communication needs* (5th ed.). Brookes.

Delaney, P. F., Ericsson, K. A., & Knowles, M. E. (2004). Immediate and sustained effects of planning in a problem-solving task. *Journal of Experimental Psychology, Learning, Memory, and Cognition, 30*(6), 1219–1234.

Duckworth A. L., Peterson, C., Matthews, M. D., & Kelly, D. R. (2007). Grit: Perseverance and passion for long-term goals. *Journal of Personality and Social Psychology, 92*(6), 1011–1087.

Duris, F. (2018). Arguments for the effectiveness of human problem solving. *Biologically Inspired Cognitive Architectures, 24,* 31–34. https://doi.org/10.1016/j.bica.2018.04.007

Eudy, R. (2019). *How do you train critical observation?* Retrieved from https://www.ej4.com/blog/the-new-business-skill-critical-observation-2

Lloyd, L., Quist, R., Windsor, J. (2009). A proposed augmentative and alternative communication model. *Augmentative and Alternative Communication, 6*(3), 172–183. https://doi.org/10.1080/074346190123312 75444

Loncke, F. (2014). *Augmentative and alternative communication: Models and applications for educators, speech-language pathologists, psychologists, caregivers, and users.* Plural Publishing.

Lovett, M. C., & Anderson, J. R. (1996). History of success and current context in problem solving: Combined influences on operator selection. *Cognitive Psychology, 31,* 168–217.

Ogletree, B. (1999). Introduction to teaming. In B. T. Ogletree, M.A. Fischer, & J. B. Schulz. (Eds.) *Bridging the family-professional gap: Facilitating interdisciplinary services for children with disabilities* (pp. 3–11). Charles Thomas.

Ross, B. H. (1987). This is like that: The use of earlier problems and the separation of similarity effects. *Journal of Experimental Psychology: Learning, Memory, and Cognition, 13,* 629–639.

Shi, M., Wang, X., YuGe, B., & Wang, L. (2015). The mediating role of resilience in the relationship between stress and life satisfaction among Chinese medical students: A cross-sectional study. *BMC Medical Education, 15*(16). http://doi:1086/s12909-015-0297-2

Stoffel, J. M., & Cain, J. (2018). Review of grit and resilience literature within health professions education. *American Journal of Pharmaceutical Education, 82*(2), 124–134. https://doi.org/10.5688/ajpe6150

Style, A. (1979). Intuition and problem solving. *The Journal of the Royal College of General Practitioners, 29*(199), 71–74.

Tempski, P., Santos, I. S., Mayer, F. B., Enns, S. C., Perotta, B., Paro, H. B. M. S., . . . Martins, M. A. (2015). Relationship among medical student resilience, educational environment, and quality of life. *PLoS ONE, 10*(6) e0131535. https://doi.org/10.1371/journal.pone.0131535

Wang, Y., & Chiew, V. (2010). On the cognitive process of human problem solving. *Cognitive Systems Research, 11*(1), 81–92. https://doi.org/10.1016/j.cogsys.2008.08.003

Zollfrank, A. A., Trevino, K. M., Cadge, W. C., Balboni, M. J., Thiel, M. M., Fitchett, G., . . . Balboni, T. A. (2015). Teaching health care providers to provide spiritual care: A pilot study. *Journal of Palliative Medicine, 18*(5) 408–414. https://doi.org/10.1089/jpm.2014.0306

■ Glossary

AAC Assessment—A process whereby AAC users, partners, and environments are critiqued to determine: (1) the need for AAC; (2) optimal aided and/or unaided AAC solutions, and 3) progress with and/or the need for adaptations to existing AAC solutions.

AAC Barriers—Factors that impede successful AAC utilization

AAC Environmental Assessment—The process of examining an AAC user's environments to determine if environmental modifications may contribute to communication success

AAC Follow-up—The final stage of the AAC process whereby AAC solutions are evaluated for their effectiveness, potentially leading to changes in the systems or reassessment

AAC Intervention—Therapeutic efforts to optimize AAC solutions with users and stakeholders in all communicative environments

AAC Partner Assessment—The process of examining an AAC user's partners to determine if interactive modifications may contribute to communication success

AAC Practitioners—Individuals who assist users with AAC solutions—can include professionals, paraprofessionals, or other stakeholders

AAC Researchers—Individuals who pose questions, gather and analyze data, and offer evidence-based findings specific to AAC practices and solutions

AAC Solutions—Aided or unaided AAC applications addressing communication deficits or needs

AAC Stakeholders—Individuals who interact with and care for AAC users

Access—How a user directly or indirectly uses an AAC device or solution

Complex Communication Needs—A term used to describe individuals with severe communication, speech, and language impairments

Device Symbol Capacity—The capacity of an AAC device to display symbol sets

Device/System Procurement—The process of securing an AAC solution

Display Capacity—An AAC device or system's ability to present symbols and messages

Emergent Literacy - A term used to describe a person's initial knowledge of encoding and decoding print

Feature Matching—The process of matching user, partner, and environmental AAC needs to potential AAC solutions

Informancy—The process of obtaining assessment/intervention information through others knowledgeable about the AAC user

Interdisciplinary Team—A team whose members maintain professional roles, yet function collaboratively and who are led by a coordinator who shares equal authority with other members

Linguistic Features—The capacity of a device or system to reflect linguistic complexity

Message Management—The creation and delivery of messages on an AAC system or device

Multidisciplinary Team—A team whose members function independently (not collaboratively) and who are led by a leader with disproportionate authority

Observation—The process of obtaining assessment/intervention information by observing users, their partners, and their environments

Operational Demands—Requirements associated with successful device or system use

Rate Enhancement Features—Methods to reduce effort associated with device/system use, for example, prediction.

Sight Words—Print evident in one's environments.

Symbol Forms—Representations of objects or concepts that can vary as to concreteness (iconicity) and form (two-dimensional or three-dimensional)

Transdisciplinary Team—A team whose members frequently release or extend roles, function collaboratively, and are led by a leader who shares equal authority with other members

Trial Run—The use of an AAC device or system prior to procurement to determine fit

Vocabulary Organization—Ways in which vocabulary can be organized for display in AAC devices or systems

Voice Options—Availability of voice alternatives provided on an AAC device or system

■ Index

Note: Page references in **bold** denote figures or tables.

A

AAC
abandonment of, 358–359
for adolescents with complex
communication needs. *See*
Adolescents with complex
communication needs
for adults with complex communication
needs. *See* Adults with complex
communication needs, AAC for
aided. *See* Aided AAC
challenges associated with, 3, 375
for communication about emotions. *See*
Emotions, communication about
communication uses of, 5
for culturally or linguistically diverse
individuals and families. *See*
Culturally or linguistically diverse
individuals and families
definition of, 4–7
grit in, 11–14, 369–370, **374**, 377
high-tech. *See* High-tech AAC
implementation of, 7
for late-stage ALS patients. *See* ALS,
persons with late-stage
low-tech. *See* Low-tech AAC
no-technology-based. *See* No-technology-
based AAC interventions
overview of, 313–314
for persons with aphasia. *See* Persons with
aphasia (PWA), AAC for
for persons with profound intellectual and
multiple disabilities. *See* Profound
intellectual and multiple disabilities
(PIMD), AAC interventions for
populations that rely on, 8–9
in preschool. *See* Preschool, AAC in

resilience in, 11–14, 369–370, **374**, 377
variables that affect, 3
AAC assessment
for bilingual children, 52
challenges in, 376
context for, 6–7
in culturally or linguistically diverse
individuals and families. *See*
Culturally or linguistically diverse
individuals and families, AAC
assessment
feature matching in, 6–7
focus of, 6
platform first mentality for, 8
purpose of, 6
settings for, 6–7
stakeholders in, 4, 6, 9
AAC environmental assessment, 7
AAC evaluation
of culturally or linguistically diverse
individuals and families, 352
goals of, 47
AAC intervention. *See also specific
intervention*
early intervention. *See* Early intervention
no-technology-based. *See* No-technology-
based AAC interventions
stakeholders in, 4
AAC partner assessment, 7
AAC practitioners, 3
AAC providers
challenge identification and prioritization
by, 375
critical observation by, 373–375, 378
grit of, 11–14, 369–370, **374**, 377
resilience of, 11–14, 369–370, **374**, 377
solution-oriented, 369–380
AAC researchers, 3

AAC service(s)
  access to, 6
  description of, 5–6
  device procurement in, 6–7
  feature matching in, 6
  "person first" process for, 8
  physical competence, 6
  "platform first" process for, 8
  schematic diagram of, **6**
  stakeholders in, 9
  system procurement in, 6
  technology, 8
AAC service delivery
  barriers to, 12
  evolving nature of, 7–11
  grit in, 11–14, 369–370, **374**, 377
  hardships in, 12
  interprofessionality effects on, 9–11
  population diversity effects on, 9
  resilience in, 11–14, 369–370, **374**, 377
  technology effects on, 8
AAC solutions. *See also* High-tech AAC;
    Low-tech AAC; No-technology-
    based AAC interventions; *specific
    solution*
  application of, 376–377, 379–380
  assessment of, 6
  problem-solving of, 376, 379
AAC team
  collaboration as, 375–376
  commitment by, 10
  composition of, 4–5
  definition of, 375
  family involvement with, 9
  follow-up by, 7
  functioning of, 375–376
  interdisciplinary, 5, 7
  interprofessionality of, 9–11
  language differences honored by, 9
  members of, 4
  multidisciplinary, 5, 7
  transdisciplinary, 5, 7
Abstraction, 372
Access
  description of, 6
  in preschool, 42–46
Acquired communication disorders, 199
Acute care hospitals
  description of, 201–202

mechanical ventilation dependency
    challenges, 203
  temporary or permanent communication
    needs, 202–203
  time constraints for, 204
  tracheostomy, 203
Acute rehabilitation facilities
  description of, 202
  mechanical ventilation dependency
    challenges, 203
  temporary or permanent communication
    needs, 202–203
  tracheostomy, 203
Adolescents with complex communication
    needs
  active participation by, 118
  case illustration of, 117–118
  communication by
    challenges to, 118–120
    supports for, 119, 121–124
    visual scene displays for, 122–134
    in workplace, 121–124
  participation by
    challenges to, 118–119
    communication effects on, 119
    in employment, 120
    supports for, 119–121
    visual scene displays for, 122–134
    in volunteer activities, 120
  video prompting, 121–122
  video visual scene displays
    benefits of, 123–124, 126, 134
    case illustrations of, 123–124, 127–128
    contexts for, 134
    creation of, 126, 130
    definition of, 122
    guided practice for, 131, 127
    hotspots in, 122–123, **123**, 126–127
    implementation of, 128–133
    independent practice for, 127, 131
    making of, 125–127
    modeling of, 127, 130
    programming of, 122–123
    recording of communication, 126–127,
      130
    research on, 124–125
    support for, 127, 130–132
    task analysis in, **125**, 125–126, 128–129,
      129

video recording, 126, 130
visual activity schedules for, 120–121
Adults with complex communication needs,
    AAC for
abandonment of, 221
access solutions for
    communication advocates, 206–207
    communication partners, 206–207
    health care systems level, 207–208
    nurse call systems, 209
    overview of, 205, **206**
    screenings, 207
    summary of, 221
    yes/no physical response, 208–209
in acute care hospitals
    description of, 201–202
    mechanical ventilation dependency
        challenges, 203
    temporary or permanent
        communication needs, 202–203
    time constraints for, 204
    tracheostomy, 203
in acute rehabilitation facilities
    description of, 202
    mechanical ventilation dependency
        challenges, 203
    temporary or permanent
        communication needs, 202–203
    tracheostomy, 203
case studies of, 215–216, 219–220
co-occurring cognitive deficits, 203–204
communication partners for, 205
delirium in, 204
eye motility in, 213
high-tech options for, 218–220
inpatient experiences of, 200–201
light tech options for
    eye-blink switches, 216–217
    laser pointers, **211**, 216
low-tech options
    eye gaze, 213–216
    eye linking, 213–216
    eye pointing, **211**
    eye tracking, **210**
    facial expressions and gestures, **211**
    head tracking, **210**
    overview of, 209, **210–211**, 211
    partner-dependent scanning, 211, 213,
    213

switch scanning, **210**
    touchscreen access, **210**
negative communication experiences,
    200
ongoing support for, 220–221
overview of, 199
time constraints for, 204
Adverse medical event, 200
Advocacy, 36
Aided AAC
    approaches to, 259–262
    effectiveness of, 262
    as evidence-based practice, 263
    limited access to, 254–255, 276
    personal access to, 262–263
    speech-generating devices, 254
    types of, 313
Aided AAC Language Modeling, 106–107
Aided language input, 264–265, 356–357
Alertness, in profound intellectual and
        multiple disabilities
    environmental stimuli effects on, 239
    fluctuating levels of, 239
    states of, 238
    stimulation effects on, 240
ALS, persons with late-stage
AAC for
    challenges associated with, 192–193
    decision-making guidelines, 186–192
    description of, 176
    eye tracking technologies, 177–178
    future for, 186
    multimodal access technologies,
        181–182
    speech-generating device, 179–181
    switch scanning, 179–181
brain-computer interface in
    auditory stimuli, 184
    challenges to, 185–186
    components of, 182–183
    invasive system, 184
    noninvasive, 183–184
    P300–based, 184–185
    research and development, 185–186
    schematic diagram of, **183**
    tactile stimuli, 184
bulbar-onset, 173
case studies of, 169, 172–173, 187–192
classification of, 171–173

ALS, persons with late-stage *(continued)*
  cognitive challenges in, 173–174
  coping with, 174, 176
  emotional challenges in, 174, 176
  Functional Communication Scale, 174, 175*t*
  King's clinical staging system, 170, **171**
  language challenges in, 173–174
  MiToS functional staging system for, 170,
    171
  motor challenges in, 173
  oculomotor abnormalities in, 174
  overview of, 169–170
  palliative care in, 176
  presentation of, 170–173
  psychosocial challenges in, 174, 176
  spinal-onset, 173
  staging scales for, **171**
  visual skills in, 178
American Speech-Language Hearing
    Association (ASHA)
  AAC as defined by, 4
  Code of Ethics, 341
  culturally responsive service delivery
    mandates by, 341
  Practice Portal, 4
Animated graphic symbols, in VIS, 284, **285**
Aphasia
  definition of, 141
  persons with. *See* Persons with aphasia
Apple Watch, 305
ASHA. *See* American Speech-Language
    Hearing Association
Assistive technology, 45–46
Asymmetrical tonic neck reflex (ATNR), **242**,
    244
ATNR. *See* Asymmetrical tonic neck reflex
Augmentative and alternative
    communication. *See* AAC
Augmented input
  definition of, 155
  early interventions, **26**
  examples of, 155
  in preschool, **49–50**, 51
  spoken language benefits of, 284
  in VIS, 284, **285**
Augmented reality, **293**
Autism spectrum disorder, students with
  conversation-based interventions applied
    to, 101
  curriculum accessibility for, 290–291

expressive language difficulties in, 283
Goal Attainment Scaling for, 298–300, **300**
prevalence of, 283
progress monitoring of, 289, 298–300, **300**
receptive language difficulties in, 283
spontaneous teaching opportunities,
    288–289
teachable moments in
  challenges in taking advantage of,
    288–289
  just-in-time technology to support,
    291–298, **293–297**
Visual Immersion System for. *See* Visual
    Immersion System
visual supplements for, 291
visual supports for, 283–286, **285**

B

Babinski reflex, **242**, 243
Background color-coding, 260
Basic-choice communicators, 157
Bilingual children. *See also* Culturally or
    linguistically diverse individuals and
    families
  AAC use by, 52–54
  preschool, 52–54
Bilingual service providers, 341
Bilingualism, 342
Brain-computer interface, for persons with
    late-stage ALS
  auditory stimuli, 184
  challenges to, 185–186
  components of, 182–183
  invasive system, 184
  noninvasive, 183–184
  P300-based, 184–185
  research and development, 185–186
  schematic diagram of, **183**
  tactile stimuli, 184
Broca's aphasia, 149, 158, 160, 163

C

CBC. *See* Conjoint behavioral consultation
CBIs. *See* Conversation-based interventions
CCN. *See* Complex communication needs
CEEDAR. *See* Collaboration for
    Effective Educator Development,
    Accountability, and Reform

Cerebral palsy, 243–244
Challenges. *See also specific challenge*
  description of, 3
  identification and prioritization of, 375,
    378
Clinician advocacy, 36
Coaching
  of parents, **28–29**
  in Project Core, 265–266
Code-switching, 345
Cognitive disabilities. *See* Students with
    significant cognitive disabilities
Cognitive-linguistic domain, for just-in-time
    assessment, **295**, 297, **302**
Collaboration as team, 375–376, 379
Collaboration for Effective Educator
    Development, Accountability, and
    Reform (CEEDAR), 94
Communication advocates, 206–207
Communication boards, 151, **152**, 211, **212**,
    214, **318**
Communication kits, 207–208
Communication Matrix, 269
Communication partner domain, for
    just-in-time assessment, **295**, 297, **303**
Communication partners, 206–207, 263, **295**
Communicative Effectiveness Index (CETI),
    164
Communicators
  contextual-choice, 158–160, **159**
  emerging, 157–158, **158**
  generative-message, 161–162
  partner-dependent, 157–160
  partner-independent, 160–162
  specific-need, 162
  stored-message, 161
  transitional, 160
Complex communication needs (CCN)
  adolescents with. *See* Adolescents with
    complex communication needs
  adults with. *See* Adults with complex
    communication needs
  barriers faced by, 339
  culturally or linguistically diverse
    individuals with. *See* Culturally or
    linguistically diverse individuals and
    families
  description of, 3, 5
  students with. *See* Students with complex
    communication needs

Comprehension
  definition of, 24
  early language, 23–24
  speech, 24
Conceptual vocabulary, 257
Concrete vocabulary, 257
Conjoint behavioral consultation (CBC), 88
Context sensitivity, 372–373
Contextual-choice communicators, 158–160,
    159
Contextualized intervention, 100
Conversation-based interventions (CBIs)
  for language, 101–102
  verbal scaffolding, 101
Core vocabulary, 256–259
Critical observation, 373–375, 378
CRP. *See* Culturally responsive practices
Cultural awareness and competence, **346**,
    346–351
Cultural broker, 351
Cultural congruence, 356
Culturally or linguistically diverse individuals
    and families
  AAC assessment
    collaborative approach to, 351–353
    cultural awareness and competence in,
      347–348
    data collection during, 355
    family members' involvement in, 355
    team-based approach to, 351–352
  AAC evaluation, 352
  AAC intervention
    abandonment of, 358–360
    aided language input, 356–357
    bilingual approach, 348–349
    collaboration for, **346**, 351–354
    cultural awareness and competence for,
      346, 346–351
    device-specific challenges, **340**, 345,
      349–350
    environmental challenges, **340**, 340–343
    goal of, 356
    implementation challenges, **340**, 343–345
    interpreter used in, 351
    language of, 344, 348
    materials or devices to enhance, 349–350
    prioritization of family and their values,
      354–357
    systematic inaccessibility to, 341
    team-based approach to, 353–354

Culturally or linguistically diverse individuals
and families *(continued)*
  bilingual service providers for, 341
  caregivers in, 354
  case studies of, 350–351, 353–354, 358
  culturally congruent practices with, 356
  definition of, 339
  devices used in
    abandonment of, 358–359
    challenges for, **340**, 345, 349–350
  ethnographic interviews and observations,
    347
  lifespan of, 357–358
  low-income families, 343
  multigenerational, 354
  overview of, 339–340
  in poverty, 343
  prioritization of, 354–357
  socio-cultural approach to, 347
  speech-language pathologists for
    collaborative work by, **346**, 351–354
    cultural awareness and competence,
      346, 346–351
    cultural biases in, 346–347
    description of, 343
    language of intervention, 344, 348–349
    team-based approach, 351–353
  values of, 354–357
Culturally responsive competencies, **92–93**
Culturally responsive practices (CRP), 81,
  96–97
Culture, 9

D

Data collection
  of culturally or linguistically diverse
    individuals and families, 355
  methods of, 7
Delirium, 204
Developmental disabilities
  language comprehension impairments in, 42
  prevalence of, 41
Developmental reflexes, 241–247, **242–243**
Device procurement, 6–7
Differentiated instruction, 100–101
Disabilities
  cognitive. *See* Students with significant
    cognitive disabilities

profound intellectual and multiple. *See*
  Profound intellectual and multiple
  disabilities
stigmatization of, 342
Diversity, 9
Door script, 78–80
Drawing, 156

E

Early Development of Emotional
  Competencies (EDEC)
  AAC decisions based on, 321–323
  biomedical signs and, 333, **334**
  case study of, 321–322, 326–331
  checklist version of, 331–333, **332–333**
  development of, 320
  family use of, 331–333, **332–333**
  field testing of, 320
  goals of, 319
  importance of communication about
    emotions learned through, 321
  meaningful activity used in, 322
  parent instruction based on information
    from, 325–326
  parental use of, 331–333, **332–333**
  sections of, 319–320
  social stories generated from, 335
  summary of, 336
Early intervention
  AAC interventions, 25–30
  augmented input and output intervention,
    26
  augmented input intervention, **26**, 30
  augmented output intervention, **26**, 29–30
  case illustrations of, 30–34
  framework for, 23–24
  language, 24
  myths about, 34–36
  overview of, 21–23
  preschool transition, 56
  stakeholders' comments about, **35**
  vocabulary, 27–29
Early learning developmental guidelines
  (ELDGs), 41
Early literacy, 54, **55**
Edinburgh Cognitive and Behavioural ALS
  Screen (ECAS), 173
Educational assistant, 291

EEG. *See* Electroencephalography
EL. *See* English Learners
ELDGs. *See* Early learning developmental
    guidelines
Electroencephalography, 184
Electromyography (EMG), 180
Electrooculography, 177
ELL. *See* English Language Learners
Emergent literacy, 5
Emerging communicators, 157–158, **158**
EMG. *See* Electromyography
Emotional competencies
    culturally appropriate, 314
    definition of, 314
    Early Development of. *See* Early
        Development of Emotional
        Competencies
    importance of, 336
    language development and, 314–315
Emotional expression, 315
Emotions, communication about
    AAC used in
        Early Development of Emotional
            Competencies. *See* Early Development
            of Emotional Competencies
        examples of, 316
        system design for, 317–320
        vocabulary used in, 317–320, 335
    cultural influences on, 319
    family preferences for, 319–320
    importance of, 321
    STEPS intervention for supporting
        case study of, 326–331
        description of, 323–325
        effectiveness of, 323–325
        guidance on, 323, **324**
        social stories generated from, 335
        summary of, 336
    unconventional behaviors used in, 316
Encouragement, 12–13
English Language Learners (ELL), 85–86
English Learners (EL), 85–86, 104–105
Environmental domain, for just-in-time
    assessment, **295**, 297, **302**
Evidence-based intervention, 23–24
Expressive language, 84, 283
Extensor tone reflex, **243**
External-stored information, 155–156
Extrinsic motivation, 370

Eye-blink switches, 216–217
Eye blinks, 208
Eye gaze, 213–216, 234
Eye gaze board, 214, **214**
Eye linking, 213–216
Eye motility, 213
Eye tracking
    in adults with complex communication
        needs, **210**
    in adults with profound intellectual and
        multiple disabilities, 234
    in late-stage ALS, 177–178
Eye transfer boards (ETAN), 177

F

Family. *See also* Parents
    AAC decision making participation by,
        56–58
    advocacy by, 36
    collaboration with, 97
    culturally or linguistically diverse. *See*
        Culturally or linguistically diverse
        individuals and families
    of preschool child
        AAC carryover to home, 58–60
        actions for, 63
        communication vision created by, 57–58
        inclusion of, in AAC decision making,
            56–60
        interprofessional collaborative practice
            for, 57
Feature matching
    definition of, 293
    description of, 6–7
    of just-in-time technologies, 292–294
Fitzgerald key, 260
Frontotemporal dementia (FTD), 173–174
Functional Communication Scale, 174, 175*t*

G

Galant reflex, **242**
Generative-message communicators,
    161–162
Global aphasia, 156
Goal Attainment Scaling (GAS), 298–300,
    300
Grasp switch, 245, **245**

Grid displays, **145**, 145–148, 314
Grit, 11–14, 369–370, **374**, 377

H

Head tracking, for adults with complex
    communication needs, **210**
High-tech AAC
    in adults with complex communication
        needs, 218–220
    advantages of, 357
    age of patient and, 357
Hillside Developmental Center, 269–275,
    270–275
Hospitalization, 200
Hotspots, 122–123, **123**, 126–127

I

IDEA. *See* Individuals with Disabilities
    Education Act
Identification and communication cards, 152,
    153
Inclusive education, for students with
        complex communication needs
    challenges impacting, 82–87
    classroom-based profiles of, 102–108
    definition of, 82
    description of, 81
    intensive interventions, **103**, 106–107
    least restrictive environment effects on, 82
    Multi-Tiered System of Supports, 90,
        93–95, 102–108
    settings, 82
    statistics regarding, 83
    summary of, 108
    supplemental support, **103**, 105–106
    universal support, **102–103**, 102–105
    variables that affect, **87**
Individualized Education Plan (IEP), 289
Individuals with Disabilities Education Act
    (IDEA), 56, 82, 341
Infants, developmental reflexes in, 241–247,
    242–243
Informancy, data collected via, 7
"Inpatient Functional Communication
    Interview," 207
Interdisciplinary team, 5, 7
Interpreter, 351

Interprofessional collaborative practice
    (IPCP), 57
Interprofessional Education Collaborative
    (IPEC), 89
Interprofessional education (IPE), 10, 89
Interprofessional practice (IPP), 81, 89, 98,
    106
Interprofessionality, 9–11
Intrinsic motivation, 370
Intuition, 372
IPCP. *See* Interprofessional collaborative
    practice
IPE. *See* Interprofessional education
IPP. *See* Interprofessional practice

J

JEPD model. *See* Job Embedded Professional
    Development (JEPD) model
Job Embedded Professional Development
    (JEPD) model, 99
Just-in-time (JIT) technology
    teachable moments supported with,
        291–298, **293–297**
    wearable technologies, **293**, 301–306

K

King's clinical staging system, 170, **171**

L

Language
    development of, 24
    in late-stage ALS, 173–174
Language comprehension, 155
Language development
    in complex communication needs
        students, 99–102
    contextualized intervention for, 100
    differentiated instruction for, 100–101
    emotional competencies and, 314–315
    in preschoolers
        AAC's role in, 56
        evidence-based interventions for, 47–52
        instructional challenges to, 46
Language input, aided, 264–265
Language interventions
    AAC, 25–30

in students with complex communication needs, 84

Laser pointers, **211**, 216

Learner domain, for just-in-time assessment, 294, **295**, **302**

Least restrictive environment (LRE), 82

Letter frequency patterns, 179

Letter recognition, **55**

Letter-sound recognition, **55**

Light tech AAC
    eye-blink switches, 216–217
    laser pointers, **211**, 216

Limited English proficient (LEP), 85

Lingraphica, 144

Literacy development
    in complex communication needs students, 99–102
    in preschoolers
        instructional challenges to, 46
        support for, 54, **55**

Low-tech AAC
    eye gaze, 213–216
    eye linking, 213–216
    eye pointing, **211**
    eye tracking, **210**
    facial expressions and gestures, **211**
    head tracking, **210**
    for older patients, 357
    overview of, 209, **210–211**, 211
    partner-dependent scanning, 211, 213, **213**
    switch scanning, **210**
    touchscreen access, **210**

LRE. *See* Least restrictive environment

M

Mechanical ventilation, 203

Megabee, 177

Message management, 7

Metacognition, 253

Miniature linguistic training, in VIS, 284, **285**

MiToS functional staging system, 170, **171**

Mobile apps, 148

Morning meeting script, 71–77

Moro reflex, **242**

Motor development, 243

MSEL. *See* Mullen Scales of Early Learning

MTSS. *See* Multi-Tiered System of Supports

Mullen Scales of Early Learning (MSEL), 25

Multi-tiered System of Supports (MTSS)
    for complex communications needs students, 90, 93–95, **102–103**, 102–108
    definition of, 90
    description of, 81–82, 107–108

Multidisciplinary team, 5, 7

Multimodal access technologies, 181–182

N

National Center for Systemic Improvement (NCSI), 94–95

Naturalistic teaching, 265

NCSI. *See* National Center for Systemic Improvement

No-technology-based AAC interventions
    communication board, 151, **152**
    efficacy of, 154–157, 163
    external-stored information, 155–156
    identification and communication cards, 152, **153**
    partner-dependent/partner-assisted, 154–155
    rating scales, 150, **150**
    self-formulated/self-generated messages, 156–157
    spelling boards, 151, **153**
    Talking Mats, 150–151, **151**
    unaided, 154

NOVAChat, 45

Nurse call systems, 209

O

Observation
    critical, 373–375, 378
    data collected via, 7

Ocular bobbing, 215

P

P300 brain-computer interface system, 184–185

Palliative care, 176

Palmar grasp reflex, **242**, 244–245

Parents. *See also* Family
    coaching of, **28–29**

Parents *(continued)*
  Early Development of Emotional
    Competencies use by, 331–333,
    332–333
  of preschool child
    actions for, 63
    communication vision created by, 57–58
Partner-dependent/partner-assisted AAC
    strategies, 154–155
Partner-dependent scanning, 211, 213, **213**
Partner-independent communicators, 160–162
Passion, 12
Patient-Provider Communication, 221
PECS. *See* Picture exchange communication
    system
Peer interactions
  in complex communication needs
    students, 83–84
  in preschool, 51–52
Peer-mediated instruction, 99, 106
Peer mentoring, 98–99, 106–107
Perseverance, 11–12
"Person first" process, 8
Persons with aphasia (PWA)
  AAC for
    abandonment of, 143
    case study of, 163–164
    cognitive demands associated with, 143
    cognitive strategies, 142
    communication board, 151, **152**
    communicators in, 157–162
    contextual-choice communicators in,
      158–160, **159**
    efficacy of, 148–149
    emerging communicators in, 157–158,
      158
    external-stored information, 155–156
    facilitative effects of, 141
    generative-message communicators,
      161–162
    grid displays, **145**, 145–148
    identification and communication cards,
      152, **153**
    information processing demands
      affected by, 142
    mobile apps, 148
    no-technology-based methods, 150–157
    partner-dependent communicators,
      157–160

partner-dependent/partner-assisted
    strategies, 154–155
  partner-independent communicators,
    160–162
  rating scales, 150, **150**
  self-formulated/self-generated messages,
    156–157
  specific-need communicators, 162
  speech generating devices, 142, 144–145
  spelling boards, 151, **153**
  stored-message communicators, 161
  Talking Mats, 150–151, **151**
  technology-based, 144–149
  transitional communicators in, 160
  unaided strategies, 154
  visual scene displays, 145–148
  written choice conversation technique
    in, 159, **159**
attention deficits in, 158
Broca's aphasia, 149
case study of, 163–164
communication in
  challenges associated with, 142
  visual scene displays for, 146–147
drawing by, 156
executive functioning deficits in, 143
language comprehension in, 155
linguistic and cognitive characteristics of,
    141
working memory in, 142–143
Persons with late-stage ALS. *See* ALS, persons
    with late-stage
Phoneme blending, **55**
Phoneme isolation, **55**
Physical competence, 6
Picture communication symbols (PCS), 156,
    262
Picture exchange communication system
    (PECS), 42–43
Plantar reflex, **242**
"Platform first" process, 8
Population
  AAC reliance, 8–9
  diversity of, 9
Poverty, 343
Preschool
  AAC in
    access challenges for, 42–46
    augmented input interventions, **49–50**, 51

barriers to, 44, 63
bilingual children, 52–54
carryover of, to home, 58–60
case illustration of, 60–63
decision-making, family inclusion in, 56–58
digital materials for, 45
early literacy skills, 54, **55**
evidence-based interventions, 47–52
family inclusion in, 56–60, 63
"input-output" mismatch in, 48
instructional challenges for, 46–55, 63
language modeling using, 48–51, **49–50**
peer interactions, 51–52
speech-generating devices, 42, 144–145, 164
teacher training in, 46–47
team members opposition to, 43–46
early learning developmental guidelines for, 41
early literacy in, 54, **55**
family
    AAC carryover to home, 58–60
    actions for, 63
    communication vision created by, 57–58
    inclusion of, in AAC decision making, 56–60
    interprofessional collaborative practice for, 57
language development in
    AAC's role in, 56
    evidence-based interventions for, 47–52
    instructional challenges to, 46
literacy development in
    instructional challenges to, 46
    support for, 54, **55**
multiword combinations in, **49**
overview of, 41–43
parents
    actions for, 63
    communication vision created by, 57–58
peer interactions in, 51–52
reading instruction in, 54, **55**
social communication in, **50**
student diversity in, 47
team members
    AAC opposition by, 43–46
    assistive technology training for, 45–46
    family life awareness by, 58

follow-up meetings for, 45
meetings by, 43, 71–72
preservice education of, 44
training of, 44–46
transition to, 41
vocabulary development in, **49**
Problem solvers
abstraction mechanism used by, 372
context sensitivity mechanism used by, 372–373
general solutions mechanism used by, 372
intuition mechanism used by, 372
relation and association discovery mechanism used by, 371
Problem-solving
algorithm deduction approach, 370–371
analogy approach to, 370–371
analysis and synthesis approach to, 370–371
direct facts approach to, 370
divide-and-conquer approach, 370–371
exhaustive search approach to, 370
factors that affect, 370
givens, goals, and operations, 370
heuristic approach to, 370
hill climbing approach to, 370–371
model of, **374**
similarity discovery mechanism, 371
solutions generated through, 376, 379
strategies used in, 370–371
Profound intellectual and multiple disabilities (PIMD)
AAC interventions for
    absence of, 230–231
    assessments before using, 233
    attitudinal barrier to, 231
    biobehavioral states conducive to, 236, 238–241
    challenges associated with, 247
    developmental reflexes incorporated into, 244
    environmental stimuli effects on, 239–240
    eye tracking, 234
    functional/intentional use of, 231–232
    preference assessment, 233–234
    prerequisites to, 232–234
    reinforcers, 232–236
    research to support, 232
    summary of, 247

Profound intellectual and multiple disabilities (PIMD) *(continued)*
  alertness in
    environmental stimuli effects on, 239
    fluctuating levels of, 239
    states of, 238
    stimulation effects on, 240
  biobehavioral states in, 236, 238–241
  case studies of, 229–230, 244–247
  communication assessments, 235–236
  communication intervention in, 230
  definition of, 229
  developmental reflexes, 241–247, **242–243**
  drowsy/sleep state, 240
  emotional competencies in, 315
  health and medical conditions associated with, 230
  language development in, 315
  preference assessments, 233–234
  support needs for, 230
Project Building Bridges, 90, 347
Project Core
  coaching in, 265–266
  core vocabulary, 256–259
  description of, 255
  evidence-based practices in, 256
  goal of, 275
  Hillside Developmental Center, 269–275, **270–275**
  naturalistic teaching, 265
  professional development, 265–269, **266–268, 272–273**
  self-reflection and observation guide, **267–268**
  summary of, 276
  universal core vocabulary, 258–262, **259, 261**, 266, 271, 273–276
Protocol for Culturally Inclusive Assessment of AAC, 348
PWA. *See* Persons with aphasia

Q

QR codes, **293**
Quadrant scanning, 179

R

Rating scales, 150, **150**
Reading instruction
  AAC strategies for, 54, **55**
  in preschool, 54, **55**
Receptive language, 283
Remnant book, 156
Resilience, 11–14, 369–370, **374**, 377
Response to Intervention (RtI) model, 82, 90
Rhyming, **55**

S

Scaffolding, 100, 318–319
Scanning Wizard software, 180
Scene cues, in VIS, 284, **285**
Schoolwide Integrated Framework for Transformation (SWIFT) Education Center, 93–94
SCI. *See* Speech communication intervention
Self-formulated/self-generated messages, 156–157
Sequenced Inventory of Communication Development (SICD), 31
SGD. *See* Speech-generating device
SICD. *See* Sequenced Inventory of Communication Development
Sight words, 5
Significant cognitive disabilities. *See* Students with significant cognitive disabilities
SLP. *See* Speech-language pathologists
Smartspeakers, in VIS, 284, **285**
Smartwatches, in VIS, 284, **285**
Social stories, 316, 335
Solution-oriented providers, 369–380
SpeakBook, 177
Special education, 255
Specific-need communicators, 162
Speech communication intervention (SCI), 25, **26**
Speech comprehension, 24
Speech-generating device (SGD)
  case study of, 164
  early uses of, 21–22, 27, 33, 36
  in persons with aphasia, 144–145, 164
  in persons with late-stage ALS, 179–180
  in preschool, 42
  in students with significant cognitive disabilities, 254
Speech-language pathologists (SLPs)
  bilingual, 341
  cultural awareness and competence, **346**, 346–351

with culturally or linguistically diverse
  individuals and families
    collaborative work by, **346**, 351–354
    cultural awareness and competence,
      346, 346–351
    cultural biases in, 346–347
    description of, 343
    language of intervention, 344, 348–349
    team-based approach, 351–353
  interprofessional education competencies
    used by, 98
  interprofessional practice competencies
    used by, 98
  in palliative care, 176
  students with significant cognitive
    disabilities access to, 254–255
Speech-output technologies, in VIS, 284, **285**
Spelling boards, 151, **153**
Spirituality, 12
Stakeholders
  in AAC assessment, 4, 6, 9
  comments by, **13**
STEPS intervention
  case study of, 326–331
  description of, 323–325
  effectiveness of, 323–325
  guidance on, 323, **324**
  social stories generated from, 335
  summary of, 336
Stored-message communicators, 161
Strategies for Talking about Emotions as
    PartnerS intervention. *See* STEPS
    intervention
Students with complex communication
    needs
  AAC use by
    augmented language input strategies,
      101
    case illustrations of, 102–108
    classroom-based solutions, 97–102
    collaborative teamwork for, 97–99
    cultural diversity effects on, 84–87
    culturally responsive practices, **92–93**,
      96–97
    expressive language associated with, 84
    inclusion of students with, 83–85
    interprofessional practice in, 98, 106
    language interventions for, 84
    linguistic diversity effects on, 84–87
    observational studies on, 83

peer interactions, 83–84
peer-mediated instruction, 99, 106
peer mentoring in, 98–99, 106–107
personnel preparation grants, 90, **91**
professional preparation for, 87–90
systems-level solutions, 87–97
teacher preparation in, 88
  cultural and linguistic diversity of, 85–87,
    96–97
  description of, 3, 5
  emotional development difficulties in, 315
  English Language Learners, 85–86
  English Learners, 85–86, 104–105
  expressive language used by, 84
  inclusive education for
    challenges impacting, 82–87
    classroom-based profiles of, 102–108
    definition of, 82
    description of, 81
    intensive interventions, **103**, 106–107
    least restrictive environment effects on,
      82
    Multi-Tiered System of Supports, 90,
      93–95, 102–108
    settings, 82
    statistics regarding, 83
    summary of, 108
    supplemental support, **103**, 105–106
    universal support, **102–103**, 102–105
    variables that affect, **87**
  language and literacy development
    augmented language input strategies
      used in, 101
    contextualized intervention, 100
    conversation-based language
      interventions, 101–102
    differentiated instruction, 100–101
    overview of, 99–100
  language interventions, 84
  linguistic diversity of, 85–87
  universal design for learning applied to,
    95, **95**, 107
Students with significant cognitive disabilities
  aided AAC for
    approaches to, 259–262
    effectiveness of, 262
    as evidence-based practice, 263
    limited access to, 254–255, 276
    personal access to, 262–263
    speech-generating devices, 254

Students with significant cognitive disabilities *(continued)*
 aided language input, 264–265
 characteristics of, 253
 communication development, 269
 communication interventions
  in classrooms, 255
  natural environments for, 265
 Communication Matrix, 269–270, **271**, **273**
 concrete vocabulary for, 257
 definition of, 253
 early communication behaviors in, 263–264
 lexicon for, 257
 metacognition impairments, 253
 prevalence of, 253
 Project Core
  coaching in, 265–266
  core vocabulary, 256–259
  description of, 255
  evidence-based practices in, 256
  goal of, 275
  Hillside Developmental Center, 269–275, **270–275**
  naturalistic teaching, 265
  professional development, 265–269, **266–268, 272–273**
  self-reflection and observation guide, **267–268**
  summary of, 276
  universal core vocabulary, 258–262, **259, 261,** 266, 271, 273–276
 speech-language pathologist access, 254–255
 systemic barriers for, 254
Study of Patient-Nurse Effectiveness with Assisted Communication Strategies (SPEACS), 207
SWIFT. *See* Schoolwide Integrated Framework for Transformation (SWIFT) Education Center
Switch scanning
 in adults with complex communication needs, **210**
 in late-stage ALS, 179–181
Symbol forms, 3
Symmetrical tonic neck reflex (STNR), **242**
System procurement, 6

Systematic Analysis of Language Transcript software, 28–29

T

Talking Mats, 150–151, **151**
Task analysis, for video visual scene display, **125,** 125–126, 128–129, **129**
TASP. *See* Test of Aided Symbol-Communication Performance
Taxonomic grid display, 145
Teachable moments
 challenges in taking advantage of, 288–289, 291–298, **293–297**
 just-in-time technology to support, 291–298, **293–297**
Teachers
 AAC preparation for, 88
 preschool, AAC training for, 46–47
Team
 collaboration as, 375–376, 379
 commitment by, 10
 composition of, 4–5
 for culturally or linguistically diverse individual and family interventions, 351–353
 definition of, 375
 family involvement with, 9
 follow-up by, 7
 functioning of, 375–376
 interdisciplinary, 5, 7
 interprofessionality of, 9–11
 language differences honored by, 9
 members of, 4
 multidisciplinary, 5, 7
 transdisciplinary, 5, 7
Test of Aided Symbol-Communication Performance (TASP), 45
Tobii-Dynavox Boardmaker, 28
Tonic labyrinthine reflex, **243,** 244
Transdisciplinary team, 5, 7
Transitional communicators, 160
Trial run, 7
Truncal incurvation reflex, **242**

U

UDL. *See* Universal design for learning
Unaided AAC, 154

Universal core vocabulary, 258–262, **259**, **261**, 266, 271, 273–276
Universal design for learning (UDL)
  complex communications needs students application of, 95, **95**, 107
  definition of, 95
  description of, 81
  qualities of, 95

V

Verbal scaffolding, 101
Video modeling, in VIS, 284, **285**, 289–290
Video prompting, 121
Video visual scene displays, 122–134
  benefits of, 123–124, 126, 134
  case illustrations of, 123–124, 127–128
  contexts for, 134
  creation of, 126, 130
  definition of, 122
  guided practice for, 131, 127
  hotspots in, 122–123, **123**, 126–127
  implementation of, 128–133
  independent practice for, 127, 131
  making of, 125–127
  modeling of, 127, 130
  programming of, 122–123
  recording of communication, 126–127, 130
  research on, 124–125
  support for, 127, 130–132
  task analysis in, **125**, 125–126, 128–129, **129**
  video recording, 126, 130
  vocabulary presentation with, 314
VIS. *See* Visual Immersion System (VIS)
Visual activity schedules, 120–121
Visual Immersion System (VIS)
  case study of, 301–306
  challenges in implementation of, 286
  definition of, 284
  effectiveness of, 286
  instructional modes in, 284
  as language accommodation, 286–287, 289–290
  as overlay function, 287–288, 290–291
  progress monitoring, 289
  spontaneous teaching opportunities and, 288–289

summary of, 306
symbol-rich classroom with, 289
teachable moments
  challenges in taking advantage of, 288–289
  just-in-time technology to support, 291–298, **293–297**
Visual Expressive Mode, 284
Visual Instructional Mode, 284
Visual Organizational Mode, 284
visual supports used in, **285**
wearable technologies, **293**, 301–306
Visual scene displays. *See also* Video visual scene displays
  in adolescents with complex communication needs, 122–134
  just-in-time programming of, **293**, 298
  in persons with aphasia, 145–148
  teachable moments supported with, **293**, 298
Visual schedules, in VIS, 284, **285**
Visual supports
  aided, 284
  in autism spectrum disorder, 283–286, **285**
  definition of, 283–284
  in Visual Immersion System, **285**
Vocabulary
  building of, 24
  conceptual, 257
  concrete, 257
  core, 256–259
  in grid displays, 314
  growth of, 24
  universal core, 258–262, **259**, **261**, 266, 271, 273–276
Voice-activated technologies, **293**

W

Wearable technologies, **293**, 301–306
Written choice conversation technique, 159, **159**

Y

Yes/no physical response, 208–209